feed your face

About the Author

Dr. Jessica Wu, a graduate of Harvard Medical School, is a board-certified celebrity dermatologist in Los Angeles and an Assistant Clinical Professor at the USC Medical School. When she's not helping Hollywood's A-list get red carpet-ready, she's dishing up advice as the Skin and Beauty Expert on EverydayHealth.com and on her daily e-Newsletter. Dr. Wu is frequently in the media and has appeared on *Good Morning America, Entertainment Tonight, E!, EXTRA*, and in the *New York Times, People, Elle, O: The Oprah Magazine, Glamour*, and *Good Housekeeping*.

feed your
face

THE 28-DAY PLAN
FOR YOUNGER, SMOOTHER SKIN AND A BEAUTIFUL BODY

PIATKUS

First published in the US in 2011 by St Martin's Press
First published in Great Britain in 2012 by Piatkus
This paperback edition published in 2017 by Piatkus

1 3 5 7 9 10 8 6 4 2

A CIP catalogue record for this book
is available from the British Library.

ISBN 978-0-7499-5745-2

Printed and bound in Great Britain by
Clays Ltd, St Ives plc

Papers used by Piatkus are from well-managed forests and
other responsible sources.

Piatkus
An imprint of
Little, Brown Book Group
Carmelite House
50 Victoria Embankment
London EC4Y 0DZ

An Hachette UK Company
www.hachette.co.uk

www.littlebrown.co.uk

To my parents, for their sacrifices and for teaching me to do things my own way

To Florin, who loves me unconditionally (even when my hair is frizzy and I have a cucumber mask on my face)

And to every woman who has purchased enough pimple cream, mineral makeup, and wrinkle-reducing serum to fill a Sephora store. There is another way. Thank you for coming on this journey with me.

Dear Reader,

A few things to note before we get started: This book is not intended to replace the advice of your own physician or health-care professional, and you may wish to consult him or her before adjusting your diet or skin-care routine, especially if you have existing health conditions.

The information you'll find in *Feed Your Face* regarding skin care, health, and nutrition is the result of observations I have made in my years of practice treating thousands of patients, as well as my review of relevant medical and scientific literature. The literature at times reflects conflicting conclusions and opinions. I have expressed my views on many of these issues; you, the reader, should understand that other experts may sometimes disagree.

No doctor can guarantee a particular result for anyone. However, I believe that you can greatly improve the appearance and health of your skin by making the right dietary and lifestyle choices. It is my hope that what you learn from reading this book will start you on the course to a lifetime of healthier, brighter skin and a younger complexion.

Dr. Jessica Wu

Contents

Introduction

Everything You Think You Know About Skin Care Is Wrong

(Trust Me, I'm a Doctor)

t's Friday afternoon in Los Angeles, and I am driving down Sunset Boulevard like a bat out of hell. Palm trees whiz past the windows of my tiny two-seater, a car I bought not so much for its awesome horsepower—though that's certainly coming in handy at the moment—but because I am not a particularly great driver. (I figured I would be less likely to rear-end someone in the cramped parking garage outside my office if I was driving something, well, *compact.*) I nearly take out a pedestrian on the corner, which is ironic considering the fact that I'm a doctor. The car bucks sharply as I jam my bare toes against the race-car-style pedal, pushing it closer to the floor. (Who can drive in stilettos?!)

In a mere 20 minutes I make it to the main entrance of Universal Studios, one of the largest working movie studios in the world, the place where some of my favorite Hollywood films have been made. But today I'm no tourist. Somewhere inside this 415-acre complex, one of my A-list patients—we'll call her Megan (doctor-patient confidentiality precludes me from divulging her real name, of course)—is smack-dab in the middle of a medical emergency.

I scour the parking lot for Kevin, the production assistant who is supposed to drive me to the set of Megan's latest movie—a raucous comedy starring several members of the "Frat Pack"—and then we're off, speeding past sound stages and set pieces, the perfectly manicured suburban homes of Wisteria Lane (home to the *Desperate Housewives*) whirring by on my left; Stage One, where Conan O'Brien filmed his short-lived version of *The Tonight Show,* is somewhere off to the right. Kevin and I fly through the back lot at what feels like 100 miles per hour (but we're in a golf cart, so we're probably clocking in somewhere around 15). Finally, we screech to a halt in front of Megan's trailer, and another assistant ushers me inside.

Megan, like most Hollywood starlets in their late 20s and early 30s, is mind-numbingly, mesmerizingly gorgeous. She's pretty much a freak of nature. But when I climb into her trailer, I see that she's hunkered down in front of a small magnifying mirror, attacking her face with two Q-tips and a bottle of rubbing alcohol.

"Dr. Wu!" she practically screams when she realizes I've arrived. "Thank God you're here. *Look* at my face."

She points to an inflamed round spot in the middle of her chin. Medically speaking, it looks like an infection of *Propionibacterium acnes.* In other words, she has a pimple.

OK, so maybe this isn't a medical emergency, but think about it: Have you ever watched a movie where the lead actress had a huge zit? Of course not. Celebrities aren't supposed to get pimples. They do, though (all the time). In fact, I get two to three "pimple emergency" calls a month from movie sets and television studios all over town. (Once I was even called to do Botox, though that wasn't an emergency, either. There's just a lot of downtime when you're shooting a TV show.) By the time I arrive, the makeup artist will invariably have tried—and failed—to cover the pimple with foundation, and the director of photography will have been instructed to change the lighting in the hope of making the zit less noticeable on screen. (Can you imagine?) But when that doesn't work, they always turn to me.

The thing is, I totally understand the urgency, and I don't mind driving across town at breakneck speed just to attend to an unexpected breakout. As a dermatologist I understand that having a pimple (or a rash or a chronic skin condition such as psoriasis or eczema) can be humiliating, especially when it interferes with your *job.* I understand that the condition of the skin affects not only how others see us, but how we see ourselves. I understand, too, because as a teenager I had really, really terrible acne.

From the age of 13 on there wasn't a day that I woke up without finding something new on my face—a new pimple, a new scab, a new reason to bury my head under the covers and go back to sleep. My mother assured me that I'd grow out of it, that all teenagers get acne. But that didn't explain why my gorgeous younger sister had a perfect peaches-and-cream complexion (and the body of a ballet dancer to boot). She never had pimples, and I ached with jealousy. Why couldn't that be me?

One morning in particular I awoke with an usually large and especially gross cluster of zits, oozing and pus filled, in the middle of my right cheek. I figured I'd just have to wear a hat or pull my hair over my face until the swelling went down, as always. And then suddenly it dawned on me: *Mom puts hydrogen peroxide on all our scrapes and scratches. How's this any different? I bet a little hydrogen peroxide will clear this right up!* I dabbed gently at my face with a peroxide-soaked Q-tip but quickly realized that the process was going to take forever. So, eager and impatient, I emptied three full bottles into the biggest pot I could find, took a deep breath, and plunged myself in, face-first.

I can still remember the smell—the sickening sweetness of it—and then, of course, the pain. It burned like crazy, and I had made my skin—now bubbling, blistered, oozing, and raw—much, much worse.

For as long as I can remember I've been obsessed with skin and skin care. I grew up in Southern California at a time when Christie Brinkley—with her surfer-girl good looks and sun-kissed complexion—was the gold standard of beauty, the woman every teenage girl wanted to look like. As a Taiwanese American (my parents moved to the States in the 1960s), looking anything like Christie Brinkley was just not going to happen for me. (I present as evidence the photo on page 4, my eighth grade yearbook picture. My pimples are covered by about a pound of makeup, and those wings look nothing like hers *obviously*.) Still, I tried face creams, acne washes, Clearasil, Noxzema—basically anything I could get my hands on at the drugstore. If I couldn't look like a swimsuit model, maybe I could at least alleviate my scarring, cystic acne.

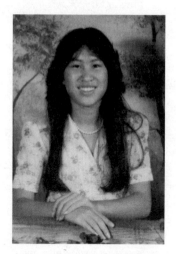

Me, in 8th Grade

It wasn't until high school that my mother finally took me to a series of (older, male) dermatologists, but each visit proved to be more frustrating than the last. One guy actually rubbed a greasy ointment on my scabby cheek and said (to this day I still remember his exact words), "There, that looks better already." Not surprisingly, my acne didn't look any better, and I kept breaking out just as I had before.

Many, many years later, I finally got some relief from my severe acne, only to develop a new problem: I was getting older, and it showed. Sun spots (which are particularly common in women of Asian descent) started to dot my hairline, clustering at the temples. A year or two after that, the tiny lines at the corners of my eyes—crow's-feet—no longer went away when I stopped smiling.

When I became a dermatologist, I gained access to an arsenal of products. Every cleanser, toner, refining mask, moisturizing sunscreen, pimple zapper, and wrinkle reducer known to man—even the stuff that wasn't on the market yet—was shipped to my office for trials and testing. But no matter what I tried, the face staring back at me in the mirror was the same: wrinkles, lines, age spots, and all. It wasn't until I turned to Botox that I got some real results (more on that later), but nothing in a bottle ever seemed to do much good.

Unfortunately, I'm not the only one who's been let down in her quest for better skin. Over and over again I've watched women get seduced by the latest "miracle" product, utterly convinced that some new cream or pill will give them the dewy complexion of Scarlett Johansson or the ethereal glow of Cate Blanchett. By the time most of my patients come to see me, they have already tried a number of different skin-care regimens and spent quite a bit of money on products that just don't work. Everyone, it seems, is consistently disappointed. I'm here to tell you why.

Secrets of the Skin-Care Industry

A few years ago I set out to create my own skin-care line—Dr. Jessica Wu Cosmeceuticals—made predominantly with Chinese botanicals such as white peony and Scutellaria extract (ingredients I had researched extensively and that I really believed in) in the hope of providing something better, something *real*, for my patients. I quickly discovered that that was easier said than done.

In the fall of 2003 I was still searching for a manufacturer to partner with, a company that could turn my vision into an actual tangible product. In meeting after meeting I explained that I wanted to use a fairly large amount of a particularly rare and delicate ingredient, an herb found only in the Fujian Province in rural China, one that grows just a few months out of every year. Admittedly, the cultivation and round-the-world shipping alone made for an arduous and expensive process, so I wasn't surprised when most manufacturers suggested an array of cheaper alternatives. Then one of those potential manufacturers told me she had a great idea, a way to utilize this special herb and still save money.

"Great," I replied. "What's your secret?"

I watched in disbelief as she held out her hand, palm up, and pretended to blow, as if she were showering me in fairy dust. "See? We just use a pinch," she said, "but you can still list it up near the top of the ingredients so that it looks like we used a lot." Needless to say, I decided to go with a different company.

Unfortunately, this kind of deception is not at all uncommon. Skin-care companies are incredibly adept at creating sleek and seductive advertisements designed to fool even the savviest consumers.

I don't mean to imply that *all* skin-care products are totally bogus. Just about everyone needs a good sunscreen, a moisturizer, and something to wash her face with. But it is very rare indeed that a product will help you in the way you've been made to believe. For example, a cream that "hydrates to fight the appearance of lines and wrinkles" (and I'm quoting, by the way, from an actual bottle) will not make your wrinkles actually disappear. In fact, most anti-aging creams do little more for your skin than an ordinary moisturizer would. They can't change the fundamental structure of your skin (which is where wrinkles start) because that would make them pharmaceuticals (for which you'd need a prescription). Similarly, an eye cream may help with temporary puffiness and under-eye circles, but it's not going to turn the clock back 10 years. Like it or not, these kinds of transformations require procedures such as laser treatments and injections or at the very least a prescription-strength product—no matter what it says on the bottle.

Deep down you probably already know this, yet the average British woman still spends over £600 a year on personal care products. Why is it that, despite being consistently disappointed, we keep falling for this nonsense, keep throwing money away on products that don't live up to their claims? Perhaps it's because . . .

skin care has always been equated with what you put on *your skin.*

Think about it: The entire first floor of most department stores is devoted to what you put on your face. So is a huge section of your local chemist. So are pages and pages of magazine ads selling creams that promise to get rid of your crow's-feet. The beauty industry is a £16 billion business in the U.K. alone, and it's built entirely on the premise that you should care for your skin from the outside in.

This is not a book about miracle products or magic ingredients. Those things just don't exist. What I'm proposing is a completely different way of caring for your skin, and it's one that actually works.

The Biggest Myth

When was the last time a skin-care professional asked you about your diet? I'm guessing never. Department store salespeople (who work on commission) certainly don't, nor do the facialists (who might pressure you into buying a basket of products that costs five times as much as the facial itself), and certainly not the doctors (who will typically dash off a prescription in a mere 5 minutes flat before scurrying off to see the next patient). Although there have been some attempts to link food and the skin before (various "acne diets" have popped up over the years), they have mostly been shot down by doctors around the world. That's because the biggest myth—what is being taught in medical schools across the country—is that food doesn't affect your skin.

This probably seems strange when you consider the fact that a high-fat diet increases your risk of heart disease, that eating lots of leafy green veggies may lower your cholesterol, and that changing your diet may even reduce your risk of cancer. We *know* that what we eat affects other organs in the body, and yet there is no medical consensus that what we eat affects our complexion.

In part that is because nutrition courses in med school focus on just two things: how to test for and treat nutritional deficiencies (such as iron-deficiency anemia and scurvy) and how fatty foods play a role in chronic conditions like adult-onset diabetes. Beyond that, nutrition just isn't part of the curriculum. And yet, had any of those stodgy old dermatologists from my childhood bothered to ask what I was eating, they would have been in for a great surprise.

My mother used to make her own soy milk.

Once a week—every week—she would soak soybeans overnight. My sisters and I would wake up the next morning to the ear-splitting sound of soybeans in the blender. Then she'd use cheesecloth to squeeze out the milk. It seemed like a hell of a lot of work just to have something to pour over Cocoa Puffs, which is what my sisters and I did on the rare occasions that we were allowed cereal for breakfast instead of porridge and pickled cucumbers, but we never had regular milk in the fridge growing up.

Dinner in my house was also traditional Chinese fare: a small scoop of brown rice, stir-fried vegetables, and a bit of meat or fish, although more often than not it was tofu. The first time I went to a restaurant with friends, I couldn't understand why everyone salted their food immediately, even before tasting it. (At my house we never salted anything at the table.) I also learned to love hanging with my best friend in the afternoons because her mother kept a huge jar filled with chocolate—we're talking full-size Snickers bars—right on the kitchen counter. (If you wanted a snack at my house, you could have some fruit.) The more I realized what everyone else was eating, the more I realized just how much I'd been missing. At home I had a seemingly limited array of foods available to me, whereas the world outside was like a smorgasbord of sweet treats and salty snacks. Oh, man, did I indulge.

At school I started getting my lunch from the vending machine in the girls' locker room; the bean burritos were my favorite. In the afternoons after P.E. I'd be back—for a bag of pretzels or a chocolate bar. By high school I was visiting McDonald's every day for a strawberry milkshake and fries. I wasn't cool enough to sit inside with the popular kids, so I took my second-hand Honda hatchback to the drive-thru. (To this day I cannot eat at a restaurant by myself. I get flashbacks of sitting alone in the cafeteria.) In retrospect, I can see that I began using food as a way of rebelling against a culture that made me "different," and all the while I was struggling with skin that battered my self-esteem.

Since doctors couldn't seem to help me with my breakouts, I figured I needed to help myself. That's when I decided to become a dermatologist . . . to find out why I had "bad" skin in the first place, to learn how I could take care of it, and to help others with the same problem. So I enrolled at Harvard Medical School. Surely I would find answers there.

In some ways I was the perfect candidate for medical school. (I was, after all, a science nerd.) In other ways I didn't really fit in. (I used to hide issues of *Vogue* in my med school textbooks, for example. I loved clothes, but it wasn't really cool to read fashion magazines at Harvard.) Plus, cosmetic dermatology was quietly frowned upon in Boston—it just wasn't the focus of "serious" medical students. In fact, when I announced to one of my advisors that I wanted to be a dermatologist and that I wanted to move back to the West Coast after graduation, he told me—and I still can't believe he said this—that I was wasting my education. I could do anything with a Harvard degree. Why would I want to be a dermatologist in an academic wasteland like L.A.? I could have a brilliant career doing brain surgery or heart transplants or curing cancer!

I went anyway. Five years in Boston was enough for me. (I just couldn't handle another East Coast winter.) So I traded the cold streets of Cambridge for sunny California, and I set out to be a different kind of doctor. I wasn't going to work in a large clinic where I was allotted ten minutes per patient—

just enough time to write a few prescriptions and look at one part of the body, if I was lucky. When I opened my own practice, I made sure to schedule enough time to treat my patients the way I would want to be treated and to ask about everything I thought might be important—questions like: Tell me about your lifestyle and what kind of work you do. (And where did you get your shoes?!) I quite literally threw out all my oppressive white lab coats because they reminded me of the rigid, old-school way of thinking I was trying to escape. And I treated absolutely everyone like a VIP. That kind of individual attention is probably why my business boomed. Suddenly I was giving advice to editors at the very magazines I used to worship (OK, *still* worship), and I had a waiting room filled with the most famous faces in Hollywood. I was no longer the dorky kid with bad skin and big glasses; I was the woman with all the answers.

Maybe it's because women in L.A. are overly concerned with what they're eating, but I also starting asking every patient, regardless of the reason for her visit, to tell me about her diet, too. Over and over I heard variations on the same theme: "I know that my diet doesn't have an effect on my skin, but I seem to break out every time I eat [fill in the blank]." It didn't take long to notice some definite patterns and to realize that I was on to something. Maybe food *did* affect the skin, despite what I had been taught. I started to read the medical literature, then did my own research, and then put my findings into practice.

The first version of the *Feed Your Face* Diet was a Word-document-processed pile of papers (held together with a binder clip) that I passed out to a few patients. Before long, family and friends were asking for it. I even gave it to my celebrity clients who, despite having access to the best skin creams, facialists, and doctors in the world, suffered from the same skin problems as everyone else. And guess what? I started to see results, *major* results. Acne cleared. Rashes subsided. Even the women I treated who already had beautiful, blemish-free complexions (who saw me for routine screenings and maintenance rather than for acne or fine lines and wrinkles) swore that their skin looked and felt more radiant and healthy than it had in years. Many of them were so thrilled, in fact, that they volunteered to share their personal stories with you.

What you're holding now is a much more complete, comprehensive, and definitely more user-friendly guide to getting the best skin of your life—no expensive products or prescriptions required. For easier reading I've divided this book into four parts, and I've sprinkled each chapter with helpful hints and real-life stories (even some from my celebrity patients). For that reason it's meant to be read straight through, so resist the urge to skip to the diet itself.

In Part I you'll learn the basic structure of the human skin as well as meet the "Skin Enemies," my top three causes of wrinkling, sagging, and breakouts. You'll also learn the basic ways that food affects the skin and discover why the link between diet and dermatology has been so controversial among medical professionals. Finally, I'll explain what everyone can do—right this second—to get healthier and more beautiful skin.

Part II, encompassing chapters 4 through 8, is intended to address a variety of skin concerns in greater detail. You'll discover not only what causes acne, rashes, wrinkles, and sun damage but how certain foods may eliminate (or exacerbate) your symptoms. (Just think how much money you'll save when eating certain foods—and avoiding others—precludes the need for expensive beauty supplies!)

Part III is where you'll find the actual *Feed Your Face* Diet, including a full month's worth of tasty meal suggestions. It has been designed to clear acne, reduce the appearance of fine lines and wrinkles, soothe inflammatory conditions such as rosacea and eczema, and reverse the signs of sun damage and aging—all while helping jump-start your metabolism and stabilize your blood sugar. You will drop pounds and inches and generally feel better in your clothes *and* in your skin. For some the diet will become a valuable addition to their existing treatment plan (particularly for chronic skin conditions like eczema). For others it may be a way to avoid turning to hard-core drugs (like Roaccutane) altogether. Even if you're happy with the skin you have now, the *Feed Your Face* Diet can help prevent signs of aging before they start. And since I've never been one for cooking elaborate meals, I've made sure every recipe is super easy to follow—no complicated techniques or special kitchen tools required. These are the same meals that I eat every day, so you can trust that they'll work for you, too.

Part IV includes two bonus chapters. You'll learn how to use food topically (I've provided some easy recipes for make-at-home skin-care products).

I've also included a chapter on the most-asked-about dermatological procedures (like Botox, lasers, and chemical peels) because even though I believe in the power that food has to change the way our skin looks and feels, at some point we could all use a little extra help. (You'd be amazed at how many world-famous yoga instructors—the kinds of women who swear by macrobiotic diets, avoid alcohol like the plague, and work out three times a day—come in to get their lips plumped and their wrinkles smoothed.) I also know these procedures can seem kind of scary, so I'll give you the scoop on what to expect (as well as tips for finding a doctor who won't make you look like an alien). I'll warn you about products and procedures I don't believe in (like certain kinds of chemical peels). I'll also discuss the dangers of overdoing it, because bad Botox is like a bad Louis Vuitton knockoff: You can spot it a mile away.

Despite all your previous disappointments and despite what you've been told, you do have the power to change the way your skin looks and feels. And you're already one big step closer because now you know the secret: The single most important thing you can do for your skin is to change the way you eat.

Now let's get started.

Part I

The *Feed Your Face*
Philosophy

1

Getting to Know Your Skin

A few years ago a young father of three came to my office with what he thought was a rash. He was a strong, sturdy guy—a construction worker—with no health problems to speak of except for this persistent itch that was keeping him up at night. His pharmacist gave him oatmeal baths, his wife bought him all sorts of lotions and creams, but nothing worked. Even as we talked, he scratched and scratched and scratched, but when I examined him, I couldn't find any rash. All the marks on his skin were self-inflicted, left over from his fingernails digging into his flesh.

There are all sorts of reasons for why someone might develop "itching of unknown cause," but it's a long and scary list (think liver problems, cancer, etc.). I didn't want to freak the poor guy out—at least not without knowing anything for sure—so we took some blood, I wrote a prescription for a soothing cream, and we sent his sample out for tests.

The next day I got a call from the lab. This was not good news: The lab *never* calls unless something is seriously wrong. As fate would have it, the young man was in full kidney failure and very, very sick. I referred him to an internist who put him on dialysis that very same day. And all he had was an itch.

t is not my intention to scare the living daylights out of you here but, rather, to point out a simple fact: Your skin is important. It's not just what keeps your insides in; how it looks is an indicator of your overall health, and it's often the first (and sometimes the only) sign of serious illness elsewhere in the body. If your liver is in bad shape, you'll get jaundice (you'll turn yellow). Pale skin and hair loss are often the first signs of anemia. People with lung disease can appear pale and sallow (because they're not getting enough oxygen to the skin). Crash dieters can look gaunt, as if their skin were sagging. In fact, every time you visit a doctor—any doctor, not just a dermatologist—he or she checks out your skin as part of the overall examination. Taking care of your skin is a big part of keeping your whole body healthy.

Here's the good news: Getting beautiful, healthy skin doesn't have to be time-consuming, expensive, or intimidating. You don't have to forgo getting a great tan. You don't have to stop wearing makeup. And you definitely don't have to keep Olga, the Russian facialist, on speed dial. But before we can talk about looking good, we have to talk about how the skin—your body's largest organ—works. Here's a look at what's really going on in there.

It's *Aliiive*! Your Skin Is Living and Breathing

Just as your digestive system takes in food, processes nutrients, and gets rid of waste, your skin takes in nutrients from the blood, produces by-products (such as oil and dead skin cells), and sends what it doesn't need back into the bloodstream. For this reason we say it has its own metabolism, and how it functions is directly related to the fuel it receives (i.e., the food you eat).

Your skin is also what we call a *microbiome;* it's teeming with microorganisms, most of which are invisible to the naked eye. Even when you think you're clean (like right after a long, hot shower), you still have bacteria, fungus, yeast, and parasites living on and in your skin (gross, but true). They're supposed to be there, of course, and normally they all live in harmony, but when that delicate balance gets disturbed (by hormone fluctuations or changes in your diet, for example), one component overgrows, and your skin reacts. Rosacea, acne, and many rashes are caused, at least in part, by bacterial overgrowth or imbalance.

Hey, Dr. Wu

Q: So, how many skin-care products do I really need?

A: Two to three products—tops—should do the trick: a cleanser, sunscreen (typically in the form of a moisturizer with SPF), and a treatment of some kind in the evening, depending on your particular needs.

Over the years I've come to realize that skin care basics often confuse people the most. In fact, the majority of questions I receive from my online newsletter* are about the simple stuff, such as the proper way to wash one's face or what to look for in a moisturizer. That's why I'll be sharing tips and tricks, as well as specific product recommendations, along the way.

*Have a question you'd like to see answered? You can write me, too. Sign up for my free e-newsletter at JessicaWu.com/newsletter.

Is It Hot in Here? Your Skin Controls Your Core Temperature

The skin maintains your core temperature of 98.6°F by controlling the amount of water that evaporates from your body. The evaporation of water from the skin is what cools you down. If it's very cold outside, you won't sweat as much because your body is conserving heat. On the flip side, if it's really warm outside, your body increases perspiration (obviously); as the water evaporates from your skin, you cool off. That's why people who live in dry heat don't feel as uncomfortable as people who live in more humid parts of the country. It could be 110 degrees outside, but if you're in, say, Athens or the Costa del Sol, the sweat on your skin will evaporate quickly because the air is dry. On the other hand, if you're in Paris in August, it might be only 85 degrees, but there's already so much water in the air that the sweat evaporates much more slowly. It's like being in a steam shower—sticky and uncomfortable.

Were you to lose large areas of your skin—in a fire, for example—you'd also lose your ability to regulate your internal temperature. That's why burn victims have to be wrapped from head to toe and kept in warm beds. There's a huge risk of developing hypothermia when you can't prevent water loss or hold in heat. That is also why a serious sunburn (as in second degree or worse, when the skin blisters and peels off) can make you shiver and shake.

Skin Enemy #1: *Inflammation*

Your skin is an important part of the immune system—it is the first line of defense against outside "intruders" such as bacteria, allergens, and foreign objects (like dirt or splinters). When the skin is breached by one of those unwelcome guests, your body sends a rush of investigative immune cells to the affected area, triggering inflammation in the form of redness, heat, and swelling. That is why your eyes will puff up during allergy season, why you'll spike a fever if you have an infection. Typically, your body's natural immune response is temporary. Once you've recovered from any trauma, infection, or allergy, the associated redness and swelling will subside. For some people with imbalanced immune systems, however, that inflammation never really dies down; and the longer their body stays inflamed, the worse it is for their health.

Recently, chronic inflammation has become a hot topic in the medical world as more and more studies suggest that it's a root cause of conditions ranging from heart disease, cancer, and Alzheimer's to osteoporosis and other diseases associated with aging. Doctors now think that cardiovascular disease, for example, is caused in part by inflammation of the arteries, not just an accumulation of plaque. Long-term inflammation can damage healthy tissue, including your arteries (leading to atherosclerosis, or hardening of the arteries) and your joints (causing arthritis).

Inflammation is also a hallmark of skin conditions such as acne, eczema, psoriasis, rashes, and even sunburn. And while you might be tempted to think of acne as a form of infection (due to the pus), it is really your body's inflammatory response that produces redness, swelling, and whiteheads. In fact, a number of the antibiotics we use to treat acne are prescribed not for their ability to kill bacteria (the dosage is too low) but to reduce inflammation.

Learning how to manage and prevent inflammation is important for your overall health and is essential for maintaining the health of your skin. And one of the most effective tools in regulating and preventing inflammation is—you guessed it—eating the right foods. Altering your diet can help modulate the effects of inflammatory conditions such as eczema and acne as well as help slow the signs of aging. Keep reading. I'll show you how.

Your Skin Is the Body's Main Source of Vitamin D

Back in the early 1900s a childhood disease called rickets, which leads to softening of the bones and skeletal deformations, was a growing national problem in the U.S. Hundreds of thousands of children, particularly in the industrialized cities of the Northeast of America, suffered from bowed legs and weak, crumbling teeth. It wasn't until the 1930s, when the U.S. government started fortifying milk with vitamin D, that rickets all but disappeared.

Vitamin D is extremely important not only in preventing rickets in children (and osteoporosis in adults) but for bone health in general (it helps your body absorb calcium from the GI tract) as well as muscle function and reduction of inflammation. Studies show that vitamin D may even help prevent both breast and skin cancer; however, there are only a few ways to get vitamin D in the body. Some foods (including milk, egg yolks, salmon, and tuna) and nutritional supplements are two ways, but the largest source by far comes from a chemical reaction that begins the minute we walk outside.

Our skin naturally contains something called 7-dehydrocholesterol. When exposed to UVB rays from the sun, this organic molecule magically becomes—drum roll, please—vitamin D. Here is where things get complicated: A small but vocal group of doctors are convinced that vitamin D deficiency is fast becoming a public health epidemic *again*. (Indeed, some studies have shown that rickets, once considered a thing of the past, is on the rise.) One possible cause? A lack of direct sun exposure. The idea is that once we all got hip to the dangers of UV light (burning, premature aging, age spots, and skin cancer, to name a few), we stopped getting enough sun to produce adequate levels of vitamin D. That's a pretty controversial notion.

Before you slather on the baby oil, you should know that studies have shown that regular use of sunscreen does not significantly interfere with your body's ability to produce vitamin D. There is also no consensus as to what constitutes an adequate level of vitamin D, and the ideal amount may be different for different people. If you're concerned about getting enough, talk to your doctor about taking a supplement. But please, don't sit in the sun unprotected. Also, skip the tanning beds altogether, which emit mostly UVA rays anyway. (Remember, it's UVB rays that produce vitamin D.)

Skin Enemy #2: **UV Radiation**

We all know that too much sun can make your skin look like a vintage leather handbag or, worse, like Magda, the scary lady from the Ben Stiller/Cameron Diaz hit *There's Something About Mary.* But UV damage is more than just aesthetic. The sun's rays penetrate deep into the skin—all the way down to your DNA. Recent research shows that UV radiation can temporarily alter the function of white blood cells, meaning that even mild sunburns can suppress the immune functions of the skin. And if you've had sunburns in the past (who hasn't?), you're already at greater risk of developing melanoma, the deadliest type of skin cancer. That's why both the American Academy of Dermatology and the American Medical Association recommend staying out of the sun between 11 AM and 2 PM as well as wearing sunscreen and protective clothing when you're outdoors. It is also why most dermatologists equate sunbathing with devil worship. But I'll let you in on a little secret: I *like* being tan. Having some color makes me feel taller, thinner, healthier, and more beautiful. UV light can even guard against seasonal affective disorder (SAD), better known as the winter blues.

That is why I'm not going to tell you to stay indoors during the day or to wear long sleeves in the summer. In my experience the less realistic the advice, the less likely you are to follow it. For example, when my osteopath told me the only answer to chronic hip pain was to ditch my high heels for flats, I told her to forget it. There's no way I'm giving up my four-inch platforms. (Besides, my husband is 6'2", and I want to be able to look him in the eye!)

The thing is, you don't have to wear a burka to be safe in the sun. Certain foods—green tea and tomatoes in particular—have been shown to boost your skin's ability to fight UV rays and sunburn, so incorporating them into your diet, especially before you hit the beach or spend an afternoon on the tennis courts, can improve the protection you'll get from sunscreen alone. For much more info on sun damage, UV-fighting foods, and even fake tanning tips, turn to Chapter 6.

Your Hair and Nails Are Part of the Skin

You may not have realized it, but your hair and nails are part of the skin, so problems ranging from dandruff to hair loss to ingrown nails should be treated by a dermatologist. More often than not, women will seek the advice of a stylist when they notice thinning hair (and end up spending a fortune on products like Kérastase, an uber-expensive professional-grade product line). Or, when they notice thickened or splitting nails, they'll head directly to a nail salon. (A manicurist might be great with acrylics, but could unknowingly file down the fungus and spread it to other clients. Gross.)

Just as your diet can affect the appearance and health of the skin, what you eat can affect the health of your hair and the look of your manicure. There's more: If your body is deprived of certain nutrients (as a result of, say, crash dieting), it bypasses "nonessential" functions such as making hair and nails and directs what nutrients it does receive to more important organs, like your heart and brain. That is why it's so important to feed your body the right kinds of foods—unless, of course, you *want* to look like Mr. Clean. (Get it? He's bald!)

Your Skin Is a Reflection of Yourself

Perhaps the most important function of the skin is also the easiest to understand. I mean, hell-*o*! The skin is your body's largest organ. It's what your man touches when he caresses your leg or kisses your neck. It's the first (and sometimes only) thing we see when we look in the mirror.

Waking up with clear, smooth skin is like having a good hair day: It can make you feel confident and sexy. But wrinkles, blemishes, and sun spots can have the opposite effect: They can sabotage your self-esteem. That's why my role as a dermatologist is not unlike being a therapist. Many of my patients come in down on themselves, depressed about how they look. Whether it's the teenager with acne who is slumped and slouched and has her hair in her eyes or the woman with sun damage who is too embarrassed to wear a strapless dress because of the blotches on her chest, my message has always been the same: You don't have to live with skin you don't like.

FROM THE FILES OF *Dr. Wu*

Patient: Anna Liza

Skin Concern: Mild to severe acne

Food Sensitivity: Dairy

In Anna Liza's Words: As a busy financial executive I spend a lot of time in airports as well as entertaining clients across the country. While I usually experience mild breakouts associated with my menstrual cycle, my acne always gets worse when I travel. I also had been suffering from chronic pain in my lower abdomen for five long years. I had seen three different specialists, each of whom ordered a battery of tests, but none could pinpoint the problem.

When Dr. Wu first gave me the *Feed Your Face* Diet—and told me to avoid dairy products—I balked. My husband is French, and we both enjoy wine and cheese. Still, I figured it was worth a try. Ten days later my skin was definitely calmer, and I'd had no new breakouts. One month later my skin was smooth and clear, and the painful cysts were gone completely. But what really surprised me was that my abdominal pain was gone, too. I had never put two and two together, never guessed that my unexplained stomach pains had anything to do with my skin!

I still travel a lot, and when I'm busy wining and dining colleagues or clients, it's always tempting to have what everyone else is having. But now that I know dairy aggravates my acne (not to mention my stomach), I don't mind skipping the cheese course or passing on creamy desserts. For me that's a small price to pay for clear skin.

Dr. Wu's Diagnosis: I wasn't at all surprised when Anna Liza told me that her breakouts worsened after traveling. From the stress of running to catch a connecting flight to the recirculated (and germ-filled) air in a crowded cabin and the subpar food, it's not at all unusual to experience skin flare-ups of all kinds, from acne to eczema, when you spend a lot of time on the go. Nor was I surprised when her skin cleared after eliminating dairy from her diet. Dairy products often aggravate acne in women of all ages. It's my stance that we all eat too much dairy anyway, even those of us who don't have acne. More on that in Chapter 3.

Putting It All Together: The Skinny on Your Skin

By now you realize that your skin is more than just something to put makeup on. And that's great, because understanding how skin functions is an important step in learning to care for it. Let's wrap up this chapter with a quick rundown of your skin's basic anatomy. For starters, you may think of your skin as having a single layer, but it's actually made of three layers, each containing several different types of cells:

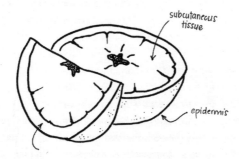

LAYER ONE: The Epidermis

The outermost layer of the skin is called the epidermis. (You can think of it as the peel of an orange.) It, too, is divided into multiple layers.

The bottom part of the epidermis is called the basal layer, and it consists of two types of cells: melanocytes, which give your skin its pigment (they're what determine if you're fair like Nicole Kidman or mahogany like Naomi Campbell) and keratinocytes, which are actively growing and rapidly dividing cells that make keratin.

Unlike your heart, brain, and other organs, your skin is constantly renewing itself. As the active living skin cells in the basal layer of the epidermis divide and multiply, the older cells get more and more crowded. They start looking for room to spread out, moving closer and closer to the skin's surface in the process. Along the way they're busy making keratin, a tough-as-nails protein that protects the outermost layers of the skin. But this must be exhausting work, because before those busy, crowded cells ever make it to the surface, they die. That top layer of dead skin cells, which is what you touch when you touch your skin, is called the stratum corneum, and it's the thickest in accident-prone areas of the body, such as the knees, elbows, and soles of the feet. Because dead skin cells contain little to no water, this top layer is prone to drying out, chapping, and even cracking, particularly in the winter months (which is why your heels may crack and your elbows and knees can look ashy).

As more and more new cells rise to the top of the epidermis, they push off the older dead cells. This is your body's natural way of exfoliating. Supporting this process (by using a body scrub or a pumice stone as well as by eating foods that fuel keratin production) will encourage new cells to come in, keeping your skin looking pink and rosy as opposed to dry and crusty.

$E=mc^2$ Did You Know . . .

There are no blood vessels in the epidermis, so the active living cells (the keratinocytes) depend on oxygen and nutrients diffusing up from the blood vessels located in the deeper layers of the skin below. Cigarette smoking and some medications constrict these blood vessels, however, allowing less oxygen and fewer nutrients to flow up to the epidermis. The result is skin that looks pale and sallow.

LAYER TWO: The Dermis

The second layer of your skin (which you can think of as the white part of an orange rind, the stuff between the peel and the fleshy meat) is called the dermis, and it contains connective tissue—collagen, elastic tissue, and hyaluronic acid—that gives the skin support and structure.

Collagen

Collagen functions like the beams in your house or the boning in a couture gown: It gives your skin its support. There are more than twenty types of collagen in multiple organs throughout the body, but the vast majority of collagen in our skin is Type I, which is the strongest. In fact, gram for gram, Type I collagen is stronger than steel.

We're all born with plenty of collagen, and at first our skin cells are busy pumping out more and more of it (which is why children have firm, resilient skin). As time goes by, however, collagen production slows, so our skin gets thinner, less resilient, and more likely to wrinkle. Eating the right collagen-boosting foods can help fight this process and keep your skin looking younger and smoother.

Don't Fall for It: COLLAGEN CREAMS

Creams that promise to fill fine lines and wrinkles with collagen are pretty much bogus because the collagen molecule is too large to actually penetrate the skin; instead, it just sits on the surface. (That's why injectable fillers such as Restylane and Juvéderm were created.) Collagen creams can make decent moisturizers, and that's good (dry skin can make fine lines more pronounced), but they won't get rid of your wrinkles.

Elastic Tissue

Pinch a piece of your skin. It snaps back in place when you let go, right? That's your elastic tissue at work. Made of a protein called elastin, elastic tissue is what keeps your skin flexible and allows it to hold its shape. As we age, elastic fibers begin to break apart, so your skin gradually loses its bounce-back ability. This is why smile lines slowly become deep creases that stay put even when you stop smiling. Over time you might notice that sleep creases take longer to go away, too (because, apparently, your face *can* freeze like that). Prolonged sun exposure can also damage elastic fibers, which is why sun-damaged skin sags prematurely. And if the skin stretches too fast (such as during pregnancy or a growth spurt), the elastic fibers snap—not unlike what happens when you pull too hard on a rubber band. That's when you wind up with stretch marks. You can help prevent snapping and sagging, however, by choosing foods that will supply your body with the building blocks of strong elastic tissue.

A CURE FOR CELLULITE?

*M*any of my more famous patients indulge in anticellulite Endermologie treatments (which incorporate suction and massage to smooth the skin) before they have to film a bikini scene or walk the red carpet in a slinky gown. (Imagine having two rolling pins that are connected to a vacuum hose rolled over your hips and thighs for forty-five minutes, and you'll get the picture.)

In the, *ahem,* interest of science, I decided to try Endermologie myself. (Did I mention this involves wearing a skintight head-to-toe bodysuit?) Although my skin did feel a bit smoother afterward, I can't be sure how much the treatments actually helped because once I knew that some stranger was going to be working on my thighs, I *really* started watching what I ate in between appointments. There is some evidence that it works, though—at least temporarily. A recent study showed that women who received the treatment twice a week for fifteen sessions lost inches, but the results are best immediately following the procedure. This may reflect a temporary improvement in circulation or a swelling of the skin (which would make lumps less obvious) rather than a real "loss" of cellulite.

You can produce a similar effect by doing your own vigorous massage at home in the shower (without the humiliation of the unitard). Try a cellulite massager to improve circulation and smooth your skin. Then towel off and apply a cellulite cream such as Bliss's fatgirlslim or RéVive's Cellulite Erasure. Both contain caffeine, which has been shown to break down fat cells.

Our skin's connective tissue (i.e., our collagen and elastin) is also partly responsible for the appearance of cellulite, the cottage-cheese-like dimpling that you might notice on your upper thighs and derriere. That's because collagen and elastin fibers sit perpendicular to the dermis. When fat expands (when you gain weight), it causes those fibers to tug on the underside of the skin, creating dimples. Women are more prone to developing cellulite than men because male connective tissue is assembled in a crisscross pattern, at a 45-degree angle to the dermis (so any dimpling appears less pronounced). Women also tend to have a thicker fat layer than men, which is more likely to bulge through the connective tissue (lucky us). Circulation problems may also contribute to cellulite in a woman's legs, hips, butt, and belly.

Hyaluronic Acid

Hyaluronic acid is a natural sugar that binds water molecules together to keep your skin plump and hydrated. It is also the "jelly" in your eyeball as well as a lubricant in your joints. The popular wrinkle fillers Juvéderm and Restylane use synthetic hyaluronic acid as an active ingredient.

Aside from connective tissue and hyaluronic acid, the dermis is also where you'll find the sebaceous glands (or oil glands)—concentrated primarily on your face, chest, back, and scalp—that secrete sebum (oil), your body's natural moisturizer. Sebum is what keeps your skin soft, supple, and waterproof. (After all, you won't melt if you walk in the rain or take a dip in the ocean, right?) Too much oil, however, can make your skin shiny and your makeup smear.

There are a number of reasons for why the sebaceous glands might go into overdrive, including stress, hormonal fluctuations associated with puberty and your menstrual cycle, and even certain foods. Overactive glands pump out lots and lots of oil, causing the pores to enlarge (which is why people with oily skin tend to have bigger pores). Excess oil on the scalp can make your hair feel greasy as well as predispose you to yeast overgrowth and dandruff. But choose the right foods, and you can modulate your skin's sebum production and control such conditions as acne and dandruff.

$E = mc^2$ Did You Know . . .

When you get inked, tattoo pigment is injected past the top layers of the skin and deep into the dermis. Since this part of the skin is constantly being patrolled for "invaders," and tattoo ink is technically a foreign substance (biologically speaking, it's not really *supposed* to be there), immune cells called macrophages attempt to gobble it up and digest it. That's why tattoos fade over time.

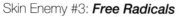

Skin Enemy #3: *Free Radicals*

You've heard about them before in countless skin-care ads and magazine articles, but what the hell are free radicals and why should we care about them?

Without getting too technical (for those of you who *aren't* science nerds), free radicals are atoms or molecules with an unpaired electron in their outermost shell. This makes them highly unstable and prone to undergo spontaneous chemical reactions in the hope of "stealing" an extra electron from a neighboring molecule.

Let's try an analogy: A free radical is not unlike a car with three wheels—you need the fourth to drive in a straight line and to stop you from wobbling and veering off course. But if you steal a tire from someone else's car, now they're left with an unstable ride. Likewise, when a free radical steals an electron from, say, a collagen or DNA molecule, those cells no longer function as intended, and that can have serious consequences. For example, it's believed that some forms of cancer are caused by chemical reactions between free radicals and DNA. According to the "free radical theory of aging," long-term free radical damage is the cause of most age-related diseases, including arthritis, Alzheimer's, and atherosclerosis. And in the skin, free radical damage causes a breakdown of collagen and elastin, leading to wrinkles, sagging, and discoloration. Put simply, free radicals are the reason that our bodies start to break down over time.

Free radicals exist all around us—they're even natural by-products of the body's metabolism, the network of chemical reactions that keeps us alive. But they're also found in abundance in pollution, toxins, pesticides, and cigarette smoke. In addition, they are produced when UV rays interact with the skin. Typically, your body can neutralize most free radical damage on its own, but if you're bombarded by such factors as UV light, pollution, and secondhand smoke, you'll overwhelm that innate ability. The net result is a breakdown of healthy cells and a face that looks old and tired.

LAYER THREE: Subcutaneous Tissue, a.k.a. the Fat Layer

Not only are we born with beautiful skin, but we're also born with a nice, thick layer of fat right underneath it. (Continuing with the orange analogy, we're talking about the meat of the fruit now, the part you eat.) This sub-cutaneous fat, which looks like the thick yellow fat you might find under chicken skin, provides a barrier between the dermis and your muscle tissue; it insulates the body and gives your face its contours. (It's why babies and children have such soft, curvy cheeks.) As we grow up, we lose some of that fat, and our faces sort of deflate; the cheeks hollow out, and the lips flatten. So where does all this fat go? Instead of gravitating to the cleavage—where we could use it—it migrates down to the belly and butt. Go figure.

Hey, Dr. Wu

Q: My dermatologist says wearing makeup can cause breakouts because it clogs the pores and doesn't let your skin "breathe." Is makeup really bad for my skin?

A: Good news, girls. Breakouts are typically caused by bacteria, hormonal fluctuations, and the foods you eat—not by Laura Mercier. In fact, some makeup can even be *good* for you. Certain cosmetics can provide SPF protection, which is great for those of us who sometimes forget to put on sunscreen. (You know who you are.) Wearing makeup may also remind you not to touch your face as often, cutting down on the transfer of germs from your hands. And as long as you're choosing the right makeup for your skin, it shouldn't make you break out. If you have oily skin, large pores, or acne-prone skin, look for a water-based makeup that is noncomedogenic. And if you're still breaking out, don't worry. In Chapter 4 you'll learn more about acne and how to fight it with skin-friendly foods.

2

What's Food Got to Do with It?

If you thought my diet was bad as a teenager, it only got worse as I got older. Because in the dead of winter, when you're hunkered down with a hundred other eager, overachieving students, deep in the bowels of Harvard's medical library—when you're seven hours in to a nine-hour cram session—the last thing you want to do is put on your coat, hat, scarf, and gloves and trudge half a mile through a snow-covered campus every time you hear your stomach rumble. You would waste an hour of study time (and get snow in your boots). So you would do what I did nearly every day for four years: Hit the vending machine.

Back in middle school I would have opted for the crisps, but as a med student I was older, wiser. A round of treatment had gotten my acne under control (at least temporarily), and even though previous doctors—even my Harvard professors—swore that chocolate wouldn't give me zits, I wasn't going to chance it by eating a chocolate bar for lunch. (OK, fine. Sometimes I did eat a chocolate bar for lunch.) But mostly I tried to choose the healthiest options. That's how instant noodles became my go-to meal, my study-time staple year after year. Occasionally I'd supplement that with pretzels. And when I was feeling fat or frumpy, I'd snack on grapes. I thought I was picking foods that were both healthy and good for my complexion. Boy, was wrong.

Food and Your Skin: A History of Mixed Messages, Myths, and Misconceptions

Did your mother ever tell you that greasy food would give you zits? Mine did. I spent roughly ten years hearing that. Even though supposedly all teenagers get acne, my pimples were apparently due to an increasingly "American" diet.

My mother wasn't the only one with this idea, however. The theory that more oil in your food would lead to more oil on your face—and therefore more pimples—was a popular notion back in the 1950s and 1960s, even among dermatologists. In fact, if you took a poll of doctors who are now between 60 and 70 years old, many of them would still tell you that fatty and fried foods will cause breakouts. Strangely, this notion seems to be in direct conflict with today's conventional wisdom. Nowadays, whether you turn to a women's magazine or an advertisement for the newest anti-acne spot treatment, you'll hear the same refrain: There is no evidence that diet has anything to do with the way your skin looks or feels. And, hey, you don't have to take my word for it. Here are some quotes.

> Scientists have been unable to find a substantial connection between diet and acne.—**Proactiv.com**

> Clinical observations have led to many attempts to improve skin disease by changing the diet, though few have stood the test of time. —*British Medical Journal*, **1989**

> Dietary restrictions—either specific foods or [whole food classes]— have not been demonstrated to be a benefit in the treatment of acne. —*Journal of the American Academy of Dermatology*, **2007**

> The truth is that no food is really bad for your skin.—**Noxzema.com**

So what do all these claims have in common? Proof that there's no connection between diet and dermatology? No. Statements like these only point to a *lack of evidence* that what you eat can affect your skin. In actuality there is very little objective data to support the notion that food and the skin aren't related. On the contrary, there is a growing body of research—albeit still in its infancy—that shows the many ways in which diet and the skin *are* related. So, what's with all the confusion?

In the last twenty years or so, doctors have started to demand that the efficacy of new treatments be proven in clinical trials or in a lab before recommending such treatments to patients. This isn't exactly a bad thing. (Otherwise, we'd be prescribing medications without having any idea if they actually worked.) The problem is that doctors are conditioned to believe medical "evidence" comes only from large-scale, randomized, and controlled trials of hundreds (and often thousands) of individuals, and it is incredibly difficult to design that kind of study to test the diet. I would know—I often conduct clinical trials that get submitted to the American Food and Drug Administration (FDA), and it's always a complicated undertaking. If I'm testing a new moisturizer, for example, each of several hundred study participants must be given not just the moisturizer to try but an entire package of products: a cleanser, sunscreen, etc., as well as a diary to record their day-to-day activities. Any deviation from the plan—like using a nonapproved glycolic cleanser or a medicated product such as Retin-A—could interfere with the legitimacy of the study. You can imagine the literally hundreds of ways an experiment centered on *food* could be compromised. In fact, unless you plan to lock a couple hundred people in cages for a few weeks so you can monitor their every bite, it's damn near impossible to do. There are just too many of what we call "confounding factors" or variables that can influence the outcome of the experiment. (See? I'm still a science nerd.)

Here's another example regarding acne. Until a few years ago there were only two major studies of record that attempted to explain the link between food and breakouts, one from 1967 and the other from 1969. In the latter, researchers attempted to test whether chocolate had an effect on acne. They fed milk chocolate candy bars to one group of college students and fed another group imitation chocolate bars (the cocoa fat was replaced with partially hydrogenated vegetable oil). Perhaps unsurprisingly the researchers noted virtually no difference in acne in the test group versus the control group. They therefore figured that chocolate had nothing to do with breakouts. But . . . both bars had the same amount of sugar. (It doesn't take a rocket scientist to see why that study yielded useless results.)

It may also be important to consider this simple fact: Conventional wisdom isn't always correct. It wasn't that long ago when doctors "prescribed" time in the sun to treat ailments ranging from acne to eczema. (And although I'm embarrassed to admit it, I can even remember when sunlamps were in vogue.) But just because we didn't yet know the dangers of UV radiation doesn't mean that it didn't exist or that we weren't seriously increasing our risk of developing skin cancer. Sometimes the "science" just needs time to catch up.

Food *Does* Affect Your Skin, Just Not the Way You Might Think

So, it turns out that dermatologists from the 1950s and 1960s (and, apparently, my mother) may have had the right idea about food and the skin, but that doesn't mean they had all the facts straight. It's not the cocoa in chocolate or the oil in French fries that causes breakouts. When what you eat manifests itself on your skin, in the form of pimples, rashes, or wrinkles, the culprit is almost always sugar—blood sugar, that is.

Virtually everything you eat gets broken down into glucose (sugar) for your body to use as fuel. That sugar travels throughout your body via your bloodstream. Too much sugar—a "sugar high"—can make you feel nervous or jittery, while not enough sugar leaves you woozy and nauseous. In an attempt to avoid these wild highs and lows, your pancreas produces insulin, which is like the yin to sugar's yang, the Siegfried to its Roy. (Glucose, by the way, is not the same thing as table sugar, so your blood sugar can still surge wildly even after eating foods that aren't necessarily sweet, such as salty and savory snacks that are full of starch.)

The glycemic index (which you've probably heard of before) is a way to measure how quickly a particular food gets broken down into glucose. Foods that are high on the glycemic index, such as sugars, starches, and simple carbohydrates (sweets, soda, and white bread, for example) are broken down very quickly, causing your blood sugar to spike sharply. Your body responds in kind, sending your insulin levels soaring high and fast. Conversely, foods with a low glycemic index, such as complex carbohydrates, proteins, and fats (whole-grain bread, lean meat, and nuts) are broken down more slowly, so your insulin will increase low and slow. Repeatedly stuffing your face with foods that have a high glycemic index forces your body to produce more and more insulin to keep up. It's like an addiction. You eventually need so much insulin to regulate your blood sugar that your body says "Forget it." This can lead to insulin resistance, which can ultimately turn into diabetes (though this happens after years of poor eating, not after one gluttonous weekend).

Aside from being generally unhealthy, sharp spikes in your blood sugar can wreak havoc on the skin. High blood sugar can jump-start oil production in the pores as well as increase the frequency of hot flashes and flushing in rosacea patients and menopausal women. Sugar molecules react with collagen and elastin to decrease firmness and elasticity (leading to the formation of both wrinkles and stretch marks), while producing by-products that leave the skin sallow and dull. Sugar also feeds the type of yeast that causes dandruff—and I'm just getting started.

Back in the library, when I thought I was making responsible choices (even if I was selecting my lunch from a vending machine), I was actually picking exactly the *wrong* things. I might as well have eaten that chocolate bar. That's because pretzels, for example, have a glycemic index higher than jelly beans. Higher, even, than a Snickers bar. They start breaking down into glucose (and cause your insulin to spike) as soon as you put them in your mouth. My other "healthy" snack, grapes, has one of the highest sugar contents of any fruit, and while there's certainly nothing wrong with eating a few grapes in a sitting (I even include grapes in the *Feed Your Face* Diet itself), I was practically eating a bushel at a time to satisfy my sweet tooth. Even seemingly healthy foods with "natural" sugars (like those found in fruit) can send your blood sugar soaring if you eat too much of them.

Things get really tricky when you consider that a great number of foods, including fruits, grains, and even vegetables, are composed of sugar, at least in part. Determining which among those foods will affect your face the most is easiest when you consider something called the glycemic load.

The glycemic load is a truer way to rate a particular food's effect on the skin because it ranks foods according to both their place on the glycemic index (how fast the carbohydrates get broken down into sugar) as well as the average serving size (how much carbohydrate is in the particular food). You can think about it like this: Sake has about the same percentage of alcohol as wine. However, a serving of sake is typically a thimble-size cup, while a wineglass can contain several ounces. In this analogy, their glycemic *load* scores, which account for the disparity in serving size, would vary greatly. The sake would have the lower glycemic load based on the amount typically consumed.

Now let's compare bagels and watermelon. Both contain carbohydrates that cause a quick spike in blood sugar (and each has a glycemic index score of 72). But a bagel has more carbohydrates *per serving* than a slice of watermelon, so the glycemic load of the bagel is 25, while the glycemic load for watermelon is just 4. Therefore, a bagel may raise your insulin (and affect your skin) more than watermelon.

Refined Foods	GI	GL	Unrefined Food	GI	GL
Baguette (white)	95	15	Potato (baked)	85	26
Corn flakes	92	24	Watermelon	72	4
Pretzels	83	16	Raisins	64	28
Rice Krispies	82	22	Sweet potato	61	17
Jelly beans	78	22	Pineapple	59	7
Doughnut	76	17	Banana	52	13
White bread	73	10	Brown rice	50	16
Bagel (white)	72	25	Grapes	46	8
Skittles	70	21	Oranges	42	5
Sugary cereal	69	18	Apples	40	6
Pancakes	67	39	Chickpeas	28	8
Healthy Choice Hearty 7-Grain bread	55	8	Kidney beans	28	7

Source: *The American Journal of Clinical Nutrition*

Here's another example: It may be hard to believe, but carrots have a relatively high glycemic index—about the same as a Snickers bar (they're both around 40). That means the carbohydrates in carrots get broken down into sugar pretty quickly; however, carrots have a very low glycemic load because they don't contain nearly as *many* carbohydrates. In fact, you'd have to eat four cups of chopped carrots to equal the amount of carbohydrates in a Snickers (and that would take a while). So the actual rise in blood sugar from a typical serving of carrots is not very high compared to a typical serving of the chocolate.

Some foods with a relatively high glycemic index score can still be good for you. It's not as if I'd ask you to give up fruits and vegetables. On the contrary, you should be eating more of them. It's important, however, to not eat too many high-sugar fruits in a sitting (such as grapes, apples, and bananas), and when you do eat them, to pair those high-sugar fruits and simple carbohydrates with proteins and fats. A whole-wheat bagel paired with peanut butter, for example, will get broken down into sugar more slowly than if you ate just the bagel. Likewise, dried fruit is best when paired with nuts (a healthy fat) and crackers should be eaten with a protein (like hummus). This principle is also why pretzels have a higher glycemic index (and load) than the chocolate bar. A Snickers has protein and fat from the nuts and the nougat, while pretzels are nothing more than simple carbs.

It's not always easy to tell which foods rate highest on the glycemic load or to remember which fruits should be paired with proteins and fats, so check out the chart on the previous page to find out where some of the most popular refined foods, as well as a number of fruits and vegetables, rank. (And if I were you, I'd stay away from corn flakes.)

FROM THE (CELEBRITY) FILES OF *Dr. Wu*

Patient: Maria Bello—Actress (*Thank You for Smoking, A History of Violence*)

Skin Concerns: Oily skin, large pores

In Maria's Words: I really believe that beauty is internal. Looking good has more to do with self-acceptance and self-love than having a certain hairstyle or fitting into a size 2. And believe it or not, my friends who are actresses in their 40s who do very little to "stop" the aging process typically get more work than women who try to look 20. I'm happy to do little things here and there to keep my

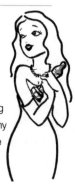

skin looking great (like photofacials, a type of noninvasive laser treatment), but I don't want to look 20. I'm actually enjoying my age.

The real key to looking your best, as I've learned from Dr. Wu, isn't tons of Botox or plastic surgery. It's about a diet that will naturally keep you hydrated while improving the skin's tone and texture. After a few months on the *Feed Your Face* Diet, my skin looks radiant and smooth (not to mention 10 years younger).

I try not to get crazy about food, though I'll admit I can get a little worked up if I have to film a scene in my underwear. In general, though, I watch what I eat for two meals and let myself go a little on the third. A typical day looks something like this:

Breakfast: Porridge

Lunch: Warm chicken salad

Dinner: Pasta with garlic and olive oil, bread, burrata (Italian cheese), and red wine

My favorite snacks are apples and peanut butter, corn chips, and low-fat mozzarella cheese sticks or string cheese.

Dr. Wu's Diagnosis: Maria has naturally youthful skin—few wrinkles, minimal sun damage—but she does have active oil glands and would like her pores to look smaller. One way to achieve that is to regulate the blood sugar (since insulin spikes can increase oil production). Adding protein (such as sausage or chicken) and fiber (like roasted vegetables) to her pasta will reduce the resulting insulin surge. She should also stick with whole-wheat pasta and cook it al dente (since the carbs in overcooked pasta will break down into sugar faster).

As a busy working mom, Maria doesn't have tons of time to shop for and prepare meals, so I'd also recommend other snacks she can eat on the go. Since apples are naturally high in fructose, she should rotate in another fruit (like fresh berries) and pair it with a protein (like almonds). As for corn chips, it's better to have a few corn chips to squelch the craving and then satisfy the hunger with a more face-friendly snack (like carrot sticks and hummus).

As for photofacials, you can read more about them (and other noninvasive procedures) in Chapter 12.

Changing the Way You Think About Food: Eating for Healthy, More Beautiful Skin

Regulating your blood sugar is an important step in managing breakouts, rashes, and chronic conditions, but it's not the only way to take control of your skin. Some foods provide natural protection from Skin Enemies such as inflammation and UV radiation, while others only worsen breakouts, flare-ups, and sensitivity. Learn which is which, and you'll have the building blocks of a diet to nourish and heal the skin.

Eat to Protect the Skin (and Reverse the Damage You've Already Done)

Research shows us that even 10 minutes spent outdoors can have a lasting effect on our skin. That's because free radicals—those nasty molecules found in pollution, toxins, and cigarette smoke—can begin a chain of chemical reactions in the body, leading to cell damage and DNA mutation. But here's the good news: Antioxidants neutralize free radicals.

No doubt you've heard about antioxidants before. Antioxidant-fortified foods and beverages (like green tea) and skin-care products (like Clinique's Super Rescue Antioxidant Night Moisturizer) have become increasingly popular as food and skin-care manufacturers alike attempt to cash in on the anti-aging potential of these miracle molecules. (A quick word of warning: Not all antioxidant products are as good for you as their advertisements make them out to be.)

Your body does produce its own antioxidants (including vitamin C and vitamin E). In fact, the epidermis—the outermost layer of your skin—has five times as many self-made antioxidants as the dermis, yet often that's still not enough to fight free radical overload. Topical antioxidants (those you apply to the skin, like those found in some sunscreens and moisturizers) are a great first step in fighting the signs of aging and preventing cellular damage, but they may not penetrate deep enough into the dermis—where collagen lives—to provide maximum protection. That's why it is essential to protect your skin from the inside out, supplementing any products you do use with a diet rich in antioxidants to help prevent age spots, wrinkling, sagging, and UV damage. Here are some of the most prevalent types and sources of dietary antioxidants:

Lycopene is found in red fruits and vegetables, including red peppers, tomatoes, watermelon, and pink grapefruit. It is perhaps the most potent of all the antioxidants and is particularly effective at blocking the damaging effects of UV rays on the skin, helping to prevent sunburn and skin cancer.

Beta-carotene is found in orange vegetables and leafy greens, including carrots, sweet potatoes, butternut squash, cantaloupe, spinach, kale, collard greens, and romaine lettuce.

Flavonoids are concentrated in berries, onions, tea (green, black, or white, not herbal), and dark chocolate.

Ascorbic acid (vitamin C) is abundant in oranges, papaya, kiwifruit, strawberries, red peppers, Brussels sprouts, kale, and broccoli.

Vitamin E is found in nuts, eggs, green leafy vegetables, avocados, and whole grains.

$E=mc^2$ *Did You Know . . .*

An antioxidant is any chemical that can neutralize a free radical, turning it from an unstable particle that damages healthy cells to a stable particle that's essentially harmless. If you eat mostly foods with *minimal* antioxidant benefit (like dairy products, meat, and processed foods), your body can't recover from free radical damage as quickly or efficiently. But load up on antioxidant-rich fruits and veggies, and you'll be providing your body with the weapons it needs to fight the signs of aging and protect itself from UV rays.

A general rule of thumb is that choosing colorful fruits and vegetables (particularly red, yellow, and green) will provide a healthy dose of antioxidants at your next meal. For more specific information about the antioxidant content of a particular food, we turn to the Oxygen Radical Absorbance Capacity (ORAC) test that rates foods (and such skin care ingredients as green tea and pomegranate extracts) based on their potential to protect against oxidative degradation. Basically, the higher the ORAC score, the higher the antioxidant activity.

But here's the problem with ORAC testing: It occurs in a laboratory using all kinds of complicated science-geek stuff. It's not clear how much relevance a high ORAC score has when it comes to how those antioxidants function in the human body—and that's important to keep in mind when you're grocery shopping, because food manufacturers just *love* to use ORAC scores in their marketing campaigns. While eating antioxidant-rich foods is a great way to protect your whole body from free radical damage, only some foods have been tested to determine their potential to neutralize free radicals in the *skin*—which is why I love the tomato.

The Tomato: A Skin Superstar

Tomatoes have more lycopene than almost any other food, making them particularly effective at preventing sunburn and UV radiation damage in the skin. In fact, studies show that eating as little as 20g of tomato paste per day (about 1¼ tablespoons) can reduce the risk of sunburn by as much as 33 percent.

The next time you're heading to the beach or spending the day in your garden, add some tomatoes to the menu. You'll counteract the effects of a day in the sun as well as help prevent wrinkles, age spots, and inflammation (not to mention lower your risk of developing skin cancer). Even when you're not lounging poolside, adding more tomatoes to your diet can protect you from the small amount of UV light you'll inevitably encounter when your sunscreen wears off—or when you forget to put it on!

You can get the same amount of lycopene found in 20g of tomato paste by eating

- 1 slice of pizza (with marinara or red sauce)
- ½ cup of V8 juice
- 6 tablespoons of salsa

Bear in mind that lycopene is better absorbed by the intestines when the tomatoes are cooked. In fact, the lycopene in tomato paste is four times more "bioavailable" than in fresh tomatoes (meaning it's four times easier for the body to absorb). The absolute best sources of lycopene (offering the most sun protection) are tomato paste and tomato sauce—so opt for pizza instead of a burger, especially if you're dining al fresco. Lycopene is also fat soluble, which means you need to pair your tomatoes with a healthy fat to get the maximum benefits. Try drizzling tomato slices with a splash of olive oil or enjoy them with some avocado.

One more thing: Lycopene may be effective at preventing sun damage, but a diet rich in tomatoes doesn't preclude the need for sunscreen altogether. Slather on a minimum SPF 30 every time you're headed outdoors.

Fatty Acids

Adding antioxidants to your diet isn't the only way to protect your skin from the elements. You also need plenty of oils and fatty acids to maintain a soft and supple complexion.

Each individual skin cell in the epidermis—every melanocyte and keratinocyte—is wrapped in a protective "bubble" of fatty tissue. This keeps the skin flexible and waterproof, and it also helps to prevent the spread of rashes and infection. Fatty acids nourish and replenish that protective layer. Without them, the skin can dry out and crack. (Fatty acid deficiency has even been linked to a number of rashes.)

Incorporate these two types of fatty acids to keep your skin supple and to prevent the appearance of wrinkles and rashes:

1. Omega-3s. The incredible health benefits of omega-3s have already been well documented, so you may already know that they can reduce blood pressure and lower cholesterol (both essential to a healthy heart) as well as reduce the risk of blood clots and strokes. Omega-3s also act as an anti-inflammatory agent in the body, lessening the effects of such conditions as rheumatoid arthritis and lupus.

While omega-3 fatty acids are not antioxidants (and therefore don't neutralize free radicals), a number of studies have demonstrated that the anti-inflammatory effects of omega-3s can decrease the redness and burning associated with UV exposure as well as lower your risk of developing certain types of skin cancer. Salmon, sardines, and anchovies, as well as flaxseed, walnuts, and almonds, are all excellent sources of omega-3 fatty acids.

2. Alpha-linolenic acid. Even though alpha-linolenic acid is not as well known as omega-3, it's equally effective at preventing dryness and irritation in the skin. Find it in soybeans, tofu, flaxseed, canola and olive oils, and walnuts.

Hey, Dr. Wu

Q: Should I be taking a supplement?

A: If you regularly skip meals, there's nothing fresh in your fridge, or you avoid whole food groups altogether (which is not uncommon if you eat a vegan or vegetarian diet or if you're lactose intolerant), then, yes, you probably should consider taking a multivitamin. But keep in mind that our bodies are made to absorb vitamins and minerals from food, not supplements. A number of studies have demonstrated the greater bioavailability of nutrients in foods as opposed to capsules. Taking a vitamin supplement should never replace the need to eat a balanced diet, and it won't earn you a "pass" to beautiful skin. You should also be aware that taking supplements willy-nilly—without any input from your doctor—could lead to unexpected complications, ranging from a minor stomachache to far more serious conditions. Vitamin E capsules, for example, have been shown to increase the risk of birth defects when taken by pregnant women. (Synthetic vitamin E also acts as a blood thinner, so it shouldn't be taken if you're already on a blood thinner such as Coumadin or aspirin or if you have a scheduled surgical procedure.) If you're considering taking a multivitamin (or any nutritional supplement), talk to your doctor first.

Eat to Build Stronger, Healthier Skin

A bodybuilder can lift weights all day long, but if he doesn't eat a diet rich in protein, he'll never build any muscle. When it comes to keeping your skin in tip-top shape, the same principle applies: You can buy the best, most expensive skin creams in the world, but without feeding your body the essential building blocks of collagen and elastin, your skin will slowly lose its resilience and start to wrinkle and sag.

As you age, the body's natural collagen production slows, so it can't keep up as more and more of your existing collagen gets broken down by stress, free radical damage, and UV light. Since you can't replace your body's natural collagen by smearing on a "miracle" collagen cream (because the collagen molecule is too large to penetrate the skin), the best way to supplement collagen production (other than with laser treatments or injectable wrinkle fillers) is by eating the right foods.

The following foods are essential for collagen formation:

Proteins. Collagen itself is a protein, so it's essential to include proteins like chicken, lean meats, and soy in your diet to keep your skin strong and flexible. The major components of collagen, however, are the amino acids glycine (which makes up 30 percent of the collagen molecule all by itself) and proline. Beef, lamb, and chicken breast have high concentrations of both of these amino acids, so they're excellent staples in an anti-aging diet. Additional glycine-rich proteins include pork, quail, bison, lobster, crab, shrimp, and scallops. You can pack more proline into your diet with cottage cheese, cabbage, and (if you're feeling adventurous) bamboo shoots.

Magnesium. Together with vitamin C, magnesium is a cofactor of collagen, which basically means it's a vital element of collagen production. Find magnesium in spinach, whole grains, almonds, cashews, peanuts, soybeans, brown rice, lentils, kidney and pinto beans, and avocados.

Copper. Another stimulator of collagen growth, copper is found in whole grains, legumes, tofu, soybeans, shellfish, cherries, and prunes.

Zinc. Studies show that zinc supports production of elastic tissue. Eat zinc-rich foods such as lean red meat (particularly beef and lamb), raw oysters and shellfish, kidney beans and lentils, and eggs to maintain your skin's elasticity.

Hey, Dr. Wu

Q: After a long day at the office (or a wild night out), the last thing I want to do is spend an hour in the bathroom getting ready for bed. Do I really have to wash my face twice a day?

A: You definitely *don't* have to wash your face twice a day, but you should always wash it before going to bed, even if you don't wear makeup. By the end of the day your face has come into contact with pollution, pollen, dirt, and about a trillion germs. If you're really in a rush, use one of those cleansing facial wipes. (I like Simple Kind to Skin Cleansing

Wipes.) Just don't use them every day. The rubbing of the fibers on your skin can be irritating, particularly if you have acne, rosacea, or sensitive skin. Plus, cleansing wipes tend to leave behind a residue even if your skin feels clean.

Whether or not you wash your face again in the morning is really up to you. My skin, for example, happens to be very oily, so if I don't wash my face in the morning, it's like an oil slick. My makeup will slide right off, and my sunscreen won't stick. But if you have dry skin, a splash of water to wash the sleep from your eyes may be all you need.

When it comes to *what* you use to wash your face, there certainly are a lot of options. I always tell my patients there are times to splurge and times to save, and choosing a face cleanser is definitely a time to save. (I mean, we're washing dirt off our faces here, ladies. No need to spend a fortune.)

If you have oily or acne-prone skin, or if you wear heavy makeup (or lots of foundation), you'll want a gel cleanser. They're water-based and tend to foam more, which helps break up oil and unclog the pores, leaving your skin feeling squeaky clean.

Creamy or milky cleansers, on the other hand, are less irritating, and they won't strip the skin's natural oils, so they're perfect for dry or sensitive skin or for people who prefer a softer, more moisturized feel. They aren't always tough enough to remove makeup, however, so if you have sensitive skin *and* you wear makeup, you may need to use a makeup remover first.

Do you need a cleanser that's strong enough to fight pimples? How about an eye cream that'll erase fine lines and wrinkles? You can find more specific information in chapters 4 to 8, which tackle common skin conditions one by one.

Eat to Soothe and Prevent Inflammation

In Chapter 1, I explained the many ways that inflammation—one of the Skin Enemies—can damage the body and affect your complexion. Luckily, you can get relief from inflammation just by changing the way you eat. Adding foods with natural anti-inflammatory potential (like omega-3s) to your diet can help calm the skin, while limiting the amount of inflammatory foods you eat may provide some relief from symptoms like burning, itching, swelling, and redness. For people with mystery rashes, certain food allergies, or chronic breakouts, cutting down on the following types of foods may alleviate your symptoms completely.

Avoid sugars and simple carbs. We already know that eating foods that are high on the glycemic index will cause a sharp spike in your insulin production, but there is also a link between elevated insulin levels and inflammation. Low-grade systemic inflammation, or chronic inflammation, is common in people with metabolic syndrome (also known as insulin resistance syndrome) as well as in people who are obese.

Elevated blood sugar can also increase the instance of *acute* inflammation by causing the bacteria on your face to flourish. When this happens, immune cells rush to the area and initiate an inflammatory response that includes redness and swelling—better known to you as a pimple. Keep your insulin levels (and inflammatory responses) in check by choosing foods that are low on the glycemic index, avoiding processed foods with lots of added sugars, and trading in sugar-soaked juices for fiber-rich fruits.

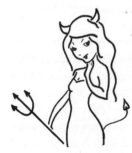

5 "Good-for-You" Foods That Actually Aren't

- Pretzels
- Grapes
- Rice cakes
- Fruit-on-the-bottom yogurt
- Raisins

Steer clear of high-fructose corn syrup. You'd be amazed to discover how many of my patients think corn syrup is healthy just because it comes from corn. While that's technically true—corn syrup is made when the starch from corn kernels undergoes a series of chemical reactions, turning it into 100 percent glucose—it doesn't mean it's good for you. (And you can guess where corn syrup sits on the glycemic index.)

High-fructose corn syrup is corn syrup that has undergone additional chemical reactions to turn the glucose into fructose, which is problematic for a number of reasons. Large quantities of fructose have been linked to obesity and insulin resistance, and may prompt the liver to produce triglycerides, which are fats that contribute to high blood pressure and high cholesterol, not to mention a thicker waistline. Both pure corn syrup and high-fructose corn syrup are very common in processed foods because they're both less expensive sweeteners than cane sugar. You'll find them in sweetened cereals, protein and meal-replacement bars, and packaged baked goods such as biscuits, crackers, and bread. High-fructose corn syrup, in particular, is used in many fizzy drinks and a number of fruit-flavored beverages. And both corn syrup and high-fructose corn syrup will send your blood sugar sky-high.

Cut down on refined grains. The process of refining flour includes the removal of bran and wheat germ (which strips the flour of its fiber and essential nutrients, including calcium, iron, magnesium, and selenium), followed by chemical bleaching. Sometimes nutrients are added back in after refinement (we call these "enriched" grains) but in very small quantities. This means that even enriched grains are nutritionally inferior to whole-grain products.

I know what you're thinking: If whole grains are so much healthier, why bother with refinement? The answer is pretty simple: Refined grains have a longer shelf life because the germ—the "living" part of a whole-grain seed— has been removed. Refined flour also tends to yield a lighter, more airy product (which is why you'll find it in everything from cakes and soufflés to white bread and Ritz crackers). Bleaching, however, is done for purely cosmetic reasons. Historically, consumers prefer flour that's bright white and "clean" looking.

Think about how a glazed doughnut melts in your mouth but you have to chew a heartier grain, such as a Ryvita cracker, for what feels like an eternity. Grains that have been stripped of their fiber (i.e., the bran) are also more easily digested, which means that your body converts them into glucose (sugar) the minute they hit your tongue. That's why foods like white toast, muffins, pastries, croissants, bagels, pasta, cereals, and white rice are so high on the glycemic index and why they'll contribute to inflammation. And remember, the more processed the grain, the higher it sits on the glycemic index. "Puffed" wheat (like Sugar Puffs) and rice cereals (Rice Krispies) are among the highest on the glycemic index charts.

FROM THE **(CELEBRITY)** FILES OF *Dr. Wu*

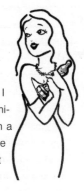

Patient: Lisa Ling—Journalist, Special Correspondent for *The Oprah Winfrey Show* and CNN, Former Co-Host of *The View*

Skin Concerns: AM Puffiness

Food Sensitivity: Salt

In Lisa's Words: I'm usually very meticulous about what I eat, though it's hard to be strict when I'm traveling (since mini-bars are a huge temptation). There are weeks when I'm on a plane 4 out of 7 days, so I also drink tons of water since plane travel can dehydrate the skin. But that means you don't want to sit next to me during a flight because I'm constantly getting up to use the restroom.

Salt is my weakness. I'm probably thin just because I crave salt over sugar. It's easy for me to avoid biscuits and pastries, but I always end up eating those salty Asian rice crackers when I'm stuck at the airport. (I am notorious for eating an entire bag.) I also love pretzels and Japanese food (which also tends to be salty).

In the last couple of years I've noticed that I'm getting puffier in the mornings. Sometimes when I wake up, I'm so puffy that I can barely see. So now I try not to eat before I go to bed. And I try *really* hard to avoid salt when I know I have to be on camera. On those days I'll have an early dinner and try not to eat at all after 7 PM.

Here's what I eat on a typical day:

Breakfast: Sliced mango

Lunch: Tuna salad with baked chips

Dinner: Kimchee and grilled fish

Dr. Wu's Diagnosis: Lisa has a flawless complexion, but a craving for salty snacks can absolutely contribute to puffiness around the eyes (as well as bloating, swelling in the legs and ankles, and overall inflammation). Although Lisa generally eats a healthy diet of whole foods, she can further lower her sodium intake by steering clear of "hidden" salt—the excess sodium that can show up in commercial salad dressings, canned vegetables and soups, soy sauce (common in Japanese cooking), and items packed in brine (such as olives or pickles).

Kimchee (or kimchi) is a traditional Korean dish of pickled vegetables (usually cabbage) and seasonings. While in many ways it's actually quite healthy, kimchee can also be high in sodium. Lisa should choose (or make) low-sodium kimchee as well as opt for low-sodium albacore (or "solid white") canned tuna in her salads, with a splash of olive oil and balsamic vinaigrette, rather than a commercial dressing.

Watch your salt. Table salt (or sodium chloride, NaCl) is a combination of two minerals that are vital to human health. Sodium and chloride are both electrolytes—compounds that are commonly added to sports drinks to aid in rehydrating the body—that carry electrical impulses (like nerve impulses and muscle contractions) from cell to cell, making them essential for nerve, muscle, and brain function. Salt is also highly concentrated in all bodily fluids, which is why your tears may taste salty and why excessive sweating can lead to salt stains on your clothing. You can have too much of a good thing, however. Aside from exacerbating inflammation, excess salt can lead to puffy eyelids, under-eye bags, swollen legs and ankles, and bloating, *and* the iodine in salt can lead to acne flare-ups. Put simply, too much salt will sabotage your skin. Yet the average British person consumes 50 percent more salt than the maximum recommended daily allowance of 2.5g. (If you have high blood pressure or a family history of hypertension, you should have no more than 1.5g/day.)

Salt not only improves how food tastes, it also extends the shelf life of processed goods by drawing out moisture and preventing bacterial growth. These are two reasons why salt—in increasingly alarming amounts—is in damn near everything we eat and is particularly prevalent in processed and prepared foods (including restaurant fare). Breakfast cereals, salad dressings, dairy products (especially cheese), and canned foods and soups are all loaded with salt. Cheerios, for example, is packed with 210mg of sodium per serving. That's more than in one ounce of salted nuts! Check the labels on packaged and processed foods, which may show salt as a percentage of your guideline daily amount (GDA) or display a 'traffic light' symbol to show whether food is low, medium, or high in salt. Foods that are high in salt have more than 1.5g of salt per 100g (0.6g sodium) and may display a red light, so try to stay away from these. Foods that are low in salt have 0.3g of salt or less per 100g (or 0.1g sodium), and may display a green light, so try to choose these foods. If the food label only gives a figure for sodium and not salt, just remember that salt = sodium x 2.5.

DOES EVERYONE NEED A MOISTURIZER?

The idea that everyone needs a moisturizer is a myth, yet it's one that many, many people believe to be true. I think that's because somewhere along the line moisturizing became equated with anti-aging (perhaps because dry skin is more prone to crack, thereby accentuating wrinkles). But using a moisturizer won't prevent wrinkles. (If that were true, we'd only have to smear Vaseline on our faces. No Botox necessary!) In fact, using heavy creams can actually clog the pores and lead to breakouts.

Unless you are on the extreme ends of the moisture spectrum (very oily or very dry), your skin will reflect the humidity and temperature of your environment, and you'll probably need to change your daily routine accordingly. That might mean switching to a lighter moisturizer—like a lotion or serum—in the summertime (or when traveling to humid climates) and saving rich creams for the winter months. If you have very oily skin, however, you may never need a moisturizer. And if you're very dry, you may need a heavy cream every day all year long.

If you're oily or acne-prone but still have patches of dry skin, choose an oil-free, water-based moisturizer with ingredients like hyaluronic acid or glycerin—not mineral oil, which can be greasy and clog the pores—and use it only on dry areas of the skin, typically the cheeks and around the eyes, avoiding the oilier T-zone. If you have dry skin (or are using a topical medication that makes you flake), you may prefer to use a heavier moisturizer all over the face. And since everyone needs sun protection (I recommend a minimum SPF 30), I always encourage my patients to choose a moisturizer/SPF combo, which is an easy way to save time and money. By the way, you can use a moisturizer with SPF at bedtime, too. Many skin care companies will try to persuade you to buy a day cream *and* a night cream even though they typically put the exact same ingredients, minus the SPF, in each. Don't fall for it.

You can start to curb your salt intake (relatively painlessly, I might add) by choosing lower-sodium seasonings (such as low-sodium soy sauce instead of regular soy sauce), swapping commercially produced salad dressings with a drizzle of olive oil and balsamic vinegar, using fresh vegetables instead of canned, and rinsing off items packed in brine, like pickles and olives, before eating. If you're planning to dine out, try looking up the restaurant's menu online. More and more eateries are posting nutritional information on the Web, so you can take your time choosing the healthiest option (without a waitress breathing down your neck). It's also a good idea to request sauces and dressings on the side (so you can control how much you use) and to avoid restaurant soups altogether. They tend to be packed with sodium.

3

What You Can Do Right Now

(Get Beautiful Skin at Your Very Next Meal)

When you think about it, the sneaky marketing tactics employed by skin care manufacturers are almost identical to those used by the food industry. Just as you can't walk through the ground floor of any department store without being accosted by an overly eager saleswoman, supermarkets are organized in a way that flaunts the stuff you don't need, urging you to splurge.

Next time you walk into your local market, take a look around. The healthy stuff—the produce section, the meat department, and the organic aisle—is always located around the perimeter of the store, forcing you to walk past all that processed junk, making you more and more likely to throw a bag of Doritos or a two-liter bottle of Coke in your basket. The same goes for the sweets they have up by the till: The longer the queue, the more likely you are to buy. You know they do that on purpose, right?

In Chapter 2 I hit you with a ton of info about vitamins and nutrients, the science behind antioxidants and free radicals, the long-term effects of chronic inflammation, as well as a long list of stuff you should and should not eat—from zinc to soy, red meat to magnesium. But you're still going to need help deciding what's for dinner.

In this chapter you'll learn the basics of eating for better skin: how to outsmart the multibillion-dollar food industry's sly and savvy marketing (by avoiding common pitfalls, like buying seemingly "healthy" foods that actually aren't), as well as how to identify skin saboteurs (like added sugars, refined grains, and salt) where you didn't even know they existed. Even if you're already pleased with your complexion, I can teach you how to maintain it (so you can continue being the envy of your friends). Whether you're 15 or 50, these are tips and tricks that everyone can use to get clearer, smoother skin, starting at your very next meal.

Know What You're Really Eating

These days many of us are relatively familiar with the ingredients in our skin-care products; we know what to look for and what to avoid. We're much less knowledgeable about the ingredients in our food, however, and we seem to have no idea how food will affect the skin. My question to you is: Shouldn't we know as much about what we put *in* our bodies as the stuff we smear on our faces?

Seriously, most of us have absolutely no idea what or how much we're actually eating. In fact, countless studies have shown that we're all guilty of underestimating what and how much we eat on a regular basis. Overweight people typically underreport their daily intake by as much as 30 to 40 percent, while people of average weight underreport by about 16 percent. One factor in this underreporting trend is our tendency to discount seemingly inconsequential food items (like a random handful of M&Ms or the creamy dressing on your mixed-greens salad) or to forget certain indulgences altogether (like a stolen biscuit from the break room at work, a midday latte, or a predinner cocktail).

We also eat for all kinds of reasons that have nothing to do with hunger or nutrition. We eat when we're happy. We eat when we're sad or stressed. We eat to celebrate and to commiserate. We ate when Denny died on *Grey's Anatomy* (*Hello,* Ben & Jerry's). And we ate when Carrie and Big got together again, for the umpteenth time. (Cosmos all around!) But mindless grazing and emotion-based eating can wreak havoc on more than just your waistline: The effects can show up on your face. Take control of what you put in your mouth by following these simple tips:

Keep a Food Diary

It's important to write down everything you put in your mouth, at least for the first few weeks of the *Feed Your Face* Diet. And spare me your whining, please. This doesn't have to be difficult or time-consuming. Right after you eat, send yourself an email or a text message. Monitor your meals with your BlackBerry or iPhone. Or, kick it old school and take notes in a pocket-size notebook. Whatever your method, keeping track of what you're eating is often the quickest way to identify the cause of an unexplained rash or sudden breakout. Usually within 2 to 3 weeks a pattern will emerge. But if you want healthy, better-looking skin for a lifetime, you'll always need to be aware of the foods you eat.

Look, I know writing down everything you eat might seem like a drag, but just think about how in tune with your body you'll become after just a few weeks. You'll learn what makes you drowsy, what makes you bloated, and what makes you break out. Got a hot date coming up? How about an important presentation at work? Avoiding your particular clear skin saboteurs in the days leading up to any important event can help ensure that you won't wake up to a big, honking zit or a sudden rash on the big day.

There's no right or wrong way to keep a food diary, but if you're wondering what one looks like, I've included a page from the diary of Nikki Sixx, bass guitar player of the rock bands Mötley Crüe and Sixx: A.M. This is a guy who partied *extremely* hard for two full decades—he famously battled severe drug and alcohol addiction. But 10 years ago he kicked all his bad habits, and now (at 52), Nikki looks and feels better than ever. (And I hope I don't kill his image here, but he's also an absolute sweetheart.)

Food Diary

Patient: Nikki Sixx—Musician (Mötley Crüe, Sixx: A.M.), Reformed Bad Boy

Notes from Nikki: *These days, I go to bed before midnight, and I always wake up before 7 AM. I don't drink, and I don't do drugs. I also have tons of water throughout the day. My food journal might be pretty boring for a rock star, but I've found what makes me feel the best and I pretty much stick with it.*

Wednesday

EARLY AM: 3 cups of coffee and a green apple

LUNCH: Grilled salmon on a bed of steamed white rice plus coffee

SNACK: Protein shake and banana

AFTERNOON: Spinach salad with ranch dressing on the side and a Diet Coke

DINNER: Homemade chicken soup

Thursday

EARLY AM: 3 cups of coffee and sliced fruit

BREAKFAST: Oatmeal

LUNCH: Steak and eggs and coffee

SNACK: Protein bar, banana, and grapes

DINNER: Chinese chicken salad and a Coke

SNACK: Protein shake with almond milk

Friday

BREAKFAST: 4 cups of coffee, oatmeal with raisins, sliced banana, and a little almond milk

LUNCH: 2 tacos and a Coke

SNACK: Protein bar and water

DINNER: Grilled chicken and coffee

SNACK: Frozen grapes (while watching a movie at home)

Saturday

BREAKFAST: 2 cups of coffee and 3-egg-white omelet with mushrooms and tomatoes

LUNCH: Clam chowder and a Diet Coke

SNACK: Protein bar and water with lemon

LATE AFTERNOON: Chilean sea bass, mixed greens salad with lemon vinaigrette dressing, water, and English breakfast tea

LATE DINNER: BIG ASS STEAK, creamed spinach, hot bread with butter, cheesecake, and cappuccino

For the most part Nikki eats a healthy, balanced diet, and it shows: His skin is amazingly smooth, supple, and wrinkle-free. By spacing out his meals and snacks, he's maintaining steady blood sugar, and by eating protein at every meal, he's helping his skin maintain its collagen. So what could he do better? I'd suggest eating more brightly colored veggies (for an antioxidant boost). He could cut additional refined grains from his diet by swapping white rice for brown. And he might consider snacking on berries rather than frozen grapes, since they're lower in sugar. Nikki is also a huge coffee drinker. I wouldn't ask him to give it up (because I know he won't), though he might want to alternate between coffee and green tea, which is packed with antioxidants and will help protect his skin from the Southern California sun.

Learn to Read Labels

Figuring out your own personal skin saboteurs is one thing, but avoiding them is another thing entirely. Nutritional labels on packaged foods are deceptive, and even the savviest of shoppers may be easily misled. For example, artery-clogging "trans fats" were declared toxic by the World Health Organization (WHO) in 2009. In fact, they're banned in Switzerland, Denmark, Austria, Sweden, Iceland, and in restaurants in New York City and California. But in the U.K., food manufacturers are not required to list trans fat content. If you're knowledgeable and have good eyesight, you may be able to detect trans fats by reading the list of ingredients, where you may find "hydrogenated vegetable oil" or "hydrogenated fats." Or, if the food is imported, it may not appear on the label at all. That means you may be eating trans fat without even realizing it, and even a little bit adds up over time.

Unfortunately, this is just one example of the dubious methods that food manufacturers use to calculate and report nutritional information. The next time you're at the supermarket remember to do the following:

Check the serving size. Among the many sneaky things food manufacturers do to confuse consumers is divide what's clearly a one-serving food into multiple servings on the nutritional label. Take, for example, a typical chocolate bar. You pick it up and read the label: 200 calories, 300mg of sodium, 25g of sugar. A closer look will reveal, however, that the chocolate bar actually contains *two* servings even though no one in his or her right mind eats only half a chocolate bar. What you thought was an indulgent snack has now become a meal: 400 calories, 600mg of sodium, and 50g of sugar!!

Get to know your grains. I've already explained the problem with refined grains, but spotting them in your local grocery store may be more difficult than you think. The next time you're shopping for cereal, pasta, or bread, stop and check the label. The first word listed should be the word *whole* followed by the grain (that is, wheat, barley, oat, rye). Don't fall for a product that's labeled "100% wheat," because "wheat" is not synonymous with "whole." The same goes for the term "multigrain," which means only that the product was made from multiple grains, all of which may or may not have been refined. (Tricky, isn't it?)

Beware of products stamped "heart healthy" or labeled with any variation of the word *Smart* ("Smart Start," "Smart Taste," etc.). Processed foods that claim—in big bold letters—to lower your cholesterol, protect your heart, or help you lose weight are typically packed with extra sugar to make up for reductions elsewhere (like less saturated fat). You know what that means: sky-high blood sugar and increased insulin. Some products that claim to be good for you actually are, but you have to read the label carefully to know for sure.

Avoid "natural flavorings." You'll find this mystery "ingredient" in just about any processed food, but increasingly it's showing up in meat and poultry and even in packages of frozen fruits and vegetables. Unfortunately, "natural flavorings" are anything but natural. The classification is actually a catchall term for any number of possible chemical additives, including citric acid and glutamic acid (the substance from which we derive monosodium glutamate, better known as MSG) that are injected into foods not only to increase taste but to counteract the effects of shipping, packaging, and freezing. The fundamental components of most of these additives are salts and sugars, which means that any food product with "natural flavorings" has the potential to aggravate skin conditions ranging from acne to eczema to sun damage to sagging.

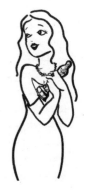

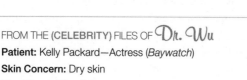

FROM THE (CELEBRITY) FILES OF *Dr. Wu*

Patient: Kelly Packard—Actress (*Baywatch*)

Skin Concern: Dry skin

Food Sensitivity: Sugar

In Kelly's Words: From the moment I found out I was

pregnant with my third child in early 2009 to the time I hit thirty weeks, I craved ice cubes. I was actually chewing 100 a day (I counted!). It wasn't until I saw my doctor and got some blood work done that we realized I had iron deficiency anemia. Although I'm normally a vegetarian, I did eat some meat (mostly chicken) during my pregnancy. Still, I wasn't getting enough iron. Once I started on an iron supplement, the craving went away.

I normally have very dry skin, but I noticed that it was softer, more glowing, and more moisturized this time around. I think that's because I drank tons of water (I usually prefer fizzy drinks and lemonade) and stayed away from sugar (although I did eat lots of guacamole). I gained 22kg during each of my first two pregnancies, but this time I gained only about 15kg!

Dr. Wu's Diagnosis: The hormonal surges associated with pregnancy can lead to all kinds of changes in the skin, from stretch marks to breakouts to a hyper-pigmentation called melasma (sometimes referred to as "the mask of pregnancy")—all of which can be made worse by eating too much sugar. Reducing her sugar intake is absolutely why Kelly noticed an improvement in her skin, but eating more healthy monounsaturated fats (like fresh guacamole) also helped keep her skin supple and hydrated.

Chewing on ice cubes, by the way, is an actual medical condition called "pica," which is defined as compulsive eating of nonfood substances. It's most frequently seen in children and pregnant women, and is often associated with iron deficiency anemia. Lentils, beans, tofu, and chickpeas are all good sources of iron as well as protein. And by eating more protein, Kelly can also help her skin hold on to its collagen and elastin, further reducing the chance of developing stretch marks and sagging.

Get Your Snack On: Eat Smaller, More Frequent Meals

Growing up in the Wu household, we ate three balanced meals a day, and that was it. We never had biscuits or crisps in the house, and I always associated snacking with unhealthy foods—foods that I ate with gusto once I was beyond the watchful eye of my mother. Years later I discovered not only that there's nothing wrong with snacking, but that regular snacking

SNACK WISELY

*N*ot so fast. Just because I've given you permission to snack doesn't mean you can nosh on just anything. The best snacks combine fiber with protein and healthy fats to fill you up and keep your blood sugar steady. Try these simple switches for common, but unhealthy, snacks:

Instead of	Try
Pretzels	Whole-grain pita chips or gluten free breadsticks
Potato chips	Whole-grain crackers with hummus
Rice cakes	Sliced apple with natural nut butter (like peanut, almond, or cashew)*
Ice cream	Strawberries drizzled with dark chocolate
Sweets	Dried cherries or strawberries (with no added sugar) and almonds
Frappuccino	Skim milk latte

*Even though apples are relatively high in sugar, when you pair them with a healthy fat like natural peanut butter, you'll decrease the resulting insulin spike.

can help keep your whole diet in check. Now I spend a few minutes on Sunday evenings packing my snacks for the rest of the week. I then stash them in the car, in my desk at the office, and even in my purse. That way I know I always have something on hand no matter what craziness pops up in my schedule (and I won't wind up bingeing on Swedish Fish). Here are just a few of the reasons that I am officially granting you permission to snack:

Regular snacking can keep insulin levels in check. Skipping meals and not eating for hours and hours can cause your blood sugar to plummet. This not only makes you lethargic, but it also slows down your metabolism and makes your body hold on to fat. When you finally do get around to eating, the body's insulin response is that much more dramatic: Your blood sugar goes through the roof (which promotes inflammation and attacks collagen and elastic tissue), and your body pumps out insulin to bring the blood sugar back down. And guess what? Elevated insulin levels have been shown to stimulate oil production and trigger the release of androgens (the male sex hormones), which aggravate acne. Supplementing your three main meals with a snack or two, however, will ensure that your blood sugar isn't all over the map. Plus, your skin will be smoother and your jeans will fit better.

Regular snacking makes you less likely to binge eat. Let's say you have a breakfast meeting at the office. Someone brings in bagels, cream cheese, and all the fixings, and you indulge. By the time lunch rolls around, you're not that hungry, so you eat a small green salad. But by dinnertime you're starving again. What's more likely in that situation? You go home and prepare a nice meal of lean chicken and vegetables, or you hit the McDonald's drive-thru near your office? If you don't eat all day (or don't eat much), you're much more likely to binge on unhealthy processed junk.

Regular snacking encourages you to eat mindfully. If you know you have to eat every few hours, you're more likely to plan your meals accordingly. Thinking ahead and packing snacks to take with you to work (or around town while running errands) does take more work, but *not* planning often leaves you with few options when you do get hungry. Suddenly it's 3 PM, and you're standing in front of the vending machine in your break room, or you wander into Starbucks and buy an economy-size muffin because that's all you can get your hands on.

Get Prehistoric: Choose Foods That You Can Hunt or Gather

You sit down to lunch at a fancy restaurant and take a moment to peruse the menu: *boeuf à la bourguignonne, coq au vin, foie gras.* Suddenly, panic sets in. *What is all this stuff?* you think. *And how am I supposed to know what's Feed Your Face friendly?* Before you decide between pasta and poultry, think: Could I hunt this? Could I gather it? You can't gather a chip. You can't hunt for pretzels. (And no, "hunting" for pretzels in the depths of your pantry doesn't count.)

This actually isn't a new idea, at least not in the weight-loss world. A number of diet plans and books have been based on the idea of eating like a caveman. But foods that you could theoretically hunt or gather needn't be *all* you eat. (For instance, I happen to think pizza—that's *real* pizza with fresh ingredients, not a stuffed-crust pie with extra cheese—makes an excellent meal, and you can't hunt or gather that.) If you're feeling confused about what will most benefit the skin, however, the hunter-gatherer test can really help you out.

GOING AU NATUREL

Choosing foods you can forage doesn't have to mean giving up on your favorites. Here are some easy ways to switch from milled or processed to whole and natural.

Instead of	Choose
White rice	Wild or brown rice
Instant porridge	Rolled or slow-cooking porridge oats
Canned veggies	Fresh veggies
Fruits canned in syrup	Fresh fruits
Fizzy drinks and artificial fruit juice	Sparkling water with fruit slices
White bread	Sprouted grain bread
White pasta	Whole wheat pasta

This method of choosing "whole" or "natural" foods—such as fruits and vegetables, nuts and seeds, and poultry and game—basically boils down to cutting processed foods from your diet. Here's why that's important for your face (and your waistline):

Processed foods contain refined grains. Remember that refined flour, even when it's "enriched," has been stripped of nearly all its fiber and nutrients, so something that used to be healthy is now, well, not. Biscuits, crisps, and sugary cereals (all made with refined flour) are quickly digested and just as quickly raise your blood sugar.

Processed foods increase insulin. As a response to all that glucose, your body pumps out more insulin. Elevated insulin levels can aggravate inflammatory conditions, which means rosacea and rashes such as eczema and psoriasis will all look worse when you eat processed foods. In addition, high insulin levels have been shown to increase your skin's oil production (making acne worse) and weaken collagen and elastic tissue (leading to wrinkles and sagging).

Processed foods are filled with hidden ingredients. Aside from increasing insulin and inflammation, processed foods are packed with fillers—sugars, artificial sweeteners, preservatives, and sodium—that extend shelf life but do nothing for you nutritionally. Plus, "hidden" ingredients make you more likely to eat something you think is healthy that actually might not be. (Take Raisin Bran, for instance. It has whole wheat, which is good, but it also has high-fructose corn syrup, which isn't.) So remember: The farther a food is from its natural state, the more likely it is to wreak havoc on your face. Hence, can you hunt it? Can you gather it?

Cut Back on Dairy Foods

For anyone with acne, as you'll learn in Chapter 4, dairy foods may be a major factor in stubborn breakouts. But as I mentioned before, it's my belief that we all eat too much dairy in general (regardless of the condition of our skin). Organic milk, yogurt, and cheese, still contain plenty of naturally occurring *cow* hormones, which can elevate insulin production (and therefore damage the skin) just as much as refined grains or sugary sweets. These cow hormones have also been shown to interact directly with our skin cells and oil glands. You can read more about the effect of dairy foods on the skin in the next chapter, but for clearer, brighter skin you can do the following:

Switch to no-fat, low-fat, and organic dairy foods. Nonfat or skim milk and dairy products have fewer cow hormones than their full-fat counterparts, so you'll get a less dramatic insulin surge after eating them. Just remember that nonfat dairy products, especially yogurt, sometimes have added sugars.

Try dairy-free alternatives. To help cut back on dairy, consider trading in skim milk for almond milk, plain yogurt for coconut yogurt, and cheese for soy cheese.

Take a calcium supplement. Dairy products are an excellent source of calcium, which is why I recommend that everyone on the *Feed Your Face* Diet take a calcium supplement fortified with vitamin D. I have trouble swallowing calcium tablets, so I take soft calcium supplements which can be chewed. You can read more about the best calcium supplements in Chapter 9.

FROM THE **(CELEBRITY)** FILES OF *Dr. Wu*

Patient: Kimora Lee Simmons—Model, Reality TV Star, Author, Fashion Designer

Skin Concern: Bumpy breakouts

In Kimora's Words: So here's the thing: I know what I'm *supposed* to be eating. My fridge is filled with fresh, healthy foods, and my family sits down for a balanced meal every night—usually it's grilled fish or chicken with veggies—because I think that's important. But the rest of the time I'm juggling three kids, several companies, and a TV show, plus meetings, interviews, photo shoots, and constant traveling. I call this the Mommy Mogul lifestyle—it's fast-paced and frenetic. Who has time for a proper meal during the day? I usually skip breakfast (and sometimes lunch) altogether.

After not eating all day, I'll hit the drive-thru and scarf down a burger before getting the girls from school. Or I'll stop at a gas station and grab a chocolate bar or swing by Starbucks and have a mocha Frappuccino with whipped cream. I also take a lot of meetings at the Beverly Hills Hotel—when I look at the menu, I want the burger and chips. And I often eat really late at night. Yesterday I had a salami and cheese sandwich at one in the morning while I was up nursing my baby.

I need help figuring out what to eat on the go. I need to know what to grab when I'm stuck at the airport or at a gas station or driving myself to a meeting at lunchtime. Otherwise, I'll wind up at Jack in the Box eating jalapeño poppers with ranch dressing. (I love creamy sauces!)

Dr. Wu's Diagnosis: Kimora has beautiful skin, but sometimes she breaks out in little bumps. That's probably because, like many women, she eats at random times during the day and relies heavily on fast food since it's, well, *fast.* But eating at irregular times, as well as eating the refined garbage found in most fast food, can increase inflammation and contribute to breakouts.

To keep her skin smooth and clear, Kimora should choose snacks she can put in her purse or in the car such as almonds and dried cherries (to satisfy her sweet tooth), edamame, or whole-grain crackers with hummus instead of creamy ranch. (If she spent just 15 minutes organizing her snacks on Sunday evening, she'd be good to go for the rest of the week.) Instead of a mocha Frappuccino at Starbucks (which is loaded with sugar and dairy), she should ask for a soy milk Frappuccino with no added syrup or whipped cream. And for those times when Kimora is eating at a restaurant (or stuck at the airport), she can use the *Feed Your Face* Guide to Eating Out (find it on page 275) to help her figure out the most face-friendly foods.

Recap of Chapter 3

Get Better, Brighter Skin at Your Very Next Meal

* Know what you're really eating. Read labels carefully, watch your portions, and keep a food diary. Eating mindfully is the first step to smooth, clear skin and a healthy, sexy body.
* Regular snacking can keep your blood sugar in check as well as prevent a late-night run for a tub of Ben & Jerry's. Just choose healthy "whole" foods (such as whole-grain crackers instead of chips) and pair simple carbs (like high-sugar fruits) with a protein or a healthy fat.
* Can't figure out what to order? Choose foods that you could (theoretically) hunt or gather and avoid processed prepackaged junk.
* Cut back on full-fat dairy foods and take a calcium supplement with vitamin D.

Part II

. . . .

Acne, Sunburn, Wrinkles, and Rashes

(Using Food to Combat a Range of Skin Afflictions)

4

Understanding Acne

(Why Some Foods May Give You Zits)

beauty editor once asked me to explain why all Asian women seem to have great skin. It wasn't the first time I'd heard this. The idea of somehow unlocking "ancient secrets from the Far East" has actually been around for decades; I get asked about it constantly—from industry insiders, girlfriends, and even patients. My own product line is based on the idea of fusing Eastern tradition with Western science (actually, that's the tagline).

Of course, not all Asians have perfect skin (certainly I am a prime example of that), but there may be some truth to the idea. We do seem to age more slowly, and studies have shown that we tend to have thicker skin and more oil glands, making us less likely to wrinkle. Then there's the nightly facial massage/acupressure routine my mother tried to teach me. And it probably didn't hurt that I was not the type of teenager to sunbathe on the beaches of Malibu; I spent most afternoons in the library.

Despite all this, I believe that lifestyle choices have more to do with having great skin than genetics. After all, it was my mother who was convinced that my breakouts were caused by an increasingly "American" diet. Whenever I got a new pimple, I'd hear the same refrain: *We never got zits in Taiwan. It's all that greasy American food.*

So, was a poor diet really to blame for my bad skin? Could my problems have been solved by shunning salty snacks or turning my back on McDonald's fries forever? Actually, the answer is yes. But before we can understand how the food you eat affects the clarity of your skin, we must first understand the nature of breakouts themselves.

The Anatomy of a Pimple

Your pores are basically openings in the skin that allow for two things: hair growth and secretion of *sebum* (a fancy word for oil) from the *sebaceous glands* (a fancy term for oil glands). Occasionally, those pores get blocked. Just like a clogged pipe won't allow your bathtub to drain, a clogged pore doesn't allow oil to escape from inside your skin. That excess oil buildup then triggers the rapid growth of something called *Propionibacterium acnes* (a scientific term so long that even doctors had to shorten it). *P. acnes,* as it's more commonly referred to, is a type of acne-causing bacteria that occurs naturally in our skin. We all have it—some of us more than others—but when it grows too quickly, you get a pimple.

There are a number of reasons—four, actually—that your pores might become clogged:

1. Dead skin cells. Have you ever squeezed the tip of your nose and watched as gooey white stuff oozes through the pores? That *stuff,* which I affectionately call "nose cheese," is actually a collection of dead skin cells mixed with a bit of oil.

Dead skin cells typically get sloughed off and replaced by new ones. Sometimes that process gets slowed down or interrupted, however. It may be because you're not washing your face enough or because you have high levels of insulin in your blood from eating too many sugary foods. (High blood insulin has been linked to an increased production of skin cells.) Regardless of the reason, if too many dead skin cells hang around on the surface of your skin for too long, they'll end up binding with sebum and clogging the pores.

2. Overactive oil glands. Everybody, regardless of gender, has both male sex hormones (androgens) and female sex hormones (estrogens). But it's androgens—

the most well known of which is testosterone—that stimulate the oil glands to produce extra oil and trigger the overproduction of skin cells, both of which lead to acne. During puberty, when your hormones basically turn you into a raging lunatic, the androgens in your body increase, which is one of the many reasons why almost all teenagers—85 to 90 percent—experience acne (not to mention unsightly hair growth and generally weird behavior). A similar spike in androgens happens just before your menstrual period, which is also why 44 percent of women experience breakouts associated with PMS. (Even though men have higher levels of androgens in their blood—and therefore more oil in their skin—they often struggle less with acne as adults because the amount of androgens in their bodies doesn't fluctuate from month to month.)

3. Propionibacterium acnes (P. acnes). The more acne-causing bacteria you have in your skin, the more likely you are to get breakouts. Production of *P. acnes* increases during puberty (yet another reason teens get pimples). Many acne treatments, including benzoyl peroxide and antibiotics, work in part by killing or reducing *P. acnes* bacteria.

4. Inflammation. So you have a clogged pore. Sometimes all that trapped oil and *P. acnes* bacteria gets to be too much for the pore to hold, and it ruptures under the skin, sending the contents into the surrounding tissue. White blood cells are sent to investigate, causing redness, irritation, and pus. That's when a clogged pore turns into inflammatory acne.

Hey, Dr. Wu

Q: What kind of face cleanser is best for fighting breakouts?
A: If you're plagued by pimples and blackheads, look for a cleanser with salicylic acid, an anti-inflammatory that will take away redness and unclog the pores. If you're more prone to whiteheads, you'll want a cleanser with benzoyl peroxide. If you have blackheads *and* whiteheads, you'll want to alternate treatments—salicylic acid one night, benzoyl peroxide the next. And if you have sensitive skin,

use a gentle nonmedicated cleanser. Harsh ingredients will irritate the skin and only make your acne worse.

Which brand of cleanser you use doesn't really matter—provided it contains the right ingredients for your skin. These days, though, it's hard to turn on the television without catching an infomercial for one of several multistep acne treatments, and all that advertising can be pretty convincing.

Proactiv, for example, a popular three-step program developed by two Stanford-trained dermatologists, claims to be the best-selling acne treatment system in the world. If that's actually true, I wouldn't be surprised. People ask me about it all the time. In fact, a number of my patients have used it at one point or another before making their way to my office. One reason Proactiv is so popular is that it's easy. You don't have to go to the drugstore and choose among hundreds of products, and you're spared the embarrassment of browsing the acne aisle. You can order it in the privacy of your home and even sign up for automatic shipments. But in my experience Proactiv is most effective for teens with pimples and pustules (whiteheads) rather than for adult or hormonal acne.

The active ingredient in Proactiv is benzoyl peroxide, which kills acne-causing bacteria (*P. acnes*) and functions as an anti-inflammatory, drying up pus-filled whiteheads. Benzoyl peroxide itself has been used for decades—as far back as the 1960s, when we had far fewer acne-fighting treatments—and it's a good alternative to topical antibiotics. But the concentration of benzoyl peroxide in Proactiv (2.5 percent) is not prescription strength, and you can get the same active ingredient in several other over-the-counter brands, including Clean & Clear, PanOxyl, Neutrogena Advanced Solutions, and Doctor's Dermatologic Formula (DDF). Benzoyl peroxide also has some potential side effects, including irritation and sensitivity (red, flaky skin), allergic reaction (itchy, bumpy skin), and, when used along with acne creams containing sulfur, such as sulfacetamide lotion or dapsone gel, it can turn your skin orange. It can also bleach colored clothing and linens, so make sure your skin is dry before sleeping on your best pillowcases or pulling on your favorite pink shirt.

If Proactiv or some other acne care system works for you without irritating your skin, then I'm all for it. Just know that it's not a miracle product, and if it *doesn't* work for you, there are still plenty of other options to choose from.

Clogged pores can also lead to multiple *kinds* of breakouts. Let's review:

Whiteheads. Also referred to as pustules, whiteheads occur when the pores become blocked by a collection of sebum, dead skin cells, and *P. acnes*. As a result, the bacteria remain trapped under the skin and begin to multiply, eventually spilling into the surrounding tissue and triggering a response from white blood cells. That's when you wind up with a pus-filled "head" on the tip of your pimple. Whiteheads, because of their associated immune response, are indicative of inflammatory acne, so they're particularly responsive to benzoyl peroxide and antibiotic treatment.

Blackheads. Contrary to popular opinion, blackheads are not caused by dirt in the pores or bad hygiene. Like whiteheads, blackheads occur when too much sebum gets stuck in the pore. But unlike whiteheads, blackheads have no accompanying inflammation—no redness, no pus. Instead, the pore enlarges, exposing all that oil to oxygen in the air. When that happens, fatty acids that occur naturally in the sebum undergo a chemical reaction called oxidation. Think about it like this: What happens to your grandmother's silver when it has been left out too long? It tarnishes. The same principle applies here.

Since blackheads aren't caused by dirt, no amount of scrubbing will get rid of them. Scrubbing the skin too hard, however, can lead to irritation, and irritation can lead to breakouts.

Go Ahead, Try It

Bioré Deep Cleansing Pore Strips, the popular "blackhead removers" that look a bit like nose bandages, *do* work. When you pull off the strip, you're removing the top layers of dead skin cells as well as oxidized ("black") oil. They won't *prevent* blackheads because they have nothing to do with your skin's oil production, but they can temporarily make your pores look smaller.

Cysts. Characterized by large, painful bumps underneath the skin, cysts occur when a blocked pore ruptures deep within the dermis rather than near the skin's surface. No matter how hard you squeeze, you won't be

UM, IS THIS ACNE . . . *ON MY BUM?*

*I*t's bad enough to suffer through a minor acne eruption on your face, but a breakout on your backside, that's just demoralizing. However, buttne, as I like to call it, is actually not at all uncommon, particularly in women who exercise a lot in tight-fitting, synthetic clothing. (Friction + perspiration = a butt breakout.) You don't necessarily have to be a fitness fanatic, though, to get acne on your ass. Some lucky people just have really active oil glands back there.

You can prevent future breakouts by wearing loose-fitting clothing, showering immediately after you exercise, and using a body scrub with salicylic acid once or twice a week. The "scrub" will exfoliate dead skin cells while the acid will help to unclog the pores. Pay attention, though, because if after a week or so you don't see an improvement, you could have a case of folliculitis, a bacterial infection of the hair follicle. If your "pimple" has turned into a large, painful bump or if it oozes pus, see your doctor. These types of bacterial infections (which include Staphylococcus, or Staph for short) will require oral and/or topical antibiotics to cure.

able to pop cystic acne. There's no "head" or opening to the surface of the skin for the contents to drain. The resulting inflammation can eat away at healthy collagen, so if you have a history of cystic acne or if your acne doesn't improve after six weeks on the *Feed Your Face* Diet, you should see your doctor. Cysts are the type of acne that most often lead to depressed and pitted scars as well as keloids, which are raised and irregular scars most often found along the jaw and neck. People with cystic acne may also benefit from adding a prescription-strength medication to their skin care regimen. (Notice I didn't say to start eating whatever you want. Sticking with the *Feed Your Face* Diet will augment the results you get from medications, so don't give up if your skin hasn't cleared as quickly as you would like. It doesn't mean the diet's not working! Some people just need extra help on their path to clear skin.)

Adult acne. Everybody knows that acne is incredibly common among teenagers, but a significant number of adults are affected, too—about 50 percent of Americans over age 25. Acne is considerably more common among adult women than men, however, affecting 26 percent of women in their forties. That means you may reach an age where you're still dealing with adolescent acne *and* starting to worry about wrinkles at the same time—while your husband or boyfriend has skin as clear as a baby's bum. (Is there no justice?)

Even if you never had acne as a teen, you can still experience acne as an adult. Women with adult acne also tend to have higher levels of insulin in their blood, elevated androgens (the male sex hormone), and higher rates of insulin resistance than those without.*

Hormonal Acne. Do you break out once a month when you're PMSing? Well, congratulations. You—along with a bajillion other women in the world—probably have hormonal acne, which tends to show up on the chin, neck, and along the jawline rather than in the oily T-zone. Don't freak out. Experiencing an occasional hormonal acne outbreak doesn't necessarily mean you have a hormonal imbalance; it just means you suffer from breakouts associated with your period, when the androgens in your body naturally spike around ovulation. It's kind of like going through puberty every 4 weeks (as if bloating, cramps, and mood swings weren't enough fun). Studies show that your body produces the most androgens during days 21 to 26 of a 28-day cycle, resulting in larger pores and increased oil production—so you can actually expect your worst acne on day 22. (Plan accordingly.) The pores are smallest, however, during days 15 to 20, right around the time you're ovulating. (Perhaps this is nature's way of giving you better skin when you're supposed to be mating?) Hormonal acne can be particularly frustrating to treat because it's often resistant to standard therapies such as medicated cleansers, topical creams, and antibiotics. There is good news, however: Birth control pills may help tame monthly breakouts. (So can eating the right foods. We'll get to that soon.)

For women who have acne and require contraception, the oral contraceptive pill Co-cyprindiol has been shown to help improve the symptoms of acne. Results can take several months, and side effects are similar to other contraceptive pills, including breast tenderness, weight gain, and mood changes. You should also keep in mind that when you come off the pill your skin might freak out a little.

---

*I hope you're paying attention, because this information is going to be really important about 10 pages from now.

Spironolactone (brand name Aldactone) is another hormonal acne treatment. Although it was originally used as a water pill (a diuretic) for high-blood-pressure patients, in lower doses it also blocks androgen receptors in your skin (which helps to tame hormonal acne). Since spironolactone works in the kidneys, it can increase urination, so I encourage patients to drink more fluids and periodically check their bloodwork to make sure the electrolytes stay balanced. Women on spironolactone must not become pregnant because of the risk of birth defects in male fetuses, so patients often take birth control pills and spironolactone together.

SEE A DOCTOR IF . . . YOU HAVE ACNE *AND* IRREGULAR PERIODS

Resistant acne—that is, pimples that don't improve within six weeks of starting the *Feed Your Face* Diet—and irregular periods may be signs of a hormonal imbalance called polycystic ovarian syndrome (PCOS), an endocrine disorder that's been linked to obesity, insulin resistance, diabetes, and infertility. (Another tip-off is increased hair growth. Lots of women have unwanted facial hair, but if you've got a 'stache like Tom Selleck, I'm talking to you.) Schedule a visit with your gynecologist, and she can take a look at your hormone levels with a simple blood test. While there's no cure for PCOS, the birth control pill, as well as other hormone-regulating drugs like spironolactone, can help reduce your symptoms.

A Word About Isotretinoin (Previously Known as Roaccutane)

Sometimes severe cystic acne can be extremely painful and debilitating, despite your best efforts at eating right. In addition, it can leave large scars and deep pockmarks. When acne is this stubborn, it may be time to bring in the big guns. While it's true that isotretinoin is a potent drug and therefore shouldn't be the first, second, or even third course of action when it comes to treating breakouts, it can also be life changing for those with scarring acne. I should know—I took it while I was in med school and was delighted to have clear, radiant skin for the first time in my life.

Brand name Roaccutane is no longer available, but there are versions of isotretinoin on the market. In the U.K., isotretinoin can only be prescribed by a dermatologist and not by your GP as it can have potentially harmful side effects. More common side effects include dry lips, eyes, and nose, and muscle and joint soreness. Some patients have also reported mood changes, including depression and suicidal thoughts, so those with a history of depression should carefully weigh the risks before starting treatment. It's also extremely important to avoid becoming pregnant during and for a month after stopping treatment, since isotretinoin has been associated with a high risk of severe birth defects (although it has not been shown to affect fertility). If you are a woman of childbearing age, you'll be required to take monthly pregnancy tests. There's also a 30-day wait before you can begin treatment, to ensure that you're not pregnant.

If taken as prescribed, with close monitoring by your doctor, isotretinoin can clear even the most severe acne, but even after a round of treatment, your acne could still come back. That's why I encourage my patients to follow the *Feed Your Face* Diet during and after treatment. Here's what you should know if you're considering taking isotretinoin:

- Some studies have shown that isotretinoin may cause folate (a B vitamin) deficiency, which can lead to anemia. So make sure you include plenty of folate-rich foods in your diet, including leafy green veggies, beans, legumes, and liver. A number of cereals are also fortified with folate.
- Isotretinoin may increase the level of triglycerides in the blood, a type of unhealthy fat. But research shows that a diet rich in omega-3s can counteract that. Make sure you're eating plenty of omega-3-rich fish while taking isotretinoin. If you're allergic or just don't like the taste, take a supplement (3g a day has been shown to reduce elevated triglycerides by 70 percent). Just be sure to check with your doctor before starting a supplement: Isotretinoin is a vitamin A derivative, which means that eating too many vitamin A-rich foods (like carrots or squash) or taking supplements with vitamin A can damage your liver.

Don't Fall for It: OVER-THE-COUNTER ACNE PILLS

If you're tempted to try the over-the-counter homeopathic acne treatment Nature's Cure, resist the urge. This is a two-part system that includes a topical benzoyl peroxide cream and an oral capsule—and it's the pill I have a problem with, mainly because it contains candida, a type of yeast (the same type that causes vaginal yeast infections). There are no scientific studies that show that swallowing any kind of yeast can improve acne. In fact, too much yeast can lead to an acne-like breakout of tiny, uniform pimples called pityrosporum folliculitis (read more about it on page 77). And, really, who needs that?

What If It's Not Acne?

Several common conditions look so much like acne that even some doctors can't spot the difference at first glance. If you have red or pus-filled bumps that spread or appear in clusters, it may not be acne at all. Treating one of these breakouts like acne, however, could make the situation worse. Here's how to tell if you're suffering from the real thing or dealing with an *acne imposter*.

Miliaria. Sometimes referred to as heat rash, miliaria typically occurs in the summer months or when you work out strenuously—basically when you perspire more than normal and the sweat glands get clogged. While it can look just like acne (small red bumps that sometimes have little white heads), miliaria typically itches, whereas acne does not. Keep the area cool and dry (so don't work out for a few days), and it should go away on its own.

Keratosis pilaris. Characterized by rough red bumps on the backs of the upper arms (though it's sometimes found on the thighs and face), keratosis pilaris is colloquially referred to as "chicken skin." It's a hereditary condition, occurring most often in families in which asthma and eczema are also common. Try using a body scrub once or twice a week and then apply a rich body cream to soften the plugged hair follicles.

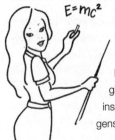

Pityrosporum folliculitis. Pityrosporum ovale is a type of yeast that occurs naturally in our skin, and it's kept in check by bacteria and other organisms that live in our hair follicles (um, *gross*). Though we're not sure why, this delicate balance can sometimes get thrown out of whack, resulting in pityrosporum folliculitis, an eruption of tiny pimples that may cover the entire face, chest, and/or back. Unlike acne, which comes in all shapes and sizes, pityrosporum bumps are all the same size. For breakouts on the chest or back, try an antifungal shampoo (like Head & Shoulders or Nizoral A-D); breakouts on the face are best treated by regulating the blood sugar, since yeast tends to flourish when blood sugar gets too high.

Perioral dermatitis. Typically located at the outer corners of the mouth and chin, the outer corners of one or both eyes, and around or below the nostrils, perioral dermatitis is a rough, flaky rash that looks like red patches with clusters of tiny bumps. It's most common in adult women (though it can occur in men and teenagers), and it's frequently misdiagnosed as adult acne and treated with harsh creams that only make the condition worse.

The exact cause of perioral dermatitis hasn't been determined. Some believe it's triggered by toothpastes or mouthwashes that contain fluoride or by fluoride treatments from the dentist, but it's also been associated with the overuse of cortisone creams and asthma inhalers (both contain steroids). Perioral dermatitis may also be caused by the overgrowth of mites called *Demodex folliculorum*, microscopic insects that live on all of us and are usually harmless. Studies show that prolonged use of prescription-strength steroids can cause an overgrowth of mites and a worsening of the rash. Strong steroid pills (such as anabolic steroids, common in bodybuilding, or prednisone, which is often used to treat asthma) can also cause an outbreak.

Since the bumps are a sign of inflammation, you can soothe your skin by avoiding refined grains and foods with added sugars. To clear up completely, however, perioral dermatitis may require an oral or topical antibiotic.

COLD SORE OR PIMPLE?

Not long ago one of my patients called me in a panic after she woke up with a small red bump on her lip. She had just started dating a new guy and was convinced she had contracted a cold sore from him. Was she contagious? Could she get rid of it? What was she going to *do*?!

A pimple and a cold sore can look identical in their early stages, and both can appear around the mouth, so sometimes it's easier to distinguish between the two by paying attention to how it feels rather than how it looks. Cold sores are caused by the herpes virus, which travels along the nerve endings in your skin. You may feel some itching, stinging, or tingling a day or two before one appears even if you don't touch it. Pimples, on the other hand (especially the larger, cystic type), can be tender to the touch, not unlike a bruise. Over the course of a few days, pimples generally dry up and heal on their own, while cold sores often blister, ooze, and scab. Impetigo, which is a contagious skin infection caused by Staph bacteria, can also cause a red, crusted bump anywhere on the face.

If you develop a bump or blister on or near your lip that you've never had before, ask your doctor about doing a culture. It's the only way to find out for sure what it is. He or she will swab the area to gather a sample, and results are typically available within 48 hours. For best results this should be done as soon as possible after the spot appears. In my patient's case, all she had was a pimple. *Whew*—crisis averted!

Rosacea. Most common in fair-skinned individuals, rosacea appears as a general redness in the central part of the face (the nose and cheeks), often in combination with small red bumps, whiteheads, enlarged pores, and dilated capillary veins on the nose, cheeks, and chin. People with rosacea often seem to flush or blush easily, especially after consuming spicy foods, hot beverages, or alcohol, as well as after a hot shower or steam bath or in hot climates in general. Rosacea is a chronic condition—there's no "magic" cure—but it can be improved by altering the diet and avoiding known triggers of the rash.

Acne cosmetica. Caused by an irritation or an allergic reaction to makeup or skin-care products—common offenders include heavy creams containing mineral oil, petrolatum, scalp oil and conditioners, and fragrances—acne cosmetica will appear as numerous itchy red bumps covering the area where the product was applied. (This could include your neck and back if you have a reaction to a shampoo.) Choosing noncomedogenic products which do not contain ingredients known to clog pores (such as mineral oil), or non-acnegenic products which have been tested on human volunteers for their potential to aggravate acne, can help decrease the liklihood that you'll have a breakout or an allergic reaction. If you do break out within a day or two of trying a new product, stop using it until you can determine the cause.

For more information about acne imposters like keratosis pilaris, pityrosporum folliculitis, perioral dermatitis, and rosacea, turn to Chapter 5.

DERMATOLOGY 911: PIMPLE EMERGENCIES

One of my patients, Stephanie, came to see me after an overzealous aesthetician tried to pop a pimple on her cheek. Nothing came out, but this Russian facialist was very determined (and apparently very strong). Stephanie had tears streaming down her face, but Olga squeezed and squeezed and squeezed. And that was a major mistake.

Somehow the facialist managed to force the infection deep underneath Stephanie's skin because the pimple quickly turned into a *huge* underground boil. One day later the entire side of Stephanie's face was swollen beyond recognition, and her right eye was swollen shut. She ended up in the emergency room on IV antibiotics. Months later I'm still treating the scarring, which luckily is getting better, but it's been a long, slow process. *This* is why we tell you not to pick your pimples. A reaction like Stephanie's is admittedly rare, but no pimple is worth that risk.

At the same time I realize that walking around with a big whitehead on your face is not only impractical, it's gross. If you have a pimple you just *have* to pop, here's the way to do it:

1. Wait until bedtime. Your skin needs time to heal itself, so don't pop a pimple before work in the morning or right before a big event, like a date. (You'll have an oozing mess on your hands that you won't be able to cover with makeup.) Besides, you can typically feel something brewing the night before; that's the time to do your dirty work. If something "pops up" during the day (sorry, no pun intended), it's better to cover it with concealer until you get home.

2. Keep it clean. You'll want to do this as hygienically as possible to prevent infection, so assemble your tools in advance. Here's what you'll need: rubbing alcohol, a sterile needle, cotton swabs, Q-tips, and a plaster—preferably a little round one. Start by swabbing the zit with alcohol. Then, using a sterile needle, *gently* lance the white tip, just enough to pierce the surface of the pimple but not enough to draw blood. After that, you can gently squeeze with two sterile Q-tips (not your fingers). If nothing comes out, stop—seriously. You don't want to force the blockage deeper into the pore, which can turn a simple pimple into cystic acne. You also don't want to squeeze so much that you start to bleed, because bleeding promotes the formation of a scab. (And wouldn't *that* be pretty.) Scabs also increase the likelihood of scarring, and they're impossible to cover with makeup.

3. Avoid pimples in the "Danger Zone." Imagine an upside-down triangle, with the point as the tip of your nose and the inside edge of your eyebrows as the two corners. The skin in this area sits about 1/8 inch above your sinuses, which are connected to your gray matter. Squeeze too hard, and instead of winding up with just a skin infection, you could spread infection to your sinus cavities or even your *brain.* (Really!) It's better to avoid this area altogether.

4. Sleep on it. Resist the urge to use a spot treatment, whether that's toothpaste (an ancient home remedy) or expensive "drying lotions." Research shows that wounds heal best when they're moist and covered; overdrying the skin just lengthens the healing process. Instead, cover the pimple with a plaster and go to bed.

There is one last resort for those moments when a simple pimple becomes a cosmetic emergency. When the lead actress in a Hollywood feature film has a breakout, for example, popping is not an option: Scabs are difficult to cover (even for professional makeup artists), and digitally correcting a pimple in postproduction is seriously expensive. Instead, I'll make a house call and inject the pimple with a diluted cortisone solution; that will bring down the inflammation within a few hours.

If you have an underground cyst (a large tender lump with no visible head) and a major event coming up in the next 48 hours (your wedding day, for example), make an appointment with a dermatologist, who can inject the pimple with a drop of cortisone to shrink the inflammation. Just make sure you see a dermatologist you trust. If not done carefully and precisely, cortisone shots can leave a depressed "pit" in the skin that can take many months to fill in.

Pimples—a Part of Life?

What if you could hop in a time machine and travel back to a time when there was no acne? Sounds like a fantasy, right? I mean, given the prevalence of acne—roughly 80 percent of teenagers suffer from breakouts—you'd think pimples were just a part of life. Recently, however, several studies of nonindustrialized societies have shown that in some parts of the world acne is virtually nonexistent. The following communities have no documented cases of acne. Like, none. Not even in teenagers.

Kitava Island in Papua New Guinea. The inhabitants of this small, isolated island community (population 6,000) raise their own livestock and do their own fishing, rounding out their diet with fruit, coconuts, and tubers. There is virtually no access to dairy products, alcohol, sugar, and salt.

Ache Indians in Paraguay. This is a population of mostly hunter-gatherers, with some farming. Their diet consists of wild game and foraged foods, supplemented by peanuts, maize, rice, and manioc, a native South American crop.

Inuit (Eskimos) in Alaska. There is virtually no acne in those who eat a traditional diet, but Inuit who live in Alaskan cities and eat a more "Western" diet experience acne at rates similar to the U.S. population.

Zulu tribe in South Africa. Like the Inuit, the Zulu suffered acne only after moving from villages to urban cities.

Rural Brazil. In a study of nearly 10,000 preteens and teenagers, researchers documented acne at rates of less than 3 percent.

Before you whittle yourself a spear and ship out to Papua New Guinea, let's put this info to use. What do all these communities have in common (besides having apparently zero need for a dermatologist)? They're hunter-gatherers with virtually no access to refined, processed, "Western" foods. In other words, they eat a low glycemic index diet. Are there other factors at play here, like pollution, overcrowding, or the stresses of city life? Sure. But does smog account for the difference between zero cases of acne in these populations and upward of *100 million* cases in America? I don't think so.

Despite the somewhat obvious connection, the idea of an "acne diet"—or using food to treat breakouts—is one of the most controversial and vigorously refuted concepts in dermatology today. Why?

As we discussed in Chapter 2, this is partly because it's incredibly difficult to conduct a large-scale medical study that centers on food and the skin, so there's little documented evidence to support the notion that "acne diets" work (though that means there's also little evidence to support the notion that they don't). Perhaps, too, it's because we're so hesitant to assign blame when it comes to breakouts. Women's magazines, television infomercials, and doctors all say the same thing when it comes to what causes pimples: It's not your fault! Everyone gets acne!

While I certainly don't mean to imply that acne is anyone's *fault* (no one deserves to get pimples), I think it's much more empowering to know that acne is caused in part by what we eat. That means you have the power to tame breakouts—without visiting a doctor, without expensive prescription medications, and without suffering years of shame, embarrassment, or guilt. So now let's take a closer look at how the Zulu do it.

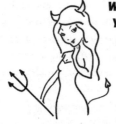

What to Avoid If You Have Acne

- Sugar and high-glycemic foods
- Milk and dairy products
- Iodine

Acne and the Glycemic Index

In Chapter 2, we discussed how foods that are high on the glycemic index can affect your blood sugar. But what does eating a cupcake or white rice or a cherry Danish have to do with *acne*?

Eating foods with a lot of sugar (as well as carbohydrates like white bread and refined grains that are broken down quickly *into* sugar) causes your blood sugar to spike. Elevated blood sugar stimulates your body to pump out insulin, which then triggers a cascade of hormonal effects, including elevated levels of androgens (the acne-causing male hormones), excess oil, and increased skin cell production, all of which lead to clogged pores and breakouts. Remember that I told you that women with adult acne tend to have high levels of insulin in their blood as well as elevated androgens? (On page 73, for those of you that need a refresher.) Recent research shows that a diet high in sugar and simple carbohydrates—a high glycemic diet—may be a major culprit.

In a study by researchers at the Royal Melbourne Institute of Technology in Melbourne, Australia, volunteers were fed a high glycemic diet consisting of 15 percent protein, 55 percent carbohydrates, and 30 percent fat—similar to a typical modern diet. After one week the volunteers experienced almost a 20 percent increase in their levels of androgens (which make your oil glands kick into overdrive). Meanwhile, a different group of volunteers ate a low glycemic diet (25 percent protein, 45 percent carbohydrate, and 30 percent fat). After just seven days this group had balanced blood sugar and lower levels of androgens. These volunteers also had lower levels of a hormone called insulin-like growth factor-1 (IGF-1), which has been shown to increase the growth of keratinocytes (skin cells) and the rate of oil production. IGF-1 also stimulates the skin cells themselves to produce androgens, which can further aggravate your acne.

Other evidence that carbohydrates are associated with acne includes a study by a group of Italian researchers, in which people with polycystic ovarian syndrome (PCOS) who had increased androgen levels *and* acne were given drugs to slow carbohydrate absorption. These volunteers experienced a balancing of blood sugars, decreased androgen levels, and clearing of their skin. (Because high levels of insulin can increase the amount of androgens in your body, the glycemic load of what you eat may be a major factor not only in acne but in other signs of hormonal imbalance, including excess facial hair and thinning hair on the scalp.)

Acne Rule #1: *Choose Low Glycemic Index Foods*

As if you needed another reason to keep your blood sugar in check, research also shows that in addition to wiping out acne, eating a low glycemic diet can help you fit into your skinny jeans: In another study by those researchers at the Royal Melbourne Institute of Technology, people with acne who were placed on a low glycemic diet had clearing of the skin, lower levels of androgens in their blood, and an average weight loss of 3 pounds a week (over 12 weeks) when compared with those who ate foods that were high on the glycemic index. What's more, the research implies that these changes may happen acutely, meaning the results are evident immediately, often after just one meal.

Studies also show that if you start the day with a low glycemic breakfast, you'll have a less dramatic blood sugar spike (and related insulin boost) at *lunch,* which suggests that the effects of healthy (or unhealthy) meals build up throughout the day. Start your day off right, and you'll have stable blood sugar in the evening. But eat a croissant or a bagel (or skip breakfast altogether), and your blood sugar and insulin will be out of whack all day long.

Step 1 in avoiding breakouts is to steer clear of sugar, corn syrup, and foods that are high on the glycemic index, including the following:

- Refined grains, such as white toast, English muffins, pastries, croissants, muffins, bagels, pasta, and white rice. Instead, choose 100 percent whole-grain products. You can look for the whole-grain stamp or read the food label; the first ingredient should say the word *whole* followed by the grain (i.e., wheat, oat, rye). If it doesn't say *whole,* it isn't a good choice. And beware of products marked *multi-grain.* They may be made with more than one grain, but that doesn't mean they're made with *whole* grains.
- Ketchup, barbecue sauce, and pasta sauces, which are often made with corn syrup. Look for sugar-free or low-sugar versions.
- Sugary sodas and sports drinks. In lieu of sugar you can sweeten beverages (and cereals) with a calorie-free sugar substitute. Or try weaning yourself off sugar gradually. For example, use just one packet of sugar in your coffee instead of two.
- Processed luncheon meats, which are often a source of hidden starches and sugars. Instead, choose fresh roasted turkey, fresh roast beef, or rotisserie or grilled chicken.

• For those days when you're *really* craving carbs, consider pairing them with protein. Studies show that eating protein and fat alongside carbohydrates (such as adding chicken to your pasta, for example) can reduce the severity of spikes in your blood sugar. Just remember that the most important factor in keeping your blood sugar balanced is still the composition of the carbohydrate. In other words, it's good to add that chicken, but it's much more important that your pasta be made of whole wheat.

Got Zits? The Link Between Milk and Acne

Your mother may have told you that greasy foods would give you zits, but did she ever tell you to stop drinking so much milk? I'm guessing not. In fact, she probably insisted you drink *more*—like, a whole glass before you could leave the dinner table. Which sounds pretty normal. After all, milk is a great source of calcium and protein, and we've been told for years that it's essential to building strong bones. But consider the fact that humans are the only species on the planet that drink the milk of other animals, and drink milk beyond infancy. There are actually quite a number of reasons why drinking milk might be considered *unhealthy*. Here's my #1: Milk may very well give you acne.

Milk is full of cow hormones. Cow's milk (even organic) contains its own hormones (including androgens) and growth factors (including bovine IGF-1), both of which survive pasteurization and homogenization. That means every time you drink milk or eat dairy products, the cow hormones are absorbed by your body and remain active in the bloodstream, so they can affect your skin (and acne) in much the same way as human hormones.

Milk can affect human hormone production. Even though milk is low on the glycemic index, dairy products have been shown to elevate insulin production to the same extent as white bread. In fact, milk is the *only* exception to the relationship between the glycemic index and insulin production. In a study by a group of Swedish researchers, people who drank a glass of milk (about 200cc's worth, or just under 7 ounces), even alongside a low glycemic meal, had an associated insulin response that was three times higher than normal. Milk also triggers your body to produce IGF-1, just like high glycemic foods.

Whey protein has androgen-like effects. Comprised of the proteins beta-lactoglobulin, alpha-lactalbumin, and serum albumin, whey protein—as it's collectively referred to—can be isolated from the whey of cow's milk and added to foods (such as cereals and protein bars) to up their protein content. You may have heard of whey protein before. In the last few years it's become an immensely popular dietary supplement, particularly among weightlifters and dieters. (It's even a major component of the Abs Diet, the weight-loss plan from the folks at *Men's Health* magazine.) I'm not convinced, though, that people fully understand what it is they're taking.

Whey protein comes from the whey of cow's milk—as in curds and whey. It's the liquid that remains after milk has been curdled and strained, and it's a by-product of cheese production. That means whey protein is not plant-based (like flaxseed or borage supplements), so it's not part of a dairy-free diet and—like milk—it contains cow hormones. The androgenic effects of whey protein include increased lean muscle mass and improved physical capabilities, so it's a bit like a "natural" steroid. (In fact, my personal trainer, a martial artist and former competitive weightlifter, tells me that drinking large quantities of milk—as much as a gallon a day—is routine for bodybuilders. Since milk is packed with androgens, it can help you bulk up naturally.) Just as hard-core weightlifters and other athletes sometimes get "steroid acne," however, some of my patients have experienced breakouts after supplementing their diets with whey protein.

Hey, Dr. Wu

Q: My boyfriend uses whey powder in his protein shakes every morning, and, believe me, milk does his body good. Shouldn't I be using it, too?

A: Not necessarily. Whey protein (which comes from cows) contains cow hormones with androgenic affects, and females just can't tolerate added androgens as well as men can. Think about it: As men get older, their androgen levels decrease and level off, so taking whey protein is kind of like turning back the clock to their teenage years—it's not really unnatural (though it can still lead to mild acne). Most women, however, have never had high levels of androgens (except perhaps during puberty), so whey protein is much more likely to cause breakouts and other unwanted side effects in women than in men.

Our bodies naturally maintain a delicate balance of hormones, but whether it's in pursuit of bigger muscles or a tighter bum, we keep coming up with ways to screw with that balance. The use of human growth hormone (HGH) injections, for example, has become rampant in Hollywood—particularly among actors and actresses in their 40s and up who are competing with hot, young 20-somethings for work. It's also wildly popular among musicians. (How do you think rap stars get so muscly?) While synthetic HGH will help you burn body fat and build lean muscle, it can have a number of unwanted side effects, including thickening of the bones in the face (à la Mickey Rourke). I have quite a few female patients of a certain age who've come in with breakouts on their chin, lower voices, thinning hair, and peach fuzz—all telltale signs that they've been injecting. Feeling good about your body is important, but it's not worth facial hair and acne. Hear me when I say: You don't need added androgens. Leave the whey protein for your man.

. . . .

Acne Rule #2: *Avoid Full-Fat Milk and Dairy Products*

- Skip out on full-fat milk and dairy products, including instant breakfast drinks, sherbet, yogurt, cheese, cottage cheese, cream cheese, and ice cream. Instead, shop for unsweetened soy milk or almond milk and soy cheeses, and swap out butter for a nondairy, trans-fat-free margarine spread. If you can't make that kind of commitment, then at the very least choose nonfat, skim, and organic milk and dairy products, which have fewer cow hormones (though they will still increase androgens in your body, stimulating your oil glands).
- Beware of "hidden" dairy products. Milk and dairy can sometimes show up where you least expect them. Processed luncheon meats, for example, are a common source of "surprise" dairy products. So are granola bars. Be sure to read the labels to avoid milk solids. Stay away from the ingredients whey and casein. Anything labeled *parve* (a kosher term) is fine.
- Get your calcium elsewhere. Everyone knows that milk and dairy products are an excellent source of calcium, so if you're cutting dairy from your diet, you'll want to account for that. You can read more about calcium supplements in Chapter 9.

FROM THE (CELEBRITY) FILES OF Dr. Wu

Patient: Kelly Hu—Actress (*X2, The Vampire Diaries*)

Skin Concerns: Food-related breakouts, pigmentation

Food Sensitivity: Salt, MSG (Monosodium Glutamate, E621)

In Kelly's Words: As a kid growing up in Hawaii, I ate lots of snacks with MSG—especially dried squid and cuttlefish—even though they made my skin bumpy and I got a little rash around my mouth. (Even now, whenever I eat MSG, I feel a tingling around my lips.) I make sure to stay away from it, especially if I'm going to be on camera. I'm also particularly sensitive to salt, which makes me feel heavy and bloated.

I don't think people are necessarily aware of the toll that making movies can take on your skin. When I was shooting *The Scorpion King* with Dwayne Johnson (a.k.a. The Rock), we were spending 10 to 12 hours a day, *every* day, filming in the middle of the desert. Since no one's going to let you take off your heavy makeup just to apply more sunscreen, we had to be really careful not to burn. On the first day of filming, Dwayne had to be buried up to his neck in sand—with only his head sticking out. Everyone was so worried about his face burning, so two assistants would run over with umbrellas between takes, trying to shield him from the sun.

When I'm preparing for a role, I drink tons of water, eat lots of fruits and veggies, and take lots of vitamins (A, B, C, and E) to make sure my skin looks its best. I also stay away from white rice, pasta, and wheat, but I'm a huge brown rice fan. I actually bring a rice cooker to use in my hotel room whenever I'm filming on location. (I don't ever want to seem like a diva, so I bring my own food to the set.)

Dr. Wu's Diagnosis: What Kelly's describing is actually a reaction to *iodine,* an ingredient in both MSG (monosodium glutamate) and salt. MSG is an EU-approved flavour enhancer, but it must be deleted as an additive. So if you seem to be suffering from "mysterious" breakouts, take a hard look at what you're *really* ingesting. That's probably the source of your pimples.

Iodine Exposure and Acne

It wasn't long ago that scientists discovered a connection between chemicals in the chlorine family (including chlorine, bromine, and iodine) and an acne-like eruption of pus-filled cystic pimples. Chloracne, as the breakouts are called, occurs most frequently in industrial or factory workers who have been exposed to dangerous chemicals as part of their jobs. Similarly, people in parts of Asia—Japan, in particular—have reported developing breakouts after eating kelp and seaweed. What do these eruptions have in common? They're both caused by exposure to iodine.

Iodine can trigger an acne-like reaction in the skin that's different from hormonal or adult acne. In fact, the connection between iodine and acne is so strong that the link between acne and dairy products was originally attributed to the iodine in milk. Cow's milk is the primary source of dietary iodine in the U.S. (Cows absorb iodine from the plants they eat.) Milking equipment and cow udders are also sterilized with iodine, so a small amount can pass into the milk supply during the milking process.

Acne Rule #3: *Avoid Foods That Contain Iodine*

- Reduce your intake of foods that are naturally high in iodine, including eggs (especially the yolks), seaweed, sushi rolls, kelp, and milk and dairy products (which you should be avoiding anyway). If you're a fan of Japanese food, opt for sashimi instead of sushi rolls. (FYI: Not all sushi rolls contain seaweed. Sushi rolls without seaweed are OK to eat.)
- Reduce your salt intake. Be thankful you weren't born in the early 1900s. Just as vitamin D deficiency became a public health epidemic in the first part of the twentieth century (leading to the mass production of vitamin D-fortified milk), iodine deficiency—which can cause thyroid problems, goiter (swelling of the neck or larynx), and even mental retardation—became a growing health concern by the start of World War I. The solution? Mass production of iodized salt, beginning in 1924.

These days iodine deficiency isn't really a significant health concern in the U.S., since prepared, processed, and packaged foods all contain plenty of iodine. (Developing nations, on the other hand, including India, Pakistan, Haiti, and Sudan, still report iodine deficiency in alarming numbers.) Some evidence suggests that Americans might even be at risk of consuming too much iodine, probably because we tend to eat too much salt in general.

The majority of salt, including table salt and sea salt, is iodized. Use it sparingly or opt instead for kosher salt, which is not iodized. Remember, you shouldn't cut iodine from your diet completely, or you'll risk some serious health complications, but reducing your salt intake can do wonders for your skin and overall health.

Don't Fall for It: HANDHELD DEVICES, LIKE THERMACLEAR OR THE ZENO MINI, THAT USE FOCUSED HEAT TO KILL ACNE-CAUSING BACTERIA

There is some scientific evidence that heat may help clear acne. Pulsed light, lasers, and radio-frequency devices (which are available only at a doctor's office) have all been shown to kill the acne-causing bacteria P. acnes as well as temporarily decrease inflammation and shrink oil glands. There are two main differences, however, between these medical instruments and a gadget you can buy at a drugstore:

1. Lasers and other medical-grade devices typically come outfitted with a fan or a chilled tip so the laser can reach deep into the dermis (where your oil glands and bacteria sit) without burning through the top layers of the skin. A store-bought device, especially one without a cooling system, won't penetrate as deeply and therefore can't be as effective.

2. Studies show that killing P. acnes bacteria alone isn't enough to stop breakouts. To treat acne most effectively, you also need an anti-inflammatory component. Even some of the antibiotics we commonly use to treat acne (substances that by definition are intended to kill bacteria) are prescribed at very low doses that are meant to reduce inflammation rather than kill P. acnes. Medical-grade lasers work because they kill bacteria *and* reduce inflammation, something handheld devices can't.

Handheld heat devices—which can cost as much as $150—are about as effective as putting a hot towel on your pimple, and even that's a bad idea. Heat only increases your body's natural inflammatory response, making a pimple red and swollen. The next time you have a blemish, try using a *cold* compress instead; it will shrink the swelling and reduce redness.

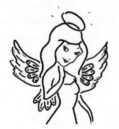

Foods to Eat If You Have Acne

Zinc-rich foods (such as red meat and lentils)
Anti-inflammatory omega-3s

Kill Acne-Causing Bacteria with Zinc

Red meat has really come under fire in the last few years for being "un-healthy," especially from the pro-vegan and pro-vegetarian crowds. While it's true that red meat is high in saturated fat and cholesterol, it's also a great source of zinc, which studies show may be even better at treating acne than antibiotics. (Sounds crazy, I know. Keep reading.)

Zinc is a natural anti-inflammatory as well as an inhibitor of *P. acnes* bacteria. Perhaps it's not surprising, then, that people with acne often have lower than normal levels of zinc in their bloodstream. In fact, most teenagers—85 to 90 percent of whom have acne—are mildly zinc deficient. (Severe zinc deficiency, by the way, is actually quite rare. It's usually seen only in the severely malnourished or in elderly hospitalized patients who are unable to eat.)

New research shows that topical zinc is as effective or better than erythromycin or clindamycin (both common topical antibiotics) in treating acne. One study in particular demonstrated that orally administered zinc, in combination with nicotinamide (also known as niacin or vitamin B_3), copper, and folic acid, helped clear acne in 80 percent of patients.

All this research means that topical and/or dietary zinc (the kind found in food, not supplements) may provide an alternative for people who want to avoid the potential side effects of antibiotics (including stomach upset, sun sensitivity, headache, and yeast infections) or who want to avoid prescription medications altogether. This is especially good news because *P. acnes* has grown increasingly resistant to antibiotic treatments in recent years.

Acne Rule #4: **Eat More Zinc-Rich Foods**

Limiting your intake of foods that are high on the glycemic index can reduce the existence of clogged pores and overactive glands. By adding more zinc to the mix, you'll be attacking inflammation and acne-causing bacteria, too. Here's how:

- Make lean red meat (beef or lamb) your main course as often as two meals a week. Aim to incorporate other zinc-rich foods such as lentils, kidney beans, and raw oysters in your diet as well (especially if you're a vegetarian).
- Phytate, a compound found in cereals, corn, and rice, can reduce zinc absorption. The same goes for casein, the main protein found in milk and cheese. Try to avoid pairing these foods with a steak or lamb entree and other zinc-rich main courses.
- Avoid zinc supplements. Excessive zinc intake can actually be toxic, leading to copper deficiency, severe anemia, and a drop in white blood cells. (I actually know of a teenage boy who wound up in the hospital after overdosing on zinc pills.) It's better to get your zinc through food.

Fight Inflammatory Acne with Omega-3s

In addition to having a high glycemic load, a typical Western diet of refined and processed foods is low in omega-3 fatty acids, the essential nutrient most commonly found in fish, wild game, and wild plants. Why should you care? Because omega-3s may actually reverse the damage caused by a diet high in inflammatory foods.

Omega-3 is a natural anti-inflammatory, so it has the potential to calm angry, broken-out skin. Omega-3 may also decrease insulin-like growth factor-1 (IGF-1), the hormone associated with increased oil production and clogged pores. And as an added bonus, omega-3s may act as a kind of natural mood booster. Studies show that omega-3 fatty acids—especially eicosapentaenoic acid (EPA) and docosahexaenoic acid (DHA), found in fish, fish oil, and algae—can relieve symptoms of depression, attention deficit disorder (ADD), and anxiety. (As you can imagine, acne is commonly associated with depression and low self-esteem. I mean, think about how it feels to wake up with a gigantic pimple—*crappy*.) But despite all these health benefits, just adding more salmon to your diet isn't enough to stop acne and inflammation. That's because the average North American diet, while low in omega-3s, is particularly high in omega-6s.

Omega-6 fatty acids, commonly found in cooking oil and processed foods, have the opposite effect of omega-3s: They promote inflammation. Omega-6 fatty acids have been linked to heart disease, cancer, and arthritis, and in the skin they can contribute to redness, swelling, and pus.

A traditional hunter-gatherer diet has a 1:1 ratio of omega-6 to omega-3, which is like eating equal parts of pro-inflammatory and anti-inflammatory food. They essentially cancel each other out. A typical Japanese diet has a 4:1 ratio. A typical North American diet, however, has a ratio somewhere between 10:1 and 30:1, which means that many of us eat thirty times as many inflammatory foods as anti-inflammatory foods. Our poor bodies—not to mention our skin—are fighting an uphill battle to soothe inflammation! You can help fight inflammation and breakouts by increasing the omega-3s in your diet, but you must also decrease your intake of omega-6 fatty acids.

(Keep in mind that not all omega-6 fatty acids aggravate inflammation. For example, gamma-linolenic acid, which is found in evening primrose oil, black currant seed oil, and borage oil, actually has anti-inflammatory properties. You can read more about gamma-linolenic acid in Chapter 5.)

IT'S NOT TOO LATE TO PREVENT AN IMPENDING BREAKOUT

OK, you lost control. Cheated. Binged. You ate a tub of Ben & Jerry's (or maybe a gigantic stack of pancakes). Here's the good news: Omega-3s, tomatoes, and dietary fiber (found in whole grains, fruits, and veggies) are all effective at lowering IGF-1 levels (the hormone associated with increased oil production and clogged pores). That means less oil and fewer zits. Incorporate them in your next meal, and you may be able to stop a big, fat pimple in its tracks.

Acne Rule #5: *Eat More Omega-3s*

- Aim to eat fish at least twice a week—cold-water fish, such as salmon, mackerel, tuna, trout, sardines, and anchovies (as well as walnuts and almonds) are all excellent sources of omega-3 fatty acids. (For a real omega-3 boost, try the nut-crusted halibut on page 264.)

- Eat more flax. Flaxseed is one of the richest dietary sources of omega-3 fatty acids around. Toss it in smoothies and on nondairy yogurt parfaits, or sprinkle it on salads.

- Decrease your intake of omega-6 fatty acids. Omega-6s, which are abundant in packaged and baked goods, as well as corn, sunflower, safflower, and soybean oils, are essential nutrients that your body needs. In fact, one recent study showed that arachidonic acid, a type of omega-6, may even help maintain skin health. The problems begin when you eat too *much* omega-6 (and not enough inflammation-busting omega-3). You can lower the amount of omega-6 in your diet by limiting your intake of dairy products, especially cheese and heavy cream, avoiding packaged and baked goods, and drastically reducing the amount of cooking oil you use. (Consider switching to an olive oil cooking spray, and you'll save a ton of calories, too.)

Hey, Dr Wu

Q: How can I erase my acne scars? I've tried a few medicated creams, but nothing works. Help!

A: There are several ways to improve the appearance of acne scars, depending on their color, texture, and size. (And if you have active acne, you should start by using sunscreen religiously. Sun exposure can darken acne scars.) Dark, discolored scars can be lightened with prescription-strength brightening creams such as Clinique Even Better Clinical Dark Spot Corrector or Boots No 7 Brightening Beauty Serum. These are especially helpful in individuals with darker skin tones who are more likely to develop dark blemishes even after their pimples heal, a condition called post-inflammatory hyper-pigmentation. If that doesn't work, a dermatologist can perform a chemical peel to help even out the skin tone.

If acne scars have left you with uneven skin texture, you may want to ask your doctor about minimally invasive laser treatments such as Affirm and Fraxel, which can smooth the skin's surface (and require only a few days of recovery time). Depressed scars can also be treated with "fillers" such as Restylane and Juvéderm, which are injected underneath the skin to lift up the scar's surface. While these treatments require little to no recovery time, they generally wear off in 6 to 12 months and must be repeated to maintain the results.

Deep or extensive scarring may require more invasive procedures such as carbon dioxide resurfacing lasers or dermabrasion. Because these treatments are more aggressive and remove several layers of skin, they require a minimum of 2 to 3 weeks of recovery time. There is also a risk of persistent redness and discoloration that can last several months depending on the area treated and your skin type.

Very large or deep acne pits may require a visit to a plastic surgeon for scar revision. In this type of surgery the scars are cut out and the healthy skin is sewn back together to allow the area to heal more smoothly. If you take or have taken Roaccutane or other forms of isotretinoin for your acne, it's important to discontinue use and wait at least 6 months before undergoing any invasive procedures. Isotretinoin can impair the skin's ability to heal properly and may lead to more scarring.

For more information about in-office treatments like lasers or injectable fillers, flip to Chapter 12.

Recap of Chapter 4

Fighting Acne with Food

* Eat foods that are low on the glycemic index. Spikes in blood sugar will increase insulin, which can raise the level of androgens (male hormones) in the bloodstream, stimulating the oil glands and leading to breakouts. If you need to, refer to the chart on page 35 to find out which foods are lowest on the glycemic index.

* Avoid dairy foods (but get your calcium elsewhere). Try soy or almond milk instead, but if you must have dairy, choose nonfat or skim milk products.
* Steer clear of iodine. You'll want to avoid seaweed, kelp, sushi rolls, and iodized salt (so use kosher salt instead of sea salt in your cooking).
* Eat plenty of zinc-rich foods. Incorporate plenty of lentils, kidney beans, and raw oysters in your diet. Red meat (beef or lamb) is a good source of zinc, too, but limit your intake to twice a week to avoid raising your cholesterol.
* Indulge in omega-3s. Omega-3s are natural anti-inflammatories, so they help calm angry breakouts. They also lower IGF-1, to help prevent clogged pores as well as reverse the effects of snacking on sugary, fatty foods. Be sure to eat plenty of fish, especially salmon, sardines, and anchovies, as well as tofu, soybeans, flaxseed, walnuts, and almonds.

5

Redness, Itching, and Flaking

(Relief from "Angry" Skin)

Not long ago I spent the evening at a charity fund-raiser in West Hollywood. (One of my patients organized the event, and she was kind enough to snag me a ticket.) It was a raucous scene—a welcome change of pace from the buttoned-up medical conferences I usually attend—and I was enjoying the music, the dancing, and the free-flowing Champagne. Suddenly I caught the eye of a handsome young actor. I'd seen him professionally (during a routine exam at my office), but the thought of his sweet, shy smile and cool blue eyes still tied my stomach in nervous knots. He waved and began making his way though the crowd.

I don't usually develop crushes on celebrities, no matter how handsome. After all, I am a doctor, a professional. I went to Harvard, for crying out loud! But this man is so charming, so charismatic, so unbelievably *dreamy,* that he usually travels with an entourage of swimsuit models and Hollywood "It Girls," all clamoring for his attention. That night, however, he was uncharacteristically alone.

We exchanged somewhat awkward hellos, and then, to my delight, he leaned forward to whisper something in my ear. "Could we . . . go somewhere?" he asked. He smelled like palm trees and expensive aftershave, a dizzyingly sweet combination.

I thought about my husband, home alone, probably reheating those noodles from last night's dinner, sitting among a pile of work papers at the kitchen counter, dripping stir-fry sauce on his tie. But I couldn't help myself. I followed the actor as he cut a path through a jam-packed dance floor, past throngs of tipsy partygoers, and led me into a dark, dimly lit hallway near the bathrooms, tucked out of view from the crowd. All I could hear was the *thud, thud, thud* of my heart in my chest. *I can't believe this is happening,* I thought. *I can't believe this is happening!* I held my breath as he leaned in and asked the question I'd been waiting to hear:

"Um, could you take a look at this rash?"

Every profession seems to have its own set of favors. Psychologists are asked to analyze dreams, accountants are begged for tax advice, and actors sign more autographs than they can count. Me? I see hundreds of cases of Mystery Rash every year—on airplanes, at weddings, any time someone can pull me aside for an out-of-office consult.

The truth is, I (usually) don't mind. Sudden skin eruptions can be kind of scary, and if I can look at a rash and reassure the person that he or she has no reason to worry, then I've done my good deed for the day. Unfortunately, most rashes need more than a quick glance to diagnose, but many people are reluctant to make an appointment with a doctor to get them formally checked out. That reluctance is what drives thousands (if not millions) of people with itchy, flaky skin to self-medicate with over-the-counter creams and pills.

Perhaps this doesn't seem like a bad thing: After all, some of the most common and effective treatments for eczema, hives, psoriasis, perioral dermatitis, and a host of other rashes and breakouts are topical cortisone creams such as HC45 and Lanacort, which are available over the counter, without a prescription. But choose the wrong pill or cream, and you can actually mask the real problem, making it not only worse but harder to treat in the long run. If you rub cortisone cream on a fungus infection, for example, the infection could spread wider and deeper into the skin. Likewise, putting cortisone on rosacea in an attempt to reduce the redness can end up causing more "broken" blood vessels if used continuously for more than a few weeks.

Here's the good news: That "masking" isn't something you have to worry about when you're treating rashes with food. In fact, there are a number of reasons why changing your diet can be a safer and more effective treatment for rashes than prescription medication. Caring for your skin with food, for example, is something you can do long term, unlike many prescription-strength drugs that should be taken for only a few weeks at a time. Pharmaceuticals can also be very expensive—especially the brand-name creams and pills—and they often come with a laundry list of potential side effects. Although I do sometimes prescribe these to my patients to help clear up a rash quickly, I also tell them that they can often use less cream and take fewer pills if they make the right food and lifestyle choices every day.

While the *Feed Your Face* Diet is certainly appropriate for people suffering from rashes of all kinds, you may have to make some adjustments to the basic meal plan based on your specific skin concerns, such as avoiding eggs and wheat if you have eczema and staying away from spicy foods and alcohol to minimize the redness associated with rosacea. In this chapter you'll learn how to tweak the *Feed Your Face* Diet to accommodate itchy, flaky skin as well as learn how to care for rashes of all kinds, from rosacea and eczema to boob breakouts, nipples rashes, and beard burn.

What Do All Rashes Have in Common?

There are about a million different kinds of rashes, but for our purposes we'll divide them into two distinct groups: chronic rashes (such as eczema, rosacea, and psoriasis) and short-term rashes (like hives, nipple rash, and perioral dermatitis). Chronic or ongoing rashes tend to languish; they can last for weeks, months, or even years. They can be difficult to treat and can flare with stress or seasonal changes. On the other hand, short-term rashes are often the result of an allergy, irritation, or infection. Figure out what you're allergic to, and the rash goes away. (On a side note, I really hate to use the term *chronic*. Many of my patients equate chronic conditions with life-threatening illnesses. And let's be honest: It sounds positively *terminal*. But fear not—ongoing (or chronic) rashes are absolutely treatable. In fact, they often respond even better to the *Feed Your Face* Diet than short-term flare-ups. Just have faith.)

In Chapter 1, I explained that inflammation—my Skin Enemy #1—is often a sign of an overactive immune system. That's important to keep in mind if you suffer from itchy, flaky skin because inflammation is the common link among all rashes. In fact, that's what a rash is: inflamed skin. (Even the name *atopic dermatitis*, better known as eczema, literally means "inflammation of the skin.") If you have an angry rash—no matter what kind of rash it is—it's a sign that your immune system is working overtime.

While common topical treatments like cortisone cream and antihistamines may temporarily reduce the symptoms of a rash (the itching and flaking), they don't treat the underlying cause. And without addressing the root cause, *chronic* rashes like eczema, rosacea, and hives will continue to be, well, chronic, while short-term rashes, particularly those caused by an unknown allergen, will just come back again and again. If you treat the inflammation, however, you can get more lasting relief, reduce your dependence on prescription medications, and help minimize recurrences. And as you learned in Chapter 2, one of the most effective ways to fight inflammation is with food.

Regardless of the type of rash you're dealing with, you can alleviate some of the symptoms by following the hunter-gatherer method of eating that we discussed in Chapter 3, which centers on choosing low glycemic foods while cutting out foods with added sugar, high-fructose corn syrup, refined grains, and excess salt. You should also try to avoid foods that contain ingredients you can't easily pronounce. Ridiculously long, scientific-sounding ingredients are usually food additives and preservatives, some of the most common triggers of inflammation and allergy.

On the other hand, eating more foods that have natural anti-inflammatory potential—particularly omega-3 fatty acids—can provide relief from burning, itching, swelling, and redness. (In fact, not getting enough omega-3s can actually make the dryness and cracking associated with many rashes worse. Omega-3 deficiency has even been linked to eczema.)

Even though all rashes have inflammation in common, some chronic rashes have specific triggers, while others (particularly short-term rashes caused by an allergic reaction or an overgrowth of bacteria) may require a round of antibiotics to clear up completely. If your doctor does recommend a prescription pill or cream, be sure to stick to the *Feed Your Face* Diet. There's a good chance it'll help you get off the pills and creams sooner and help prevent the rash from coming back. Your skin—and your body—will be better off in the long run.

THE REAL SCOOP ON CORTISONE

*C*ortisone creams, when used inappropriately, can "mask" the real cause of certain kinds of rashes or even make them worse. But does that mean they should be avoided entirely? The short answer is no. In fact, over the course of this chapter I'll even recommend it for certain types of flare-ups. But getting cortisone treatments right can be tricky, so here's what you need to know:

The Good: Cortisone creams are often used to treat rashes of all kinds. Mild versions, such as HC45 and Lanacort, can be found in any drugstore and can relieve redness, swelling, itching, and flaking regardless of the cause of the rash—and often in a matter of days.

The Bad: Many of my patients are actually afraid to use cortisone creams—even when I recommend them—because they've heard the risks associated with topical steroids. The truth is that cortisone creams (especially the most potent prescription-strength versions) can be potentially harmful. Continual long-term use can lead to something called tachyphylaxis, which is basically cortisone addiction. The skin gets so used to having cortisone around to control any inflammation that if you suddenly stop using it, the skin "rebounds" by becoming angrier and itchier than ever.

The Ugly: Cortisone is a type of steroid—not anabolic, the type used by bodybuilders to build muscle tissue, but catabolic, which breaks down tissue. If you abuse cortisone cream, it can break down collagen and elastic tissue, which can lead to thinning of the skin and, in severe cases, stretch marks. I once treated a young woman who bought a super-strong cortisone cream from a pharmacy in another country. She used it all over her body, several times a day for more than ten years, whenever she had an itchy rash. By the time she came to see me, her skin was one big stretch mark from her neck to her knees. It's an extreme case, but it's why I urge my patients to use cortisone sparingly, even the milder, over-the-counter versions.

How to Use Cortisone Safely: Despite the horror stories, you shouldn't be afraid of cortisone. It's sometimes the only thing that will break the itch/scratch cycle and get your rash under control, fast. In severe cases I might even prescribe cortisone pills or administer a cortisone shot, but that's only when a rash is unresponsive to topical treatments.

At home you can reduce the risk of steroid atrophy (severe thinning of the skin) by using cortisone creams only during bad flare-ups and only for up to 2 weeks at a time, and then giving your skin a break for at least a week. Use the mildest strength available and save the prescription-strength creams for really stubborn patches. It's also a good idea to go light on areas where the skin is already thin, such as the groin, face, and underarms. (Imagine stretch marks in those areas—not cute.) If your doctor recommends a prescription-strength cream and you have rashes in these delicate areas, be sure to ask how and when you should apply it.

Calming "Chronic" Rashes: Rosacea, Eczema, Psoriasis, and Chronic Hives

Relief from Rosacea

Not long ago one of my patients—a well-known pop star—came to see me because she noticed that her face seemed unusually red and broken out. She's fair-skinned with rosy cheeks, but lately the redness had been getting worse. I asked about her basic skin care routine, and she swore that it hadn't changed. She was using the same mild cleanser, oil-free moisturizer, sunscreen, even the same makeup. She was following the same relatively bland vegetarian diet (she's always watching her figure). She also wasn't taking any new medications, nor was she spending any more time outdoors than usual (after all, it was December). Still, her face was bright red with scattered whiteheads and tiny spider veins.

When we still hadn't nailed down the cause of the redness, I made her walk me through exactly what she'd been doing every day. It turned out that she had recently moved into a home with a steam shower in the bathroom. For the past month she'd been spending up to an hour a night in there in order to relax and unwind after a jam-packed day in the recording studio. Unfortunately, the steam is also what most likely triggered her first rosacea attack.

Rosacea is an incredibly common disorder, affecting about one out of every ten people in the U.K., usually in middle age. It causes a general reddening of the skin—like a blush that lasts a little too long—as well as what may look like tiny broken capillary veins on the nose, cheeks, and chin. Unfortunately, there's a lot we don't know about rosacea (including exactly what causes it). What we do know is that people with rosacea have very sensitive blood vessels in the face. At the smallest provocation the vessels "swell" or dilate. As more and more blood flows through them (and they grow larger and larger in size), they become more visible (hence those "broken" capillaries and the general redness). The more you flush and blush, the more the veins stretch out, kind of like pantyhose that become stretched and saggy after too many wears. Eventually they become permanently enlarged and won't go away.

Rosacea seems to run in families, especially among fair-skinned people. (Take a peek at the faces of your older relatives to see where you're headed.) In your teens and 20s you may notice that warm weather (or a steamy shower), spicy foods, and alcohol make you feel flushed and hot. In your 30s and 40s, you might begin to develop tiny bumps and pustules that look like pimples (a sign that bacteria or microscopic mites may be further irritating the pores). For this reason rosacea is routinely mistaken for mild acne (though it does not cause blackheads or clogged pores the way acne does), and it typically worsens with heat, skin irritation, or after eating spicy foods, whereas acne does not. (Adult acne in women is also most likely to occur in monthly cycles along with the hormonal ebb and flow of the menstrual cycle, while rosacea flares are unpredictable.) If rosacea is allowed to progress far enough, the inflammation and irritation can trigger the skin cells to thicken and grow out of control. In its most extreme form, the nose can become bulbous and deformed (though this occurs more often in men, and, thankfully, it can be prevented if you take care of your skin at the earliest signs of redness).

Despite the fact that you do have the power to help your skin by eating face-friendly foods and avoiding my Skin Enemies, I often meet new patients who have been told by other doctors to just live with the redness, that there's nothing that can be done. This makes me sad (and it really pisses me off). That's like telling those with a family history of heart disease to eat all the bacon, red meat, and French fries they want because they're already doomed to an early death. But just as you can reduce your cholesterol and your risk of heart attack by eating less saturated fat and adding omega-3s to your diet, you can find relief from the flushing and blushing associated with rosacea by avoiding certain foods that have been known to cause flare-ups and choosing other anti-inflammatory foods that will fight the rash.

$E = mc^2$ Did You Know . . .

About 50 percent of Asians (and some people of non-Asian descent) lack the enzyme necessary to metabolize alcohol. As a result, many people have a huge problem with flushing when they drink. Not only do their faces turn red, but in severe cases they can experience facial swelling, headaches, and heart palpitations. Alcohol can also aggravate rosacea, causing permanently enlarged veins on the face, especially on the nose, cheeks, and chin. The best way to avoid symptoms like these is to abstain from alcohol altogether. But if you want to enjoy a drink or two, here's how to minimize the damage:

• Avoid the worst offenders. Beer and wine—especially red wine—contain higher levels of alcohol by-products like acetaldehyde that cause flushing, so choose mixed drinks made with distilled alcohol, such as gin, vodka, or whiskey.

• Go sulfite-free. If you must drink wine, look for sulfite-free, organic, or "biodynamic" wine. (There should be an indication on the label.) Sulfites, which act as preservatives, can also cause flushing and redness.

• Stay cool. People with rosacea are sensitive to heat and alcohol, so stay away from hot Irish coffee and steaming cups of hot cider (with or without added booze). Instead, order your drink on the rocks.

What Not to Eat When You Have Rosacea

Rosacea is one of the few skin conditions that's already been linked to food by medical researchers and doctors alike. In fact, a recent survey by the National Rosacea Society not only cited a variety of foods that have been known to cause rosacea flare-ups, but also found that 87 percent of participants reported reductions in their flare-ups and generally improved skin after modifying their eating habits.

Regulating your blood sugar by eating every few hours is an important first step in treating rosacea, especially for menopausal women, because skipping meals and low blood sugar in general have both been shown to increase the frequency of hot flashes and flushing. On the other hand, eating a low glycemic meal will suppress hot flashes for up to ninety minutes. To further alleviate the symptoms of rosacea, *avoid* the following foods:

Spicy foods. These include salsa, hot sauce, peppers (like jalapeños and habañeros), red or cayenne pepper, horseradish, and Mexican food. Spicy foods are by far the number one food-related trigger of rosacea. (More than half of the participants in the above study reported flare-ups after eating hot peppers, chili, and salsa, for example.) Less common triggers include black "table" pepper and paprika. Rarer still are onions, garlic, and mustard. Start by avoiding the most obvious offenders (the stuff that's most likely to make you sweat) to determine what your skin is most sensitive to. And if you're a fool for spicy foods, don't fret. Experts at the National Rosacea Society recommend substituting red pepper or chili powder with two parts cumin and one part oregano for a kick of flavor. And instead of traditional salsa, try a fruit-based variety. (Peach and mango salsas are widely available and seriously tasty.)

Monosodium glutamate (MSG). Perhaps best known for its presence in take-out Chinese food, monosodium glutamate, or MSG, is a popular additive found in everything from crisps to such condiments as barbecue sauce and salad dressing. (You might remember this information from Chapter 4.) Because it can be lumped under the term *natural flavorings* on nutritional labels, it's sometimes difficult to detect in prepared and processed foods. To avoid it, you'll have to read those labels carefully.

Vinegar. Histamine is a substance your body releases in response to an allergy or irritation, which can include certain foods. Since histamine causes swelling and increased blood flow, it can aggravate the swelling and inflammation associated with rosacea. For that reason you'll want to avoid foods containing histamine, as well as fermented foods, including vinegar and soy sauce. Don't think you're getting a lot of vinegar in your diet? Think again. Vinegar is a popular additive in crisps, pickles (it's in the brine), sushi rice, and—especially—commercial salad dressings. For rosacea patients I recommend substituting the classic oil-and-vinegar combo with herb-infused olive oil, which you can find at specialty markets or make yourself with fresh herbs. You'll get a burst of flavor without the flare-up.

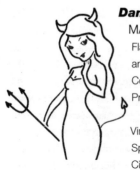

Danger: THE FOLLOWING FOODS
MAY AGGRAVATE ROSACEA

Flavored crisps, especially Cheese, BBQ,
and Sour Cream and Onion

Commercial salad dressings

Prepared chicken stock or bouillon cubes (look for
brands with no MSG)

Vinegar

Spicy salsa and hot peppers

Cinnamon-flavored chewing gum

Cinnamon oil. You'll find cinnamon oil in everything from chewing gum and breath mints to mouthwash and toothpaste, as well as in noninjectable lip plumpers—glosses and lipsticks designed to "plump" your lips up like Angelina Jolie. (These work by irritating the lips, making them swell.) In addition, oral cinnamon supplements have been reported to cause sudden severe worsening of rosacea in type 2 diabetics who take them to lower blood sugar and cholesterol.

Vitamin B_6 and B_{12}. If you take a multivitamin, check the ingredients. High doses of B_6 and B_{12} (twenty to forty times the recommended daily allowance) have also been reported to trigger rosacea. Keep in mind that this doesn't mean you should avoid these vitamins entirely; they're essential for healthy brain function.

SEE A DOCTOR IF . . . YOU HAVE SEVERE, PAINFUL LUMPS OR BOILS

If your rosacea has progressed to this point, you may need a prescription-strength cream or a short course of antibiotics to calm the flare-up. It's best to wean yourself off these types of medications as soon as you can to avoid side effects like yeast infection, abdominal pain, and sun sensitivity. You should also be sure to continue the *Feed Your Face* Diet, both during and after pharmaceutical treatments, to help prevent another painful episode.

Treating Rosacea with Topical Foods and Herbs

While you're treating your rosacea from the inside out (with a somewhat modified version of the *Feed Your Face* Diet), you can also treat it from the outside in. A number of topical foods and herbs can help you maintain calm, clear skin and reduce the likelihood of a flare-up. You can use them in combination with any prescription-strength products your dermatologist recommends. Some of the safest and most effective include the following:

Licorice. The active ingredients in licorice include glycyrrhizin, glabridin, and licochalcone A, all of which have been shown to reduce inflammation and soothe irritation. You can get the same skin-soothing benefits from creams that contain licorice. Many of my rosacea patients have good results with Eucerin Redness Relief, which research shows can reduce redness due to mild to moderate rosacea when used daily for 4 weeks.

Oatmeal. Not the cereal—colloidal oatmeal, which is made from whole oats. Oatmeal is a potent skin protector that can relieve irritation and itching. It also contains a compound called avenanthramide, which has powerful anti-inflammatory effects. There are many different colloidal oatmeal products on the market including a moisturizing cream and a daily face wash from the Aveeno brand.

Feverfew. This herb, which comes from the same family as marigold and chamomile, has been used (in oral capsule form) to treat headache and inflammation for years and years. Problem is, *topical* feverfew can actually irritate the skin because of an active ingredient called parthenolide. Luckily, science has found a way to remove that offending chemical. The new, improved version of the herb—called feverfew PFE (parthenolide-free extract)—has been shown to reduce redness associated with rosacea as well as redness and dryness associated with sensitive skin. It has even been shown to calm razor burn and skin irritation from shaving your legs! You can get all these benefits from the feverfew PFE in Aveeno Ultra-Calming Daily Moisturizer.

Avoiding Common Rosacea Triggers

You know the phrase "You are what you eat"? Well, when it comes to rosacea, you are what you *do*. Certain behaviors and lifestyle choices (beyond just what you eat) can also trigger an outbreak. That's why reducing your exposure to the following known triggers is the third and final step in caring for rosacea:

Steer Clear of Extreme Temperatures

- Long, hot showers and baths. Excessive heat can cause your face to flush and rosacea to flare, so turn the temperature down and use lukewarm water when washing your face. If you're one of those people who insists on a scalding-hot shower, at least avoid letting the water hit you directly in the face.
- Saunas and steam baths. If, like my pop star patient, you like steam showers, turn the temp down as low as you can or consider avoiding them altogether. (I asked my patient to lay off the steam for a while, and her face cleared up in a week.)
- Hot towels at the day spa. Although many facialists are well-informed about rosacea, some can go a little overboard with the hot steam. Ask your aesthetician to use a cool mist and lukewarm towels.
- Bikram yoga or "hot" yoga, which is practiced in a room heated to 105 degrees.
- A seat in front of the fireplace. You may love the smell of chestnuts roasting on an open fire, but sitting too close to the hearth can flare your rosacea, too.
- Steaming cups of coffee, tea, or soup. Let heated beverages cool before drinking or switch to iced tea and iced coffee. Even better, drink chamomile tea (iced or lukewarm). It is a natural anti-inflammatory and will help calm the redness and irritation.

Limit Your Sun Exposure

Too much sun can damage already fragile blood vessels, adding fuel to your rosacea fire. Try to shield yourself from the sun as much as possible. At a minimum, wear wide-brimmed hats or baseball caps, and use an SPF 30 sunscreen that protects against UVA rays. (For more information about protecting yourself from the sun, see Chapter 6.)

Survive Hot Weather

In warm climates and during the sweltering summer months, it's important to stay as cool as possible. Try these tricks:

- Take charge of the air conditioner controls in your home or office. When you're in the car, angle the vents toward your face.
- Try sucking on ice cubes throughout the day. It may sound weird, but ice cubes will cool you down and help calm your skin. (And they're better for your waistline than ice cream.) Many of my patients actually travel with ice cubes stored in a thermos or insulated coffee cup.
- If you don't feel like packing your own ice, ask your Starbucks barista for a cup of crushed ice to have after your morning coffee.
- If ice is too boring, try frozen blueberries, a sweet antioxidant-filled treat that will help keep you cool.

Just as warm weather and hot showers can aggravate your rosacea, so can very cold climates. Going from the cold outdoors to a warm room will send blood to your face, causing the same flushing and dilated blood vessels you might experience after spending a day at the beach. To reduce the effects of extreme cold weather, keep your face covered (choose a soft scarf that won't scratch or itch), rewarm slowly, and—no matter how tempting—don't immediately plunge into a hot tub.

Skip Abrasive Skin-Care Products

Be gentle! People with rosacea have ultrasensitive skin. Rubbing and scrubbing will cause irritation and make the condition worse. Avoid rough washcloths and instead cleanse gently with your fingertips. Always choose skin-care products that are designed specifically for sensitive skin, and be careful with ingredients like glycolic acid, salicylic acid, and vitamin C, which can irritate the skin and make redness worse. Also, use Retin-A sparingly and carefully. While it can prevent breakouts, it can also worsen redness.

Hey, Dr. Wu

Q: *Every year when the weather gets warmer, I get a bright red rash right under my breasts at the bra band line. It gets worse as the temperature rises, and it lingers all summer long. I've used baby powder, "medicated" powder, and even nappy rash cream, but nothing seems to work. Is there something I can do to get rid of it once and for all?*

A: Just when you thought it was safe to show off that new bikini, your chest breaks out in an unsightly rash! The condition you're describing is called miliaria. (It's also known as prickly heat because it can sting or feel prickly.) It's most common in the summer months, especially in humid climates. Miliaria occurs when the sweat glands become blocked. Instead of making its way to the surface of your skin, the sweat leaks into the surrounding tissue, causing irritation and tiny, itchy red bumps. Additional friction from tight clothing can aggravate this condition, which is why it often occurs under the bra band (or at the waistband of your pants).

The best treatment for heat rash is to keep your body cool and dry. When it's sweltering outside, stay in an air-conditioned environment if possible. Once the sweating subsides and the sweat glands unblock, the rash should go away on its own within several days. To prevent new outbreaks:

- Shower immediately after strenuous exercise.
- Avoid using thick, greasy lotions that can "trap" heat.
- Wear loose clothing made of natural fibers, such as cotton and linen; they'll absorb sweat better and help it evaporate more quickly.
- Avoid underwire bras, which can rub and irritate sensitive skin.
- Look for exercise clothing that lets your skin "breathe."

Sometimes fungus or yeast infections can resemble a heat rash, so if your skin doesn't look better in a week, make an appointment with a dermatologist. The doctor may recommend a prescription-strength cream or do additional tests to make sure you don't have an infection.

Understanding Eczema

Atopic dermatitis, more commonly known as eczema, is a condition that produces an itchy red rash that can become dry, cracked, or crusted. It often starts in childhood, typically on the insides of the elbows and the backs of the knees. In adulthood it often migrates to the neck, chest, and back (although it can appear anywhere on the body). Eczema can come and go for years, and it often flares due to stress, dry winter weather, and exposure to harsh detergents and soaps.

People with eczema have what I call "leaky skin" or an impaired skin barrier, meaning the skin is more permeable than usual. As a result, water evaporates from the skin much more quickly than from the average person, leaving it dry, flaky, and dehydrated. At the same time, ingredients that wouldn't bother most people can seep into and irritate the sensitive skin of people with eczema, causing classic signs of inflammation: red patches and itchy bumps.

If you're struggling with eczema, I feel your pain. I've dealt with the itching and flaking my whole life. As a child, it was so bad that I had to walk around with a thick, greasy cream on the backs of my knees. I couldn't sit down (for fear of ruining the furniture), and I remember missing more than one birthday party as a result. As I got older, my eczema localized to the eyelids, neck, collarbone, and upper back. It tends to flare in the winter, when I'm stressed, or when I eat more wheat than usual, which is just one of the foods that can aggravate eczema.

SEE YOUR DOCTOR IF . . . YOUR RASH IS OOZING OR CRUSTY

Open, uncovered areas of the skin—such as nicks, cuts, razor burn, and eczema—can leave you more susceptible to Staph, which is short for the bacteria *Staphylococcus aureus*. Since Staph infections can cause unsightly and painful skin infections, including folliculitis (pimples with whiteheads), abscesses (boils caused by deep infections), and impetigo (red patches that crust over and ooze), it's important to catch them early. In recent years there's also been an increase in a particular type of Staph called methicillin-resistant Staph aureus (MRSA), which is aggressive and very contagious. If you notice painful "pimples" that don't dry up and heal within a few days, a sudden eruption of pimples or blisters in one area of the body, or pimples that ooze pus and crust over—especially if they're accompanied by swelling of the surrounding skin or fever—it's time to see your doctor. He or she may prescribe an oral or topical antibiotic as well as medicated soap to clean the infected area.

What Not to Eat When You Have Eczema

Histamine, which causes itching, redness, and inflammation, is a substance our bodies release when we're exposed to an allergen, from ragweed and pollen to certain medications and foods (like peanuts or milk). For some reason people with eczema have higher levels of histamine in the blood than those without—even when they haven't been exposed to something they're allergic to (hence the inflamed, itchy skin). Toss in the fact that somewhere between 30 and 60 percent of people with eczema actually do have food allergies, and you can see why it can be so challenging to treat. If you have eczema, you can help soothe the skin by avoiding the following foods:

Eggs. Studies show that intolerance to eggs (especially the yolk) is relatively common in people with eczema, and about 50 percent of eczema patients who avoid eggs report improvement in the look and feel of their skin. If you have eczema, you should avoid eggs even if you don't think you have an actual food allergy. Once your skin improves, you can slowly introduce them back into your diet to test your personal sensitivity.

Gluten. Celiac disease is an autoimmune condition that triggers an allergic reaction to gluten, a protein found in such grains as wheat, barley, and rye. Symptoms include abdominal pain, diarrhea, bloating, and, in some cases, an intensely itchy, blistering rash called dermatitis herpetiformis. Some people, however—including those with eczema and psoriasis—may be sensitive to gluten even if they don't actually have celiac disease.

If you have eczema, you should avoid most bread, pasta, and cereal. You don't have to give up bread and pasta *completely,* just switch to gluten-free varieties. (FYI, gluten-free crackers are delicious with hummus.) Be aware that gluten is also a thickening agent, so it can show up in seemingly unlikely places, such as ice cream, canned soup, gravy, ketchup, and other condiments. (It'll be listed as "modified wheat starch" on the label.) On the other hand, starches like corn, potatoes, rice, sweet potatoes, quinoa, and chickpeas (the primary ingredient in hummus) are all naturally gluten-free. (Phew!) Just be aware that these foods can still cause spikes in blood sugar, so you'll want to eat them in moderation.

SEE YOUR DOCTOR IF . . . YOU HAVE ECZEMA AND AN UPSET STOMACH

If your eczema flares only after eating a particular food or if you have gastrointestinal symptoms along with the rash (such as upset stomach, vomiting, or diarrhea), you may have a *true* food allergy. Ask your doctor about getting tested—he'll prick the skin and/or perform blood tests to determine your sensitivity to the most common allergy-causing foods, including milk, eggs, wheat, peanuts, and soy.

Foods containing histamine. Histamine is the substance our bodies release when we're exposed to an allergen, but some foods already contain histamine. These foods can cause a reaction that's technically different from a true allergy, but carries with it the same symptoms (including itching, rashes, or hives). Perhaps it's not surprising, then, that reducing the amount of histamine in your diet may help improve the condition of your skin.

The following foods are either naturally high in histamine (like fermented or pickled foods) or they stimulate your body to release excess histamine, which is the case with some fruits and vegetables. But before you strike them from your diet completely, grab your food diary. (I told you it would come in handy.) Do any of the following foods show up in the pages? Rather than avoiding *all* foods with histamine, see if you can make a link between one or more of these foods and your most recent flare-up.

Tofu

Soy sauce

Aged cheese (like blue or
    Parmesan)

Canned fish (fresh fish is fine)

Sausage and salami

Egg whites

Citrus fruits

Strawberries

Chocolate

Champagne, beer, and wine

Cobalt and nickel. Eczema of the hands (also known as dyshydrotic eczema), which appears as itchy red patches of skin, tiny clear blisters, and cracks on the hands and fingertips, is quite common in people who wash their hands frequently, particularly health care providers, restaurant workers, and gardeners. (But it can also affect the feet.) Studies show that these people also tend to experience flare-ups when their diets are high in cobalt and nickel. If you have hand or foot eczema, avoid Brazil nuts and cow's liver (not exactly a hardship, I'd say) and eat the following cobalt-rich foods in moderation: flaxseeds (no more than 2 tablespoons per day), sunflower seeds, garbanzo beans (also known as chickpeas, the main ingredient in hummus), mixed nuts, chocolate milk, chocolate cake, and clam chowder. Beware that many homeopathic and herbal remedies are also high in cobalt and nickel, so always read the label before starting a new treatment or supplement.

FROM THE FILES OF *Dr. Wu*

Patient: Diena

Skin Concern: Severe eczema

Food Sensitivity: Dairy

In Diena's Words: I had been struggling with eczema for two years when it finally got so bad that makeup could no longer hide it. I tried steroid creams and oral steroids to control the inflammation, but nothing worked. Eventually, the swelling spread down my neck. I didn't even recognize myself.

I made appointments with all kinds of doctors: An allergist told me I was allergic to twenty-eight of the thirty basic environmental factors in L.A., yet he had no solutions other than heavier doses

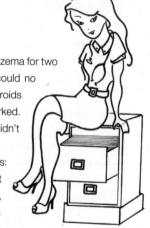

of steroids. A doctor at UCLA said my ANA numbers were high (ANA stands for Antinuclear Antibody Test, which is used to diagnose autoimmune disorders like lupus), but it wasn't an autoimmune disease. A rheumatologist even suggested chemotherapy.

When I heard the word *chemo,* it was as if I suddenly woke up. I realized I hadn't even considered alternative medicine, and at this point there wasn't anything I wasn't going to try. Within days I met with a macrobiotic counselor, who methodically explained what was going on in my body—a diet lacking in vital nutrients plus irregular eating and occasional overeating had thrown my entire digestive system out of whack.

Working with my counselor, I started on a strict diet. For the first few weeks I cut out all dairy, sugar, baked goods, and processed foods, and focused instead on eating tons of fresh organic vegetables, beans, and fish. Within 1 month the swelling, redness, and itching were gone. But my skin didn't just return to normal, it looked better and brighter than ever before.

Dr. Wu's Diagnosis: The first time Diena came to my office, she told me she was a strict vegan but that she occasionally allowed herself ice cream or frozen yogurt. It wasn't until her condition worsened that she started *really* paying attention. She was actually eating frozen yoghurt two to three times a week. Though frozen yogurt is a lower-calorie treat than ice cream (and there are certainly worse foods to indulge in), for someone with an undiagnosed dairy sensitivity like Diena's, it can trigger a huge inflammatory response. But by cutting out sugar, baked goods, and processed foods (and loading up on fish and vegetables), she was able to calm her angry skin. Diena is the perfect example of a woman who thought she had a handle on what she was eating but really had no idea.

Foods to Soothe Eczema and Inflammation

When it comes to treating rashes with food, it's not always about what you can't have. Research shows that adding the following foods to your diet may reduce the itching and redness associated with eczema:

Yogurt. People with eczema not only have leaky skin but they also have a leaky GI tract barrier, meaning their intestines are more vulnerable to being invaded by food particles and by-products that might trigger an allergic reaction. Yogurt, it turns out, can increase the amount of "good" bacteria in your body, which can help promote a more normal intestinal lining. Studies also show that yogurt (eaten daily for four weeks) may reduce the itching and burning associated with eczema.

If you'd like to add more yogurt to your diet, just remember to choose a low-fat, low-sugar variety since sugar is known to aggravate inflammation. Likewise, avoid fruit-on-the-bottom yogurt, which is loaded with added sugar and sometimes high-fructose corn syrup. And if you suffer from breakouts *and* eczema, you might consider taking a probiotic supplement instead since dairy has been linked to acne.

Fish. You already know that fish, especially salmon, is good for your heart and your complexion in general, but it's also rich in something called docosahexaenoic acid, or DHA, which is a specific type of omega-3 fatty acid that researchers think may be particularly helpful for people with eczema. In a study published by the *British Journal of Dermatology,* patients who took about 5g/day of DHA had improvement of the skin after 8 weeks as well as an increase in the amount of omega-3s in their blood.

While taking seven capsules of fish oil a day, as the study participants did, may not be realistic (or appetizing, for that matter), even moderately increasing the amount of DHA in your diet can only be a good thing. Just stick with fresh fish because canned fish typically has about half the omega-3s and DHA of fresh fish, and it's higher in sodium. You may notice, too, that lots of foods, from eggs to orange juice, now come fortified with omega-3s, but that doesn't mean they contain DHA—so you'll have to read the label. If you're a vegetarian, you can swap the fish for an algae oil supplement (which is also high in DHA).

Zinc. Recent studies have suggested that people with eczema have a low concentration of zinc in their blood. While the exact link isn't clear, we do know that zinc is a powerful anti-inflammatory as well as an important part of our skin's immune system. (And now you know that people with eczema tend to have immune systems that are totally out of whack.)

Increasing the amount of zinc in your diet is also an important step in caring for acne, so I'm going to repeat below the information from Chapter 4. (If you read that chapter, this'll just be a refresher.)

To increase the amount of zinc in your diet, be sure to do the following:

MERCURY POISONING: AM I AT RISK?

As more and more people shun red meat in favor of low-cholesterol fish, and sushi becomes a staple of a more mainstream diet, the general public has become increasingly aware of the dangers of mercury poisoning. (Who can forget the controversy when actor Jeremy Piven cited mercury poisoning as the reason for his sudden departure from the Broadway production of *Speed the Plow*?)

Mercury poisoning, although rare, can cause a range of serious health complications, including fatigue, kidney failure, and even cardiac arrest in extremely severe cases. It can also cause an itchy, bumpy rash that clears only after eliminating seafood from the diet or undergoing chelation therapy, a treatment that "traps" the mercury in your system and removes it from the body. Although I do see a few cases a year, the threat of mercury poisoning is pretty low. (You have to eat a *lot* of fish to be at risk—at least several servings of high-mercury fish a week for weeks on end.) But for others, especially pregnant women and children, the threat is slightly greater. To reduce your exposure to mercury, you should avoid eating fish that are naturally high in mercury, such as shark and swordfish, and limit the amount of low-mercury fish you eat to a couple of times a week. The FDA also recommends that you eat tuna no more than once a week since it contains a moderate amount of mercury.

If you have a bumpy red rash that won't go away *and* you eat a high-seafood diet, ask your doctor about getting a blood test to rule out mercury poisoning. Although it's rare, the rash may be your first and only sign.

- Make lean red meat (beef or lamb) your main course as often as twice a week. Aim to incorporate other zinc-rich foods, such as lentils, kidney beans, and raw oysters in your diet, too (especially if you're a vegetarian).
- Phytate, a compound found in cereals, corn, and rice, can reduce zinc absorption when eaten at the same meal. The same goes for casein, the main protein found in milk and cheese. Try to avoid pairing these foods with a steak or lamb entree and other zinc-rich main courses.
- Avoid zinc supplements. Excessive zinc intake can actually be toxic,

leading to copper deficiency, severe anemia, and a drop in white blood cells. (I know of a teenage boy who wound up in the hospital after overdosing on zinc pills.) It's better to get your zinc through food.

Dietary hempseed oil. Hempseed oil is pressed from the seeds of non-drug varieties of cannabis, which means it doesn't contain THC, the hallu-cinogenic found in marijuana. (So, no, I'm not about to give you an excuse to get high. Sorry.) It is packed, however, with protein and anti-inflammatory omega-3s. Studies have shown that dietary hempseed oil may improve the itching and dryness associated with eczema as well as improve hydration of the skin (when used regularly over the long term). Try it on salads (in place of olive oil) or mixed into hummus or smoothies. Just remember that hemp-seed oil must be refrigerated, and it's not meant to be cooked, so you can't use it to, say, sauté your veggies.

Evening primrose oil (supplement). Though the research has been conflicting, I've been recommending evening primrose oil to my eczema patients for several years now, and the results pretty much speak for them-selves. (Indeed, the most recent study on evening primrose oil found that after four to eight weeks it does help reduce itching, redness, swelling, and crusting.) That's because it contains something called gamma-linolenic acid, which is an omega-6 fatty acid with anti-inflammatory properties. (Other sources of gamma-linolenic acid, or GLA, include black currant oil, borage oil, and hempseed oil.) Studies have shown that taking 320 to 480mg/day of GLA, divided into two or three doses throughout the day, can help relieve eczema rashes. Look for high-quality forms of the supple-ment, which should be packed in light-resistant containers and marked with an expiration date.

While evening primrose oil doesn't bother the majority of my patients, side effects including stomach upset and headaches have been reported. You also shouldn't take evening primrose oil (or other omega-6 supplements) if you have a seizure disorder. And if you're planning to go under general anes-thesia for surgery, you should stop taking evening primrose oil at least two weeks before due to the possible increased risk of seizure. As always, talk to your doctor before beginning any new supplements.

Treating Eczema from the Outside In

One of the most effective treatments for eczema (other than altering your diet) is really pretty basic: Using a good-quality moisturizer—even in areas where the skin appears "normal"—can restore your skin's natural barrier, relieving the dryness, tightness, and itching. (This is especially important in the dry winter months, or if you live in an arid climate with low humidity.) Limit your showers and baths to 10 minutes (long, hot showers will dry out the skin), then immediately apply a rich body lotion made with ingredients like argan and jojoba oils (found in Nivea Pure & Natural Body Moisturizer for Very Dry Skin), shea butter, oatmeal, or glycerin. Try to avoid moisturizers with added fragrance, as these can irritate your skin.

If you have a severe flare-up and the skin becomes extremely sensitive, you can also try smearing on a little olive oil. Seriously. Olive oil has no additives or preservatives, it won't burn or sting, and you can safely use it as many times a day as needed. Warning: You will look a little greasy and it can clog the pores. If you're prone to breakouts, choose an oil-free moisturizer with glycerin or hyaluronic acid instead.

THE BEST LAUNDRY PRODUCTS FOR SENSITIVE SKIN

Okay, so doing laundry isn't exactly glamorous, but I find it strangely relaxing. Plus, there's just enough time during a wash and rinse cycle to watch *Entourage* or flip through *OK!* magazine. Problem is, using the wrong kind of laundry detergent or fabric softener can wreak havoc on sensitive skin, so it's important to know the right products to purchase.

If you have dry, sensitive skin or eczema rashes, you'll want to avoid laundry detergents (as well as the harsh chemicals used by dry cleaners) that may aggravate your skin condition. Instead, choose a detergent with the word *free* in the label, which means the product has been formulated without dyes or fragrances. They won't be hard to find: These days more and more detergents use environmentally friendly plant-based ingredients.

Green detergents don't always clean as well as some of the so-called leading brands, but they're gentler on your skin. And if you have tough stains, you can always try presoaking or pretreating with additional detergent. My favorite green laundry products are these:

Seventh Generation Free & Clear Natural 2X Concentrated Laundry Liquid. Rather than animal-derived surfactants, which are common in most other detergents, this detergent contains gentle coconut-derived surfactants and plant enzymes to create the bubbles and foam that break up dirt. (Animal surfactants can create a residue on clothing that irritates dry skin.) Seventh Generation also makes a chlorine-free bleach that I often use.

Method Squeaky Green Free & Clear Dryer Cloths. These dryer cloths are free of fragrance and dyes, and they're made with plant ingredients (unlike most dryer sheets, which are made with animal tallow or beef fat, and can leave a tacky residue on clothing and skin). They also leave your clothes feeling super soft.

Boob Breakouts and Nipple Eczema

Even though eczema is most commonly found on the inside of the elbows and backs of the knees, sometimes it can appear on the nipples—and that can be kind of scary. I mean, when it comes to "the girls," knowing what's normal and what's not can be kind of difficult, since it's not as if we have much opportunity to contrast and compare. While the vast majority of rashes on the chest aren't serious (including nipple eczema), some may require medical attention. Here are the most common types of rashes that might spring up on your boobs:

Nipple eczema. If one or both of your breasts appears red and itchy, you may have a case of nipple eczema, which is particularly common in women who also have eczema rashes elsewhere on the body. Nipple eczema is often aggravated by friction from clothing (such as snug-fitting exercise wear), but it can be resolved by using a mild cortisone cream. If the rash doesn't go away after two weeks, however, or if you notice any nipple discharge, feel a lump, or the rash seems to be spreading quickly, see your doctor.

Mastitis. Usually associated with breast-feeding, mastitis is an infection that occurs when bacteria enters the skin through tiny cracks in the nipple and spreads through the milk ducts into the surrounding tissue. Symptoms include warm, red, swollen, and tender breasts with cracked nipples. Sometimes these can be accompanied by fever and/or pus. If that's the case, it's time to call your doctor.

Paget's disease of the breast. This is a type of breast cancer that affects the skin of the breast, often including the nipple and/or areola. It may appear as a red, discolored, or flaky patch, often on one breast only, that may or may not itch. This condition is usually associated with an underlying cancer deeper in the breast tissue, although you may not detect any lumps. See your doctor right away if you do feel a lump, notice any discharge, or if the flaky patches seem to be spreading. Your doctor can perform a skin biopsy to determine the exact cause.

Bumps on the areola. The oil glands around the nipple—called Montgomery glands—can become enlarged and clogged, which can sometimes cause a little pimple to form at the edge of the nipple. If you think you have one, don't squeeze it. That'll just force the clog deeper or, worse, turn the pimple into a nasty boil or cause an infection. Try to have patience; it should go away on its own in a week or so.

Extra nipples. Yes, that's right, some people have extra nipples, which are technically known as "supernumerary" nipples. They're usually smaller than the "main" nipples and tend to appear on the chest somewhere below the normal ones. Males are more likely to get these extra nipples (super-hunky actor Mark Wahlberg has one), and for some reason they tend to show up on the left side of the body. Not to worry, though. Extra nipples are relatively common (about 5 percent of us have a spare), and they're usually harmless. If your extra nipple is tender, growing, or changing, however, consult your doctor.

Soothing Psoriasis

Psoriasis is a chronic condition that produces patches of intensely red, inflamed skin covered by thick, scaly, or flaky blisters, bumps, or spots. Unlike eczema, which often affects the insides of the elbows and the backs of the knees, psoriasis normally shows up on the outside of the elbows and knees, though it can spread anywhere on the body, including the scalp. We don't know exactly what causes psoriasis, but it does seem to run in families.

There's a bit of a stigma attached to psoriasis: It's thick and scaly, more obvious and "angry-looking" than other rashes, including eczema, and it appears as though it may be contagious (even though it isn't). Perhaps that's why so many people with psoriasis feel self-conscious or even depressed about the condition of their skin.

In recent years "biologic" drugs, which are regular injections that can control inflammation, have become an increasingly popular treatment for psoriasis despite their potential effect on the internal organs and immune system as well as their exorbitant cost. (Biologic treatments can cost between £8,000 and £10,000 a year in the U.K.) As an alternative to such serious drug therapy, I encourage my patients to manage breakouts first with topical treatments and diet and lifestyle changes. Just as some people with severe acne need a heavy-duty treatment like isotretinoin, however, some psoriasis is severe enough to require doctor-administered therapies. The good news is that avoiding the following foods (especially during flare-ups) can not only reduce the severity of psoriasis and the need for prescription-strength drugs, but can also improve the effectiveness of any drugs you may opt to take.

What Not to Eat When You Have Psoriasis

Gluten. Like people with eczema, psoriasis sufferers are often sensitive to gluten, a protein found in such grains as wheat, barley, and rye. Choose gluten-free varieties of bread, pasta, and cereal, and avoid foods made with "modified wheat starch," which is often found in ketchup and other condiments, canned soup, and even ice cream. (You can read more about gluten sensitivity on page 112).

Alcohol. We all know that alcohol gets absorbed into the bloodstream. (Think about it: If you're pulled over on suspicion of drink-driving, the police will measure your "blood alcohol concentration.") But alcohol can also be secreted through your sweat glands, which is why you might reek of booze after a night of heavy drinking. The alcohol is literally coming out your pores.

The amount of alcohol in your blood peaks between 30 minutes and 2 hours after drinking, while the amount of alcohol in your sweat is highest two to three hours after that. So you'll smell the worst about two to four hours after downing that last shot. Why is this relevant (besides using the info to time your showers)? It means that alcohol doesn't just affect the liver, it also affects the skin.

Doctors have known for a long time that drinking increases your risk of developing psoriasis, but it can also make existing psoriasis worse if you drink while having an outbreak. Until recently we figured that was because heavy drinkers might be less likely to be compliant with their medications or that alcohol interfered with the effectiveness of those medications. But new research shows that alcohol can increase inflammation in the skin, which may explain why people with psoriasis experience more flaking and itching when they drink. Alcohol can also increase the production of skin cells, which can worsen thick, scaly patches.

If you have psoriasis, you should reduce the amount of alcohol you drink as much as possible and avoid it entirely when you're experiencing a flare-up. I realize that might sound like a drag, but your skin will thank you.

Attention Psoriasis Sufferers:

Eat More Fish!

You already know that omega-3-rich fish can reduce the rashes and redness associated with eczema. The same holds true for psoriasis. But the type of fish you eat is just as important as the quantity. In a study by the Department of Dermatology at Westminster Hospital in London, participants who ate 6 ounces per day of oily fish (such as salmon, sardines, and trout) had even more improvement in their skin than patients who ate white fish, such as cod or haddock. Even though this study tested the effect of eating fish every day, you can still get the anti-inflammatory benefit of omega-3s by eating fish just twice a week.

Smoking. In a study by Oregon University School of Medicine, researchers found that female smokers have three times the risk of developing psoriasis as nonsmokers, and the risk climbs even higher in women who smoke a pack or more a day. Smokers (both men and women) also tend to have worse outbreaks than nonsmokers and typically don't respond as well to psoriasis treatments.

Almost everyone knows that cigarettes come with a laundry list of associated health problems, so I'll spare you the antismoking speech. If you can't break the habit, at least try to cut back when your psoriasis flares up.

Calming a Case of Hives

Hives, also known as urticaria, are smooth, pink (often itchy) welts that spring up when something triggers your body to release histamine. Most often that "something" is something you ingested (which could include medications, preservatives, herbs, and supplements), but hives can also appear after extreme exercise, exposure to excessive heat or cold, or after touching something you're allergic to. My sister, for example, will get a hive if her skin comes in contact with a single cold raindrop. (This makes living in a rainy city like London or Seattle pretty much out of the question.)

Hives can be as small as a pea or as large as your entire abdomen. They can be individual bumps or merge into one large mass. And they can pop up anywhere on the body, including your scalp, the palms of your hands, and even in your ears. All hives, however, come and go within 24 hours. You may continue to break out in "new" hives for up to 6 weeks or longer, but each individual welt will disappear by day's end. (If you have the same red bumps for more than a day, chances are they're not hives.) Since they come and go so quickly, hives are not considered a chronic rash, but there is a condition known as "chronic hives," which we'll get to momentarily.

It's not always easy to identify the cause of hives, particularly if they're a result of some unknown food allergy or sensitivity to a popular preservative. After all, think of how many hundreds, if not thousands, of different ingredients exist in the various foods you eat over the course of a few days—especially if you eat packaged and processed foods. (Mr Kipling Mini Victoria Sponge Cakes, for example, have thirty-five different ingredients!) It's also possible to develop new food allergies at any point in time, so you may suddenly find yourself itching after eating something that has never bothered you before.

What Not to Eat When You Suffer from Frequent Hives

Whenever a patient comes in with a new case of hives, I ask her to begin keeping a diary of absolutely everything she eats or drinks—every vitamin, herb, fizzy drink, snack, medication, illicit drug, or diet drink. (Why illicit drugs? I once knew someone who traced his hives all the way back to the pesticides used on the marijuana he smoked. You never know.) Then when the hives show up again, we review what she ingested 24 to 48 hours before the attack. Sometimes an obvious source jumps out, but most of the time it takes several cycles to spot a pattern. If after several outbreaks we still can't find the source of the hives, I'll refer the patient to an allergist who can perform more extensive testing.

The most common hive-inducing food allergens are shellfish, eggs, cheese, nuts, milk, berries, and alcohol, but sometimes hives occur only when certain foods are eaten together. For example, I know a number of people who can eat shellfish alone or alcohol alone, but put the two together—like a shrimp dinner with Champagne—and they'll wind up in the emergency room. Aspirin, nonsteroidal anti-inflammatories like ibuprofen (Motrin, Advil), and homeopathic or herbal supplements are also common hive triggers, especially if they're new to your diet. If you have recurrent hives, you'll also want to avoid foods that contain histamine or that trigger your body to release histamine.

The majority of hives aren't severe enough to require hospitalization. If you get a few small hives here and there that disappear on their own, there's really no need to seek medical help. If it happens more than a few times a year or lasts longer than a few weeks at a time, though, you should start paying attention. Every exposure to an allergen makes you a little more sensitive, so the next outbreak could be more serious. Start keeping a food diary if you experience an outbreak (*ahem,* you should be doing this already), and talk to your doctor about your hives at your next regular appointment.

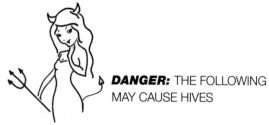

DANGER: THE FOLLOWING
MAY CAUSE HIVES

**Foods high in histamine
(especially fermented or pickled):**

Tofu

Soy sauce

Aged cheese (i.e., blue or Parmesan)

Canned or smoked fish (fresh is fine)

Sausage and salami

Champagne, beer, wine

Sauerkraut

Eggplant

Vinegar and mayonnaise

**Foods that stimulate your body
to release histamine:**

Egg whites

Citrus fruits

Strawberries

Chocolate

Seafood and shellfish

Alcohol

Milk

Nuts

Aspirin, ibuprofen (Motrin, Advil)

Topical Treatments for Hives

Since hives are caused by excess histamine, the best treatment for ordinary occasional hives is an *anti*histamine (like Benadryl), which will block the body's histamine response. If you have only a few small hives, try Benadryl cream or pills, but choose the kind labeled "dye-free." Pink dye, ironically, is a known trigger of hives. (I once had to make a house call at the Beverly Hills Hotel after one of my patients took a pink Benadryl to prevent swelling after I performed a lip injection. Poor thing, she ended up swelling three times as much as normal because she was allergic to the dye.) Remember that antihistamines tend to make people drowsy, so avoid them when you need to be alert or awake or when you need to drive. And if you already take over-the-counter or prescription meds, you should speak with a doctor before starting on an antihistamine since the combination can heighten the drowsiness. (You don't want to be hopped up on Night Nurse *and* an antihistamine, for instance, unless you plan on falling asleep at the dinner table.)

SEE A DOCTOR IF . . . YOUR HIVES SEEM MORE SEVERE THAN USUAL

Harmless hives can sometimes escalate into something called angio-edema, which is a type of allergic reaction that causes swelling of the lips, tongue, throat, and gastrointestinal tract. If the inflammation is severe enough, it can even cause your throat to close, interfering with breathing and swallowing. Head to the ER immediately if any of the following occurs:

- Your hives start to spread up the neck or onto the face.
- You have any swelling of the lips or tongue.
- You have itching of the throat, difficult breathing, or hoarseness.

If you've ever had angioedema, ask your doctor about getting an EpiPen, which is an injectable dose of epinephrine (adrenaline) that will instantly open the airway and help you breathe.

As an alternative to Benadryl pills, you can try the Benadryl Extra Strength Itch Relief Stick, a topical, nongreasy, roll-on antihistamine liquid that comes in a plastic tube the size of a thin marker or highlighter. Just dab the hives with the stick, and a clear, quick-drying liquid stops the itching within a minute. Lots of my patients carry a tube in their purse all the time, not just for hives but for mosquito bites and other itchy skin emergencies.

Other nonprescription options to reduce swelling and itching include Claritin, a nondrowsy antihistamine pill, and topical cortisone creams (like HC45 or Lanacort) for their anti-inflammatory properties. In a pinch you can also try calamine lotion, which will soothe and cool the skin to reduce itching. It's not as effective as cortisone cream or an antihistamine pill, but you probably have some in your medicine cabinet.

For more stubborn hives your doctor can prescribe a cortisone pill or a prescription-strength antihistamine such as Atarax. Anti-ulcer pills such as Zantac, Tagamet, and Pepcid can also help reduce swelling and hives since they have antihistamine-like effects. Studies suggest that acupuncture can also be an effective treatment for hives because it stimulates the body's own natural ability to fight inflammation.

While antihistamines are certainly useful in the short term (and it's a good idea to keep Benadryl on hand if you have a tendency to get severe hives), it is possible to get hooked on them. Before you know it, you've been taking them for years. Antihistamines also don't eliminate the *cause* of hives; they only address the reaction. That's why it's particularly important to try to pinpoint the food (or other substance) that causes your breakouts. Avoiding certain foods may not completely cure hives in every case, but it can lessen the need for medications, which can be expensive over the long term and may cause side effects—from drowsiness, in the case of Benadryl, to weight gain and increased blood sugar, in the case of cortisone pills.

Chronic Hives

If you suffer from hives for over six weeks at a time, you probably have what we call chronic urticaria, which can be incredibly difficult to manage and can come and go for years. Research shows that for people with chronic hives, food additives, naturally occurring histamines, and other natural substances found in fruits, vegetables, and spices can trigger extended reactions. (We call these substances pseudoallergens because they can give you hives even if you don't have a true allergy.) But here's the good news: Getting rid of the pseudoallergens in your diet can minimize both the occurrence of hives and the length of the outbreaks.

In a study by German researchers, participants were fed an (admittedly bland) diet of only rice, potatoes, bread, butter, salt, olive oil, and plain coffee and tea for three days. Then, for another three weeks, they were told to avoid processed food, artificial ingredients, food additives, preservatives and dyes, as well as natural foods known to release histamine, including eggs, fruit, alcohol, pasta, seafood, tomatoes, spinach, olives, artichokes, peas, sweeteners, modified starches, and basically any ingredient they couldn't easily pronounce. The intention, thankfully, wasn't to strike all these foods from the diet *forever*. Avoiding certain foods for a month or so can allow the body to recover from prolonged irritation and inflammation. In fact, many people reported improvement in their skin after just one week. After three weeks participants could begin to add "restricted" foods back into their diet one by one, watching to see which might trigger an outbreak. One in three people with chronic hives had significant improvement without any help from medications or creams.

If you have chronic hives, you may want to try a similar experiment at home. While I wouldn't recommend the German diet, you can try avoiding the foods on the "Danger List" (page 126). Restricting your diet for a few weeks will give your body a chance to "detox" from inflammatory foods as well as make it easier to determine which of those foods tends to cause your hives in the first place. Although a strict diet can certainly be hard to follow, learning to manage your outbreaks without the use of antihistamines is better for your skin (and your body) in the long term.

Don't Fall for It: GREEN- OR BLUE-TINTED "REDNESS-CORRECTING" CONCEALER

Way back in the third grade we learned that red is opposite green on the color wheel. But that doesn't mean that heaping green gunk on red, flaky skin will even out your complexion. (It's more likely to make you look like the Wicked Witch of the West.) All you need to cover redness is a good-quality (flesh-colored) concealer. Personally, I love Nars concealer, which stays put all day and doesn't crease. It's pricey, but one tube will last all year. Or try the Rimmel Hide the Blemish Concealer stick available at your local chemist.

Pinpointing the Cause of Short-Term Rashes

Taming Yeast Beasts

Yeast (which feeds on dead skin and oil) is always present on our bodies, but it doesn't usually cause problems for most people. Hormonal fluctuations, stress, extreme temperatures, and overactive oil glands can all cause yeast to multiply, however, and that can lead to the development of "twin" skin conditions: seborrheic dermatitis, which causes dry, flaky patches on the nose, ears, eyelids, and scalp (where it's more commonly referred to as dandruff), and pityrosporum folliculitis, a bumpy acne-like rash of whiteheads that may appear on the neck, chest, and back. (You can distinguish folliculitis from acne by paying attention to the size and uniformity of the bumps. Folliculitis causes tiny bumps and whiteheads that are nearly the same size, unlike acne.) I call these twin conditions because (a) they're both caused by an overgrowth of the same type of yeast, and (b) many people experience flare-ups of both conditions at the same time, so you might have dandruff *and* tiny breakouts on the face and body. While there's no definitive cure for either condition, you can control the itchy, flaky symptoms. Here's what I recommend:

Eat to maintain steady blood sugar. Although eating foods that are low on the glycemic index and regulating your blood sugar by eating frequent small meals are important tenets of the *Feed Your Face* Diet in general, they're especially important for people struggling with yeast infections, because yeast flourishes when the blood sugar is too high (which means you'll suffer from itchy, flaky skin for a prolonged period of time). You can also fight yeast overgrowth and the resulting inflammation by eating anti-inflammatory foods such as omega-3s (just like eczema and psoriasis sufferers), as well as by balancing the carbs you eat with proteins and healthy fats. Remember, if you pair a whole wheat bagel with peanut butter, for example, the resulting blood sugar spike will be less dramatic than if you eat the bagel by itself.

For a flaky scalp, try an over-the-counter shampoo such as Original Source Mint and Tea Tree Daily Refresh Shampoo, which contains mint to cool an itchy scalp and tea tree oil to fight yeast. If that doesn't work, you can upgrade to a medicated shampoo that contains pyrithione to control yeast, such as Head and Shoulders or Nizoral A-D antifungal shampoo. Feel free to use your regular conditioner, and style your hair as you normally would.

For red patches and/or itching on the eyebrows and ears, try an over-the-counter cortisone cream. If you have severe itching on large patches of crusty, red skin or if the flaking doesn't clear up within a week or two, stop using the cortisone and talk to your dermatologist about stronger, prescription-strength topical treatments such as Diprasone lotion or Betta-mousse, a cortizone-containing foam that dissolves quickly and won't mess up your hair.

FROM THE FILES OF *Dr. Wu*

Patient: Ariane

Skin Concern: Pityrosporum folliculitis

Food Sensitivity: Challah bread, alcohol, juice

In Ariane's Words: I was diagnosed with type 2 diabetes at age 12, and ever since I've been taking daily insulin shots to regulate my blood sugar. While I do watch what I eat, every Friday I bake challah bread (made with flour, yeast, oil, sugar, and salt) for the Jewish Sabbath. It's not only a tradition; challah bread is my favorite food. In fact, I love it so much that I used to eat it for breakfast *and* lunch every day. And that's when the rash started. My skin became rough, and I was waking up with ten to twenty new whiteheads every morning. When I noticed that my blood sugar was also going up, I finally made the connection. Now I know that if my blood sugar gets kind of erratic, I'll break out in bumps within three or four days. Before, I had even tried taking Diflucan, a prescription-strength anti-yeast pill. Now I know that controlling my blood sugar is what keeps my skin clear.

Dr. Wu's Diagnosis: Ariane has a cute figure (she looks great in skinny jeans!), but she also loves dessert. Perhaps surprisingly, cheesecake is one of the better ways to satisfy her sweet tooth: It has some fat in it, which makes the resulting blood sugar spike less dramatic (so she'll need less insulin). On the other hand, a piece of angel food cake will send her blood sugar sky-high, since it has hardly any fat at all. Even if you don't have diabetes (and your body can produce enough insulin to regulate your blood sugar all on its own), a brief period of elevated sugar—such as after a carb-loaded meal or sugary snack—may be enough to trigger a yeasty rash. That's why I tell people, "If you're going to splurge, a Snickers bar (with protein-packed peanuts and fatty nougat) is better than a straight-sugar treat like Jelly Bellies."

Getting Rid of Chicken Skin

Keratosis pilaris, also known as chicken skin, affects approximately 50 percent of adults—including yours truly. The rough, pink bumps on the backs of the arms (and occasionally the upper thighs) are caused by dead skin cells that plug the hair follicles. It's a hereditary condition, so there's no permanent cure, but you can minimize the bumps by following these tips:

- Resist the urge to pick and squeeze. Unlike acne, keratosis pilaris bumps can't be popped, but you could end up with scabs and even scars if you don't resist the urge to scratch and pick. Instead, use a body scrub once or twice a week. I like Bliss Fat Girl Scrub (despite the name), which contains Himalayan sea salt to exfoliate and glycerin to hold moisture in the skin. Rub in a circular motion to loosen tough plugs of dead skin, and be careful to avoid any scabs. Rubbing too hard can make the red spots look darker, so be gentle!

- After showering, apply a rich body cream. Look for such ingredients as lactic acid and urea found in Eucerin Dry Skin Replenishing Cream 5% Urea with Lactate and Carnitine, and La Roche-Posay Iso-Urea Smoothing, Moisturizing, and Anti-Roughness Body Milk. Both are available at chemists without a prescription and will help to soften plugged hair follicles.

- If your skin is rough and dry, try adding omega-3s to your diet (such as salmon and flaxseeds). If it's red and inflamed, avoid foods containing histamine. (Refer to the list on page 126.) Studies have shown that topical oils, including wheat germ oil, sunflower oil, and evening primrose oil, may also help reduce keratosis pilaris.

- If the condition persists, a dermatologist can prescribe Hydro-40 foam, which contains a stronger dose of urea to dissolve stubborn bumps. If your skin smoothes but the red spots remain, noninvasive laser and light treatments can help fade the discoloration.

Could You Have an Oral Infestation?

Perioral dermatitis literally means "inflammation of the skin around the mouth," and that's exactly what it looks like. This common condition typically starts as a cluster of tiny red bumps on one side of the mouth; if left untreated, they eventually spread to the other side of the mouth, then up around the base of the nostrils, and finally to the outer corners of the eyes. Though it may come with some redness and flaking, it is routinely misdiagnosed as acne even by dermatologists. Acne medications will only irritate the rash, however, and makeup will make the problem more obvious.

No one knows exactly what causes perioral dermatitis. Some researchers think it may be related to rosacea. Others believe the inflammation is caused by a teeny-tiny parasite called Demodex, which looks like a mini caterpillar, with eight stumpy legs and a tail. The Demodex burrow down headfirst into the hair follicles (leaving just their tails poking up out of the skin), and it's the wiggling around that causes the itching and redness. Sounds nasty, but it's actually perfectly normal; even people who don't have perioral dermatitis have Demodex on their skin. It's also not contagious, so you don't have to worry about passing on the rash to people around you.

You can help soothe the inflammation associated with perioral dermatitis by avoiding foods that are high in sugar and by eating more foods with omega-3s, but it often won't go away on its own. Actually, it can spread and get worse. If you think you have an oral infestation, be sure to mention it to your doctor, who may prescribe an oral or topical antibiotic. The key to quick and appropriate treatment is to find a physician who will thoughtfully listen to your symptoms and thoroughly examine the rash since the condition is so often mistaken for acne. Your doc may need a mental nudge to get the diagnosis right.

$E = mc^2$ Did You Know . . .

If you need to get rid of the redness of a rash or acne quickly, try this trick: Put a drop or two of Murine eye drops on a cotton swab and apply it to your spots. You know how Visine "gets the red out" of your eyes? It can do the same thing for your skin by temporarily constricting the blood vessels. This technique should be used only occasionally, though—certainly not daily. Routine use could backfire and cause the blood vessels to rebound, actually increasing redness.

How to Recognize Beard Burn, the Other "Kissing Disease"

You may love the way he looks with a few days of stubble, but getting up close and personal with your man's beard can leave you with a nasty rash. Beard burn is that irritation that develops around your mouth, cheeks, and chin after a steamy make-out session, caused by his coarse facial hair rubbing against your delicate skin. Mild episodes can look a bit like sunburn, but some women can develop deep redness, flaking, itching, and sometimes even open sores. Not to worry—there are some things you can do to protect yourself. You can play hard to get until he shaves, or you can follow these tips:

- Get immediate relief from beard burn with an over-the-counter antihistamine pill (such as Benadryl), which will reduce inflammation, stop the itching, and control allergic reactions. If you've been kissing and feel a little chafed, take one tablet before going to sleep.
- Soothe the skin with a chamomile tea compress. Chamomile is a natural anti-inflammatory, so it has the power to reduce redness, itchiness, and swelling (and it's a great alternative to cortisone). Brew a cup for two minutes and then put the tea bag in a storage container and place it in the fridge. After about two hours, when the tea bag is cold, apply it directly to the red parts of your face.
- Get your guy in the habit of using a moisturizer, preferably one with glycerin; it will help soften his skin and hair without feeling greasy. Be sure to choose one that's fragrance-free since he probably won't appreciate smelling like a girl. Try Vaseline's MEN Body & Face Lotion and offer to demonstrate how to rub it in. I guarantee he'll love the extra attention.

SEE YOUR DOCTOR IF . . . YOU HAVE A RASH *AND* COLD OR FLU-LIKE SYMPTOMS

Just as a chronic rash can signify some underlying cause of inflammation (like a food allergy), a rash accompanied by cold or flu-like symptoms—including sore throat, chills, fever, or allover aches and pains—can signify some larger illness or infection occurring in the body. If you have a rash that "hurts," it's time to see your doctor.

Recap of Chapter 5

Relief from Angry, Itchy Rashes

* Rashes are caused by inflammation. To soothe the skin, choose foods that are low on the glycemic index and avoid excess sugar, salt, and refined grains.
* Be careful with cortisone. While it'll provide fast relief from itching and redness, cortisone can be harmful if abused. Stick with the mildest version that works for you, and don't use it for longer than two weeks at a time without checking with your doctor.
* Keep a food diary. If you're suffering from recurrent hives, eczema, or Mystery Rash, keeping track of exactly what you eat can make it easier to nail down the cause of your itchy, flaky skin.
* Avoid foods that contain histamine. Pickled or fermented foods (including tofu, soy sauce, Champagne, and vinegar) all contain histamine, the substance that causes itching, redness, and inflammation in the skin. Avoid foods on the "Danger List" (page 126), especially if you suffer from hives.
* Eat more anti-inflammatory omega-3s. Oily fish like salmon are packed with DHA, and tofu, flaxseeds, walnuts, almonds, and

soybeans are great sources of omega-3s, which can fight flaking and itching, especially if you're dealing with eczema or psoriasis.

* Steer clear of foods with ingredients you can't pronounce. Scientific-sounding ingredients are typically additives and preservatives, the foods most likely to cause inflammation and allergy.

* Don't be afraid to get your Mystery Rash checked by a doctor. Hey, that's what we docs are here for. If your rash doesn't improve after a week or two on the *Feed Your Face* Diet, give your dermatologist a call.

6

To Tan or Not to Tan

(Protecting Yourself from the Sun)

When my father was a young man coming of age in Taiwan, his family hired a matchmaker to find him a suitable wife (which was pretty much normal practice in those days). The matchmaker—a wise woman, indeed—told my dad that if he wanted to know what a woman would look like in twenty years, he should take a peek at her mother. So over the next few months my father stared intently at the various mothers he met. Was her skin fair, smooth, unblemished? Luckily, he found someone—*my* mother—who is truly beautiful on the inside. (And to this day she is commonly mistaken for someone ten years younger.)

I love that story, but it's about much more than just my mother and father. It demonstrates the effect of what dermatologists call "intrinsic" aging, which is the idea that the condition of your skin is determined by heredity. If you take a look at *your* parents' skin or the faces of your older siblings, you'll get a clue as to how your skin may look when you're older. Heredity is only part of the story, however, when it comes to how your skin will age over time. The other part is what we call "extrinsic" aging, which refers to the effects of what you *can* control: environmental factors, cigarette smoke, and—a major component—sun exposure. While you can't go back in time and change the genes you were born with, you can slow down the aging process by protecting your skin from the sun.

What Happens When You Spend Time in the Sun?

Most people are at least somewhat familiar with the concept of ultraviolet radiation (UV rays), the type of energy emitted by the sun. Even though UV rays aren't visible to the human eye, they travel easily through glass and can even penetrate some types of clothing. (Actually, the name "ultraviolet" literally means *beyond violet,* because UV light has a shorter wavelength than violet light, the last visible color of the rainbow.) There are a number of positive applications of UV light: Forensics labs use it to identify DNA evidence at crime scenes (just like on *Law & Order*); it can even be harnessed for air purification. But when it comes to the skin, UV rays can do much more harm than good. UVA rays—the "aging" rays—penetrate deep into the skin, causing discoloration, wrinkles, and skin cancer, including melanoma, the deadliest type. UVB rays—the "burning rays"—lead first to tanning and then to a painful burn, while long-term exposure has been linked to basal cell and squamous cell skin cancers. (There are also UVC rays, but we don't generally worry about them because they are almost completely filtered out by the earth's atmosphere.)

In addition to causing wrinkles and sunburn, UV rays react with the cells in our bodies, producing unstable particles called free radicals. These act a bit like PacMan on steroids. Free radicals gobble up DNA, "corrupt" healthy cells, and damage proteins like collagen and elastin that are meant to keep our skin firm and smooth. There are other sources of free radicals besides UV rays (your body even produces free radicals as a byproduct of metabolism), so some of the damage can be absorbed. However, when the skin is bombarded by excessive UV rays (as well as cigarette smoke, heavy pollution, and other toxins), the damage becomes too much for the body to neutralize on its own. And that's when sun damage starts to accumulate.

Hey, Dr. Wu

Q: I'm not a beach bunny, and I don't spend a lot of time outdoors. Why should I worry about sun damage?

A: Whenever I'm getting to know a new patient, I ask (among many, many other things) how much time she typically spends in the sun. And lots of women respond with something like "Oh, I'm *never* in the sun." But even if you're not lying out poolside, you may be a victim of what we call incidental sun exposure: the dose of UV rays you get every day, when walking to and from your car, checking the mail, or driving. Since UV rays can penetrate light-colored clothing, I often notice faint tan lines under the bra straps—even among my more "sun-conscious" patients. And while most windshields are made of laminated glass (which does cut out some UV rays) the sun can still shine pretty bright through those side windows. It's not uncommon to develop "sun spots" on the left side—or driver's side—of the face. A general rule of thumb is this: If it's bright enough to wear sunglasses, it's bright enough to develop discoloration, wrinkling, and sunburn. That's why daily protection is so important—even in the winter.

Sunburns Are Real Burns, So Know the Risks

OK, here's my dirty little secret: I like looking tan. Although some of my dermatology colleagues may attack me for this, I happen to think many of us look better—taller, thinner, healthier—when we have a little color. (So I *never* wear a skirt without at least a little bronzer on my legs.) Still, many of my patients are shocked when I tell them to keep biking, playing golf, or taking their kids to the park. They expect me to wag my finger or scold them for spending time outdoors. Maybe that's because so many other doctors do.

One of my patients, an assertive, successful businesswoman, told me she was once humiliated—in public—by a dermatologist. Apparently they were both attending a summer pool party, and when she showed up with a glistening tan, he launched into a full-blown lecture (in front of a roomful of guests) about how she was going to turn into a shriveled prune and die of skin cancer. Now, I can be bossy (I grew up ordering around two younger sisters), but I can't imagine chastising a patient like that, much less someone I'd just met!

I don't like to lecture my patients about the sun. Scare tactics and humiliation just aren't my style. I am very clear, however, about the risks associated with UV exposure, and I take sun protection very seriously. While I don't personally have as much time to spend outdoors as I would like—I often stare longingly at the joggers and cyclists when I'm driving to the office on Saturday mornings—I do wear sunscreen every day (Dr. Jessica Wu Cosmeceuticals brand), I eat foods that provide added UV protection, and when I am in the sun, I'm very careful not to burn.

Sunburns are actual burns with very real consequences. A first-degree burn will cause inflammation of the skin, leaving you red, tender, and swollen, while a more severe second-degree burn, the kind that blisters and peels, signals DNA damage and the death of skin cells. Repeated injury (from multiple burns over time) makes that damage harder and harder to fix. Your cells will begin to grow abnormally and clump together, leading to rough, leathery skin and scaly patches. Burns also suppress the skin's immune system, which can lead to cancer. But if you think you can just slather on SPF 50 and head to the beach worry-free, you're mistaken.

Hey, Dr. Wu

Q: *I'm always so pale by the time beach season rolls around—seriously, I could pass for a character in the* Twilight *saga—and I worry about getting burned. Will getting a "base tan" protect me from sun damage?*

A: It's a common misconception (popularized by the tanning bed industry) that getting a "base tan" before going out in the sun will protect your skin. While getting a gradual tan outside may prevent you from *burning,* it doesn't protect from the other types of UV damage: excess melanin pigment (sun spots and melasma), damage to collagen and elastin (wrinkles and sagging), and DNA damage (which can lead to skin cancer). Getting a base tan at a tanning salon is even worse because you'll get a huge dose of UVA (aging) rays without the burn to signal when you've had too much. (At least when you're out in the sun, you'll cover up and head indoors when you start to turn red.) Forget trying to get a base tan. The best way to protect yourself from sun damage is to wear sunscreen and protective clothing and to supplement your diet with foods that provide extra UV protection. And, hey, since when did looking like a member of Edward Cullen's family become such a bad thing?

Why SPF Isn't Enough

You might think that a high-SPF sunscreen is enough to protect you from aging, wrinkling, and skin cancer. Well, think again. SPF (or "Sun Protection Factor") only refers to the amount of protection you'll get from UVB (burning) rays. So what about UVA (aging) rays—the kind that lead to saggy skin and cancer? In the U.K., many sunscreen packages display a UVA star rating. The stars range from 0 to 5 and indicate the amount of UVA protection as a proportion of the UVB protection. But be aware that if you use a sunscreen with a low SPF, it may have 5 stars, not because it is providing lots of UVA protection, but because the ratio between the UVA and UVB protection is about the same. That's why it's important to look for a high SPF (between 30 and 50) as well as a high UVA protection (4 to 5 stars).

In addition, many sunscreen manufacturers are now complying with the 2006 European Union (E.U.) sunscreen recommendations, which means that you will start to notice new changes on sunscreen labels. In addition to the SPF number, sunscreens will also be categorized as providing low to very high protection. Sunscreens with a SPF below 15 will be labeled "Low Protection"; those with a SPF of between 15 and 29 will be labeled "Medium Protection"; those with a SPF of between 30 and 50 will be labeled "High Protection", and those with a SPF of above 50 will be labeled "Very High Protection". Furthermore, according to the E.U. Recommendation, the UVA protection for each sunscreen should be at least a third of the labeled SPF. A product that achieves this requirement will be labeled with a UVA logo (the letters "UVA" printed in a circle). The bottom line is: look for a sunscreen with a SPF of between 30 and 50 (High Protection), a rating of 4 or 5 stars, and the UVA symbol.

THE BEST MOISTURIZERS WITH UVA AND UVB PROTECTION

Sunscreen should be a part of every woman's morning makeup routine, but who has time to slop on 4 or 5 different lotions or creams? That's why I recommend using a moisturizer/sunscreen combo; you'll save time and money without sacrificing your skin. Here are my favorites:

For oily or acne-prone skin:

Clarins UV Plus Day Screen High Protection SPF 40
Soltan Ultra-Light Texture Suncare Lotion SPF 50+

For combination skin:

Clinique Sun SPF 30 Face Cream

For dry skin:

Shiseido Extra Smooth Sun Protection Cream SPF 38

For sensitive skin:

Blue Lizard Australian Sunscreen Sensitive SPF 30+

What Does Sun Damage Look Like?

One of the most common reasons that people come to see me is for advice on getting rid of their "age spots." And what I always tell them is: no fair blaming your age!

When was the last time you really studied the skin on your boobs or your behind? (Go ahead and take a peek. I'll wait.) Chances are the delicate skin in these private areas is soft, smooth, and flawless—similar to what it looked like the day you were born. Now compare that to the skin on your chest and the backs of your hands, two areas of the body that are typically drier, blotchier, and more wrinkly. Despite the difference in appearance and texture, all the skin on your body is the same "age." What's not the same is the amount of sun your hands, face, and other exposed areas get on a day-to-day basis (unless, of course, you're a nudist). Put simply, UV rays are a primary cause of aging.

Sun damage comes in lots of shapes and sizes. Here's what you're likely to see if you spend too much time in the sun:

Freckles. Freckles may be cute (on Julianne Moore and Lucy Liu, for example), but when I see a young child with freckles on his face, it pains me. That's because freckles—*all* of them—are caused by your skin's response to UV rays. While it's true that some people are more susceptible to *getting* freckles (it's more common in people with fair skin and red or blond hair, for example, and the tendency to get freckles can be hereditary), they're still triggered by the sun. And, contrary to popular opinion, no one is born with them.

When you step outside, UV rays stimulate your skin's pigment-making cells (the melanocytes, located in the bottom layer of your skin) to pump out more skin pigment (melanin). That's why freckles tend to pop up in places where the sun hits you—particularly the nose and cheeks. In your younger years you might have had freckles only in the summer when you typically spent more time outdoors. But as you got older, they may have spread to the tops of the arms, legs, and exposed parts of the trunk. (Since men often spend time outdoors without a shirt, they may develop freckles on their chest and back.) Freckles, which are typically flat, round, light tan to brown spots, can also clump together to form larger, darker "sun spots" that can range in size from your fingernail to as large as a ten pence coin. These spots—which are sometimes called "liver spots" even though they have nothing to do with the liver—typically don't fade in the winter since the pigment has fallen deeper into the skin, so they are more permanent and harder to treat.

Dark patches on the face (melasma). Caused by a combination of heredity, a surge in hormones (brought on by pregnancy or birth control pills, for example), and sun exposure, melasma causes large dark patches on the face, typically on the cheeks, forehead, and upper lip (so you could spend a day at the beach and wind up with a suntan mustache). It's when all three of these factors are present at the same time (in a sort of sick trifecta) that your skin cells become stimulated to pump out more melanin. In addition, some researchers think that heat can worsen the condition.

The first time you develop melasma, the patches may fade on their own. Repeated sun exposure combined with amped-up hormonal activity, however, can make the spots appear darker and sink deeper into the skin, which also makes them harder to remove. New spots (less than 6 months old) may disappear with a botanical skin lightener such as Clinique Even Better Clinical Dark Spot Corrector or Boots No 7 Brightening Beauty Serum. Older, darker patches may require a prescription-strength retinoid cream (like RETIN-A). Really stubborn cases of melasma may require an in-office procedure such as a series of chemical peels. (You can read more about these procedures in Chapter 12.)

$E=mc^2$

Did You Know . . .

Most women don't have time to stop and reapply sunscreen (or makeup) halfway through a busy workday when their SPF protection has worn off and their foundation looks like a drippy mess. But a quick way to refresh your look, soak up excess oil, and reapply SPF is to use a mineral powder. Mineral makeup is made of finely ground minerals, including zinc and titanium, the main ingredients in some sunscreens. While the powder won't give you *even* SPF coverage—so you shouldn't rely on mineral makeup for all your sun protection—it is great for a midday touch-up. My favorites include Laura Mercier Mineral Powder, L'Oréal True Match Minerals, and Sheer Cover by Leeza Gibbons.

Precancerous growths (actinic keratosis). When you're in your teens and early 20s, you can spend hours in the sun and still have skin that looks smooth and even. That's because young, undamaged skin sloughs off evenly every 4 weeks or so, revealing a layer of healthy, "fresh" skin cells underneath. But by the time you hit 30, this renewal process has begun to slow down: Dead skin doesn't slough off as quickly; instead, the cells sit on the surface of your skin and clump together. After prolonged UV exposure, that clumped-together skin can begin to form rough, scaly, precancerous growths called actinic keratosis (AK), which are brown and crusty and may feel tender or produce a stinging sensation. AKs are most often found on the face, hands, and chest, where people tend to get the most sun exposure. It's estimated that as many as 10 percent of them progress into squamous cell skin cancer.

If you already have AKs, a dermatologist can remove them in a variety of ways, such as freezing them with a liquid nitrogen spray, "peeling" them with a chemical solution, or sloughing them with a prescription cream.

Atypical moles (dysplastic nevi). These are precancerous moles, which may be large or raised, with irregular pigmentation and/or indistinct borders. I call them "funny moles" because they look, well, kind of funny. But the real concern with atypical moles is their potential to develop into melanoma skin cancer. It's estimated that if you've had at least one dysplastic nevus, you already have a 5 percent chance of developing melanoma. And if you have a family history of atypical moles or a parent or sibling with melanoma, then the chance of developing melanoma yourself shoots up to 50 percent.

Seeing a dermatologist once a year for a full-body exam is a good way to ensure that you don't have any precancerous growths. (Actually, it's a good idea in general.) But performing self-exams is important, too (just as you should regularly check your breasts for lumps). And if you already have atypical moles or a family history of melanoma, you should see a dermatologist at least twice a year to have them monitored.

Skin cancer. Skin cancer is one of the most commonly diagnosed type of cancers in the U.K. According to the British Association of Dermatologists, more than 70,000 new cases of skin cancer are diagnosed every year.

There are three main types of skin cancer: basal cell carcinoma (affecting the cells of the basal or bottom layer of the skin), squamous cell carcinoma (cancer of the keratinocytes), and melanoma (the most deadly type, affecting the melanocytes, your skin's pigment-producing cells).

Although melanoma is less common than basal cell and squamous cell cancers, it's the most common type of cancer found in young people (ages 20 to 39). Fortunately, it can also be one of the easiest cancers to detect and cure if it's discovered early. Once melanoma metastasizes (spreads to another part of the body), however, the prognosis is very poor. More than 10,000 cases of melanoma are diagnosed in Britain every year.

During a routine skin examination a dermatologist can typically tell you whether or not a mole or growth is harmless. If there's any doubt, however, or if she suspects a skin cancer or precancer, she will remove a part or the entire portion of the mole (in a procedure called a biopsy, which usually involves a local anesthetic to numb the surrounding tissue) and then send samples to a pathology laboratory for examination. Some physicians may also examine the mole with a dermoscope; it allows them to see internal structures not visible to the naked eye. But examination in a lab is the only way to tell for sure.

What types of moles or growths should you be worried about? Moles that crust and bleed (such as a sore that does not heal), a thick patch of scaly skin that's growing, and dark brown to black spots, especially if they change shape, size, or color.

Wrinkles. Don't worry, ladies. I've got a whole chapter devoted to wrinkling and sagging. We'll get there (in Chapter 7 if you're feeling impatient).

BRONZE BEAUTIES NEED SUNSCREEN, TOO!

If you have a peaches-and-cream complexion, you're probably (hopefully) well acquainted with the sunscreen aisle. But what if you tan easily and have more pigment in your skin, like Eva Longoria, Halle Berry, or Angela Bassett—do you still need sun protection? The answer is an emphatic yes!

Even if you've been blessed with a natural bronze glow, the sun's UV rays can still cause blotches, wrinkles, and skin cancer, including melanoma. While melanoma is less common in women (and men) of color, it can occur in any race or ethnic group. I've removed skin cancers from Hispanic, Asian, Middle Eastern, and African American patients, all of whom were surprised that they had even been at risk. Both sunscreen and yearly exams are important since studies have shown that melanoma in skin of color tends to be more aggressive and has a lower survival rate.

Follow these tips to make sure you (and your skin!) stay healthy and beautiful:

• Darker skin tones can look pasty and ashy when slathered in thick sunscreens containing zinc or titanium, so choose light lotions or gels that dry invisibly. I recommend Kiehl's Ultra Light Daily Moisturizer SPF 50, Soltan Ultra-Light Texture Suncare Lotion SPF 50+ or Clarins UV Plus Day Screen High Protection SPF 40.

• If you don't have time to reapply your makeup during the day, touch up with a mineral powder to boost your SPF before going outside again. Try MAC Mineralize SPF 15. (By the way, MAC has an especially great color selection for olive and darker complexions.)

• In darker-skinned individuals, melanoma is more common on the hands, feet, and lips (called acral-lentiginous melanoma). If you see a new or changing mole in these areas, see a dermatologist right away. It's always better to be safe than sorry.

The Vitamin D Controversy

Freckles, moles, and free radicals aren't the only things your skin produces when you spend time in the sun. Every time you walk outdoors, UVB rays react with an organic compound in your skin (7-dehydrocholesterol) to produce vitamin D. While some researchers believe that sunscreen can interfere with that process (since high SPFs can block UVB rays), the most recent research shows that sunscreen doesn't significantly interfere with the body's ability to produce vitamin D. But that's where things get complicated, especially for medical professionals.

Here's what doctors agree on: Vitamin D is essential for good health. It helps the body absorb calcium for strong bones and muscles, and recent research suggests that vitamin D also plays a role in preventing colon, prostate, and breast cancer as well as diabetes (types 1 and 2), hypertension, and multiple sclerosis. Since a number of cells (including the skin cells) contain vitamin D receptors, it's possible that there are additional uses and benefits of vitamin D that we don't yet know about. And here's another thing: Many of my patients tell me they feel healthier when they've had a little sun—and so do I. Perhaps that's our body's way of telling us that it *needs* vitamin D, just as you might crave red meat during your period since your body loses a lot of iron when it's that time of the month.

What's not clear is how much vitamin D we actually need. According to the U.K. Department of Health, most people should be able to get the vitamin D they need by eating a varied and balanced diet and getting some sun. However, it does recommend that you should take vitamin D supplements if you are pregnant or breast feeding, if you cover up your skin for cultural reasons or are confined indoors for long periods of time, or if you have a darker skin tone.

Contrary to what dermatologists have been telling patients for years, some scientists are even advocating sitting in the sun *without sunscreen* to get vitamin D. Crazy as that sounds, there may be some sense in it. After all, our bodies were built to make vitamin D, and it's more than a small group of researchers who recognize the benefits of vitamin D. Australia, for example, is streets ahead when it comes to education about sun protection. In the early 1980s, Australia premiered the "Slip, Slop, Slap" public health campaign, which reminded people to slip on a shirt, slop on sunscreen, and slap on a hat whenever they went outside. (At that same time U.S. citizens were bombarded with ads to use "Bain de Soleil for the St. Tropez tan.") Over the next twenty years the rates of basal cell and squamous cell skin cancers dropped in Australia. However, vitamin D deficiency actually increased. These days, Australian medical groups recommend small amounts of sun exposure for people who don't spend a lot of time outdoors (like office workers).

How much vitamin D your body makes depends largely on where you live. For example, if you live above 40 degrees north latitude (in Northern Europe, for example), then the sunlight isn't strong enough to make vitamin D in the winter, from November through February. On the other hand, if you live below 34 degrees north latitude (somewhere like Los Angeles), then spending just a few minutes a day outdoors will give you all the vitamin D you need, regardless of the season.

Another indicator of vitamin D production is the UV Index, which measures the strength of ultraviolet radiation on any given day. (You can look up the UV Index in any basic weather report.) One recent study showed that when the

UV Index is 3, a fair-skinned individual will produce an adequate amount of vitamin D by exposing the hands and face (without sunscreen) for just 10 minutes a day (it would take an hour to burn). In the summer, when the UV Index might be 7 or 8, you might need only three to four minutes outside.

So what does this all mean? A little sunlight *can be* good for you, but that's not an excuse to get a rotisserie tan or use a sunbed every other week. You can get enough UVB to make vitamin D well before developing a sunburn. If you do burn, you've overdone it. The body will break down the excess vitamin D (so it won't even be stored for use later), and you'll have increased your risk of skin cancer and premature aging. After no more than a few minutes in strong sunlight, you'll want to apply a sunscreen with UVA and UVB protection. (I recommend a minimum SPF of 30.) And if you have a lot of sun damage, a previous skin cancer, or a family history of melanoma, get your vitamin D from food or a supplement, not the sun.

Unfortunately, very few foods in nature contain vitamin D. The flesh of certain fish (such as salmon, mackerel, and tuna) and cod liver oil (yuck) are among the best sources. Small amounts of vitamin D are also found in beef liver, cheese, and egg yolks. Other foods, including some brands of orange juice, yogurt, margarine, breakfast cereals, and especially milk, are fortified with vitamin D. Scientists have even discovered that zapping different kinds of mushrooms with UV light makes them produce large amounts of vitamin D (though you probably won't find these at your local supermarket yet). The easiest way to increase your vitamin D, however, is simply to take a supplement.

If you choose to take a calcium supplement, which is recommended for anyone following the *Feed Your Face* Diet, then you can knock out your calcium and vitamin D requirements in just one dose. (The best calcium supplements include vitamin D because it helps the body absorb calcium.) You can read more about calcium and vitamin D supplements in Chapter 9.

If you opt to take vitamin D on its own, without the calcium, be aware that too much vitamin D can cause nausea, vomiting, constipation, and a buildup of calcium in the body (which can lead to heart rhythm abnormalities and kidney stones). If you are taking vitamin D supplements, you are advised not to take more than 25mg per day, as anything above this amount could be harmful. As with any supplement, talk to your doctor before you start.

THE REAL DANGERS OF SUNBEDS

*T*he cast of MTV's *Jersey Shore* may be a bunch of tanorexics, but the dangers of sunbed use are no joke. The reality is that sunbeds emit harmful UV rays which damage the DNA in our skin and can cause skin cancer. Recent research has revealed that using sunbeds before the age of 35 can increase your risk of developing malignant melanoma – the deadliest form of skin cancer – by 75 percent. Consequently, The Sunbeds (Regulation) Act was passed in the U.K. in 2011 to prevent anybody under the age of 18 from using tanning salons and sunbeds, and it is recommended that anybody with fair skin, lots of moles, or a family history of skin cancer should avoid any use of sunbeds.

Most sunbeds use primarily UVA rays, so they won't increase your vitamin D level since it's UVB rays that produce vitamin D in your skin. While UVA rays may not burn you, they do cause premature aging and skin cancer. In fact, according to a study from the International Agency for Research on Cancer (IARC), a branch of the World Health Organization, men and women who have *ever* used sunbeds have a 15 percent greater risk of developing melanoma. Don't be fooled: There is no such thing as a safe sunbed. Avoid them at all costs.

Using Food to Fight Free Radical Damage: How Certain Foods Can Protect Us from the Sun

By now you should be pretty familiar with the concept of free radicals and understand the importance of wearing a sunscreen with UVA and UVB protection. But here's the thing with sunscreen: It wears off and it sweats off. Sometimes, you might even forget to reapply it after taking a dip in the pool. So what's a girl to do?

The answer is simple: Eat more antioxidants.

An antioxidant is any chemical that can neutralize a free radical, turning it from an unstable particle that damages healthy cells to a stable particle that's essentially harmless. There are all kinds of antioxidants.

Some occur naturally. Your body produces its own antioxidants to neutralize the free radicals created by metabolism, for example, but the rest are supplied by the foods you eat. If you eat mostly foods with a minimal antioxidant benefit (such as dairy products, meat, and processed foods), your body can't recover from free radical damage as quickly or efficiently. That means more wrinkles, discoloration, and sun damage. (In fact, these foods have been shown to increase inflammation, which can actually make sun damage worse. Think about it: The first signs of sunburn are redness, swelling, and pain—all hallmarks of inflammation.) On the other hand, if you load up on antioxidant-rich foods, particularly fruits and veggies, you'll be providing your body with the weapons it needs to fight the signs of aging and protect itself from UV rays.

Have you ever been outside on a bright winter day and wound up with an unexpected sunburn? By eating foods with antioxidant potential, not only can you supplement your daily sunscreen, but you can also provide extra UV protection for those days when you forget to put it on in the first place (like on a brisk yet bright 30-degree day). And since the chemical reactions triggered by the sun continue for days on end, eating a high-antioxidant diet is a way to protect yourself before, during, and long after sun exposure. This is one of the many reasons the *Feed Your Face* Diet is so effective at improving the look and feel of your skin.

We're just now beginning to understand the real power of antioxidants in food. For example, we all know that vitamin C is good for us; it's an antioxidant so, by definition, it fights free radical damage in our bodies. However, the vitamin C in an apple contributes only 0.4 percent of the total antioxidant activity that occurs when you eat the fruit. So where does the other 99.6 percent come from? It turns out that fruits and vegetables contain a complex mixture of chemical substances (including polyphenols and flavonoids), each one working to fight free radicals in its own way. It's the *combination* of these compounds that makes the fruit so powerful—much more powerful than any one single vitamin or antioxidant you can take in pill form. That's why you can't truly substitute a vitamin or supplement for a diet rich in fruits and vegetables.

What to Eat for Added UV Protection

Imagine a young tomato plant sitting in an open field, baking under a blazing California sun. Instead of shriveling in the heat, the little fruit thrives. Why? Because it's filled with carotenoids and polyphenols—two classes of powerful plant-based antioxidants whose primary function is to protect chlorophyll from photodamage. (Rough translation: They keep fruits and veggies from getting sunburned.) As it turns out, these antioxidants can do the same for your skin.

You'll find carotenoids in a wide variety of brightly colored fruits, vegetables, and even in the skin or shells of some animals. In fact, it's the carotenoids that give these foods their color. Lobsters, for example, contain a type of red-colored carotenoid called astaxanthin. In live lobsters the carotenoid is mixed with proteins and other substances, so the animals appear reddish brown or green. But when you boil a lobster, those proteins break down, leaving only the bright red astaxanthin. (Voilá, a bright red lobster on your plate!) Carotenoids are also responsible for the pink feathers of the flamingo. (Flamingos are born—er, hatched—with gray feathers, but adults range in color from light pink to bright red because they eat a diet high in beta-carotene. A healthy flamingo will have a vibrant color, while an unhealthy or malnourished bird will appear white or pale.) The two most common carotenoids in the human diet are beta-carotene (found in orange foods like carrots and pumpkins) and lycopene (found in red foods such as tomatoes and red peppers). Carotenoids are why you've probably heard that eating a diet of brightly colored foods is so good for your health.

The other class of UV-protective antioxidants—polyphenols—was once briefly known as vitamin P. They're commonly found in fruit, vegetables, nuts, seeds, flowers, and bark. Some of the most important dietary sources of polyphenols include onions (which contain a type of polyphenol called flavonols); cacao and grape seeds (proanthocyanidins); tea, apples, and red wine (flavonols and catechins); citrus fruits (flavanones); berries and cherries (anthocyanins); and soy (isoflavones).

For a dose of carotenoids and polyphenols and maximum UV protection (especially for those days when you're headed to the beach or playing a round of golf), supplement your diet with plenty of the following foods:

Tomatoes

Unlike beta-carotene, which can actually turn your skin orange (many years ago, people took beta-carotene in a failed attempt to get tan) as well as increase your risk of lung cancer (if ingested in high doses), there are no side effects associated with lycopene, the main carotenoid found in tomatoes. That's one reason the tomato is a mainstay of the *Feed Your Face* Diet.

In a recent study, volunteers added 40g (about 2½ tablespoons) of tomato paste a day—taken with 10g (about 2 teaspoons) of olive oil—to their normal diet. After four weeks they reported 20 percent less sunburn and by 10 weeks had 40 percent less sunburn even when they were exposed to a dose of UVB rays. (BTW, when I explained this to a friend of mine, she gasped in horror. "You mean they *burn* people for, like, scientific research?" Which is true, kind of. In studies involving UV exposure, scientists shine a special UVB-emitting lamp in gradually increasing strength until they determine a volunteer's specific, shall we say, burn threshold. That way they can determine whether someone's inherent UV protection has increased after eating certain foods. But they focus the beam only on a small patch of skin, the size of a matchbox, not the whole body.)

All red fruits and vegetables, including peppers, apricots, papaya, pink grapefruit, guava, and watermelon, contain this super antioxidant—lycopene, like all carotenoids, gives red foods their color—but more than 80 percent of the lycopene consumed in the U.S. is derived from tomato products. The amount of lycopene present in tomatoes can vary significantly, however, depending on the type of tomato and its ripeness. Typically, the redder the tomato, the more lycopene it has. But lycopene is the most *bioavailable* (or easily absorbed) when the tomatoes have been cooked because the processing of tomatoes (into paste, juice, soup, and sauce) helps release lycopene from the plant cells. In fact, research shows that the body absorbs four times more lycopene from tomato paste than from raw tomatoes. And since lycopene is a fat-soluble nutrient, mixing cooked tomatoes with a natural fat, such as olive oil, helps your intestines absorb it even more. (Just avoid products like ketchup and barbecue sauce. They do contain lycopene, but they also tend to have added sugars as well as artificial colors and flavors, which cancel out the benefits.)

Not long ago two of my patients—Hank and Sarah, who happen to be married—were headed out of town to host a lavish anniversary party at a beautiful resort in Mexico. "I know you're going to be out in the sun," I told them, "so wear plenty of sunscreen, but remember to eat some cooked tomatoes, too! They'll save your skin."

A few days later, as they boarded the plane at LAX, a friend asked Sarah what she was doing with tomato paste in her purse. "Dr. Wu says it's good for your skin," she told her. "It gives you added protection from the sun." Well, bless her heart, the very next day the friend showed up at the pool with tomato paste slathered all over her face. While there is some evidence that topical lycopene can help protect against UVB rays, sunburn, and skin cancer, studies clearly show that for the best sun protective effects, you have to eat the tomatoes, not smear them on your skin!

Hey, Dr. Wu

Q: What if I hate tomatoes? Can I just pop a lycopene supplement?

A: It's generally better for your skin (and your body in general) to get your nutrients from whole foods rather than supplements. If you don't like tomatoes, however, or if they aggravate your rosacea, you can at least choose the right *kind* of supplement. Synthetic lycopene supplements, which contain only lycopene, don't provide the same UV protection as tomato paste or "natural" supplements, which are derived from tomato extract. One commercially available supplement, Lyc-O-Mato, is extracted from organic tomatoes and contains, in addition to lycopene, other plant nutrients such as phytoene, phytofluene, tocopherols, and beta-carotene. This may explain why it works better than synthetic lycopene.

Eggs

It's not just fruits and veggies that have free radical-fighting potential. Eggs, especially organic eggs, contain high concentrations of antioxidants, too. In a German study, researchers found that the concentration of carotenoids in the skin increased 20 percent after just one week of eating two hard-boiled organic eggs per day. Of course, egg yolks also contain cholesterol, so you'll want to limit yourself to about one egg a day or fewer if your diet also includes red meat and seafood.

Green Tea

Growing up, we only had hot green tea with dinner—even if we were in the middle of a Southern California heat wave. When we went out to eat, it was only at Chinese restaurants, where each table had its own pot of the stuff. So when I got to college, I rebelled and took up drinking coffee instead— right up until the caffeine started to make my hands shake (not OK when I make my living holding needles and lasers very close to people's eyeballs).

Turns out, rebelling was kind of silly. Not only is tea the second most popular drink in the world (next to water), it's filled with loads of skin-saving properties. Green tea in particular has a high concentration of catechins, which have anti-inflammatory, anti-aging, and antioxidant effects to help fight free radicals created by the sun, pollution, cigarette smoke, and stress. Consider this: Men in China are, statistically speaking, the heaviest smokers in the world, yet they have relatively low rates of oral, bladder, prostate, and colon cancer. Perhaps it's no coincidence that the average green tea consumption in China is about one cup a day per person. (The stats are similar in Japan, where drinking green tea is also part of the culture.)

When it comes to the skin in particular, topical green tea has been shown to thicken the epidermis (the top layer of skin) as well as inhibit the enzyme that causes uneven skin pigmentation, resulting in less blotchiness and discoloration. Research also shows that green tea can protect the skin from sunburn and skin cancer after exposure to UV light. In fact, one recent study showed that applying green tea directly to the skin 30 minutes before UV exposure greatly reduced the resulting sunburn and DNA damage caused by UVB (burning) rays. In yet another study, participants were given 250mg of green tea polyphenols twice a day (one cup of green tea has between 50 and 100mg of polyphenols). Six months later they reported significant improvement in overall sun damage, redness, and broken capillary veins, suggesting that green tea can actually *reverse* the sun damage you already have.

Given these promising effects, different formulations of green tea extracts are being researched extensively for future inclusion in facial creams and sunscreens. The hope is that even if you forget to reapply your SPF 30 or it rubs off after sweating or swimming, you'll still get some of the residual antioxidant effects of the tea. But while scientists work to develop a formula that penetrates deep enough into the skin to provide real protection, I'll be ordering the Tazo Green Shaken Iced Tea (unsweetened) whenever I go to Starbucks.

Hey, Dr. Wu

Q: I took a day off from work to go to the beach. It was the first day of summer, OK? And now I have a telltale sunburn when I was supposed to be at home ill. Help!

A: A sunburn is a real burn, so start treating it right away to minimize the damage to your skin and to hide the evidence when you go back to work (you naughty girl). Follow these tips as soon as you see or feel the burn:

- Head indoors as soon as possible. If you're stuck outside, reapply sunscreen, put on a hat, and slip on a dark-colored T-shirt to reduce your risk of further burning.
- As soon as you can, take a cool shower to bring down the temperature of your skin. Then apply aloe vera gel, which contains natural anti-inflammatory ingredients and is water-based, so it cools as it evaporates. Avoid heavy, greasy creams and lotions, which can "trap" heat. And if you can't shower right away, buy some cold yogurt at a convenience store and apply it to the sunburned areas; the coolness and milk proteins help to soothe the burn.
- Pop an aspirin or ibuprofen pill to help reduce swelling, redness, and discomfort.
- Apply cold compresses every few hours. Use a washcloth or handkerchief soaked in cold green tea to calm inflamed skin, reduce pain, and minimize swelling.

- Drink plenty of fluids. Sunburn can cause dehydration, so be sure to drink plenty of water or a low-calorie sports drink to help replace electrolytes. If you have fever, chills, nausea, or large areas of blistering, it's time to see a doctor. These are signs of sun poisoning, which can make you really unwell.

Chocolate

Finally, a reason to eat chocolate—guilt-free! (Well, almost.) Researchers in Germany have found that drinking cocoa with a high concentration of flavanols—the type of antioxidant found in cocoa beans—can protect the skin from sunburn (25 percent less redness after UV exposure!) and other signs of sun damage. And after drinking high-flavanol cocoa for twelve weeks, participants in this same study had better circulation to their skin and improved skin hydration, as well as smoother skin overall.

Now that doesn't mean you can gorge yourself on Cadbury Mini Rolls and expect to wake up looking refreshed and radiant. (Actually, you can expect the opposite.) That's because the *type* of chocolate you eat makes all the difference when it comes to its effect on your skin. Milk or semi-sweet chocolate—the kind found in Mini Rolls—has a high sugar content, so it can trigger inflammation. While you can't buy the specially made high-flavanol cocoa used in the above study, you can get a skin-soothing boost by adding a bit of high-quality dark chocolate to your diet.

Chocolate is measured (or graded) by the amount of raw cocoa it contains. Basically, the higher the percentage, the greater the antioxidant quality. High-grade dark chocolate (made with at least 70 percent cocoa) also has less added sugar, so the higher you go, the more bitter it will taste. Choose the highest cocoa percentage you can, and since chocolate is relatively high in calories and fat, limit yourself to—at most—about 100 calories of the sweet stuff a day.

Red Wine

In Europe, melanoma is actually more common in the rain-drenched northern states than in the sun-soaked countries of the Mediterranean. Darker skin tones and heredity may have something to do with protecting Italians and Greeks from UV rays, but I think it also has a lot to do with the diet and lifestyle. People in this part of the world commonly observe the midday siesta (when the sun shines the brightest), eat a diet rich in tomatoes and olive oil, and drink lots of red wine. And according to recent research, red wine can protect you from sunburn even *after* you've spent a day at the beach.

In a recent German study, a group of volunteers was asked to drink 6ml of Châteauneuf-du-Pape (a popular Côtes du Rhône) for every kilogram of their body weight—that's about 12 ounces for a woman who weighs 10 stone—right after being exposed to a dose of UVB light. The volunteers in the second group—who received no wine—reported sunburns across the board. But the wine drinkers didn't. Why? Because polyphenol antioxidants, which protect against redness, swelling, burning, and blistering, are concentrated in the skin of grapes; this is also why red wine, which is fermented along with the skins, has more antioxidants than white wine.

DERMATOLOGY 911:
FOODS THAT FIGHT SKIN CANCER

*R*esearch shows that between 40 and 50 percent of Americans who live to age sixty-five will be diagnosed with either basal cell or squamous cell skin cancer at least once in their lifetime. The good news is that you can help prevent new and recurrent skin cancers by choosing your food carefully. If you have noticeable sun damage or a history of severe sunburns, a family history of skin cancer, or a previous skin cancer diagnosis, you'll want to follow these tips:

Eat less fat. Studies show that a high-fat diet—particularly one high in fatty meat, fried foods, and fried take-out food—is linked to a greater risk of developing basal cell and squamous cell skin cancers, especially if you've had skin cancer before. In fact, if you've had a previous skin cancer *and* you eat a high-fat diet, you'll have increased your risk of developing another squamous cell skin cancer by 400 percent. On the other hand, a low-fat diet (where

20 percent of your total calories come from fat) has been shown to reduce the incidence of actinic keratosis precancers and skin cancer in those with a previous history of skin cancer.

Avoid dairy foods. Studies show that a high intake of whole milk, cheese, and yogurt can make people who had a previous skin cancer three times more likely to develop squamous cell skin cancer.

Eat more leafy greens. People who eat lots of greens have a 50 percent lower risk of developing squamous cell skin cancer.

Drink red wine. In people who already have actinic keratosis precancers, half a glass of red wine a day has been shown to reduce AKs by 27 percent.

Eat more fish. One serving of oily fish every five days has been shown to reduce the incidence of new precancerous growths by 28 percent.

Fish and Fish Oils

Research shows that fish oils can boost the skin's natural immune system and ability to fight off cancer as well as reduce inflammation—a contributing factor in sunburn and sun-related rashes.

In one recent study, participants who took 3g of mixed omega-3 fatty acids per day (administered in five capsules taken twice daily) more than doubled their body's natural SPF after six months. Another study showed that taking 4g of fish oil for four weeks provided the equivalent of SPF 1.15 (as well as lowered triglycerides—an added benefit). While fish oil doesn't replace the need for sunscreen (an SPF of 1 is, of course, relatively low), if this added protection was provided over a lifetime, one could lower one's risk of skin cancer by as much as 30 percent!

Because fish oil can thin your blood, it could cause excessive bleeding in people who have certain blood disorders. The American Heart Association recommends that people taking more than 3g/day of omega-3 fatty acids should consult their doctor first. Also, be sure to let your doctor or dentist know that you're taking fish oil before undergoing any procedure. He or she may want you to stop taking it for a week or two to reduce the risk of bleeding or bruising.

Heliocare Supplements

Extracted from a South American fern called *Polypodium leucotomos*, these oral dietary supplements (available at most chemists) have been shown to protect the skin from UV rays that sneak past sunscreen, so they can ward off damage to collagen and DNA. Take one pill thirty minutes before going in the sun and then another one every three hours for as long as you're outdoors.

FROM THE (**CELEBRITY**) FILES OF *Dr. Wu*

Patient: Kris McNichol—Former Actress (*Little Darlings, Empty Nest*)

Skin Concerns: Brown spots, sun damage

Food Sensitivity: Peanut butter

In Kris's Words: I was 15 when the movie *Little Darlings* (starring Tatum O'Neal and Matt Dillon) was filmed, and I needed to smoke cigarettes for the role. So Matt taught me how—how to hold the cigarette and how to inhale without coughing. I noticed a change in my skin within months; it was very dry, and I lost color in my cheeks. But by the time filming ended, I was hooked. I wound up smoking about half a pack a day between the ages of 15 and 20.

Growing up, I was also completely irresponsible about protecting my skin from the sun. When I was a teenager, my friends and I would compete to see who could get the darkest tan. I'm one-quarter Lebanese, so I'd always win. But just to make sure, I'd mix a few drops of iodine in a bottle of baby oil and lather myself up.

At 20, I discovered a new love: tennis. I wanted to be good, but I knew I'd have to quit the cigarettes. So I went to the Schick Institute where, for an hour a day, I'd get a tiny electric shock every time I was asked to light up. It seems kind of barbaric now, but a week later I was cigarette-free. And even at the age of 20, I noticed a difference almost immediately: I looked (and of course felt) healthier. It was the impetus for a total life change. I stopped going to McDonald's and gorging myself at the Craft Services table. I drank more water. For years I even hosted the annual Kristy McNichol Celebrity Tennis Tournament.

These days I'm a bit of a workout junkie. I exercise twice a day, alternating among running, hiking, tennis, and yoga. I eat tons of pomegranates, which makes my skin look rosy and vibrant, and avoid peanut butter since it makes me break out in red bumps. I'm also diligent about sun protection—especially since I've noticed some brown spots on the left side of my face. Being retired has truly given me the opportunity to take care of myself—and I'm so glad because I look and feel better now than at any other time in my life. I think, cliché as it may sound, I'm living proof that it's never too late to change your life or your skin.

Dr. Wu's Diagnosis: These days Kris really does take excellent care of her skin. For someone with a history of sunburns and an outdoorsy lifestyle, however, she needs to increase the amount of tomatoes and other red veggies in her diet for a boost of UV protection. Luckily, this is pretty easy to do: Throw some sun-dried tomatoes or red peppers into any salad or add grilled tomato slices to any sandwich. Even better, incorporate some tomato paste into soup or pasta. (Remember: Cooked tomatoes pack more lycopene than uncooked ones.) She's smart to have nonfat milk with her cereal, as listed in her diary, but she can protect her skin even more by switching to iced green tea instead of Coke or Cherry Coke. And while there's nothing wrong with an occasional vodka tonic, Kris could get an additional antioxidant boost by opting for red wine or a Bloody Mary.

Sometimes "Faking It" Can Be a Good Thing: The Secrets to a Flawless Fake Tan

Back in the 1920s a group of scientists attempted to develop a sugar substitute—dihydroxyacetone (DHA)—that children with diabetes could eat without disrupting their glycemic control. It failed miserably. People who tried it claimed it tasted terrible, and it stained the sides of their mouths a brown color that didn't go away for days. Voilá! Self-tanning creams were born (and they still smell sickly sweet).

It may have taken decades to perfect the formula, but modern self-tanners are an excellent option for people who want that sun-kissed look without the risk of burning, wrinkling, spotting, or getting skin cancer. And after years of practicing on myself—I told you I like looking tan—I've become a bit of a self-tanning expert. Here's how it works: DHA chemically reacts with the proteins in the top layer of the skin—the dead cells of the epidermis—turning it brown. Since DHA and a similar substance, erythrulose, are the only two ingredients approved by the FDA for temporary tanning, you'll find them in every formulation, whether you use a cream at home or get a spray-on tan at a salon. The concentrations and combinations of DHA and erythrulose vary from brand to brand, however, so you may need to experiment to find one that gives you the most realistic tan (with the least offensive smell). Tanners have gotten a bad rap because they can make the skin look blotchy, uneven, and even orange. (Oh, the horror!) But there are secrets to a great tan:

- Exfoliate! DHA reacts only with the dead skin cells in the outermost layer, but areas of dry or flaking skin will "grab" more DHA, making the tan look uneven. Exfoliating with a washcloth, loofah, or body scrub will help smooth your skin for a more uniform application.
- Moisturize. After exfoliating, moisturize all the rough and dry patches on your body, especially the elbows and knees. Otherwise those areas will absorb more pigment, and you'll look as if you've been kneeling in the dirt. If you're using a tanning lotion on your face, don't forget to moisturize your cheeks, which tend to be drier than your T-zone.
- Watch your spots. Freckles and sunspots also absorb more DHA, so they can get darker with tanning creams. While that's not at all dangerous, it can be a pain in the you-know-what when you're trying to hide those spots in the first place. If that's the case, you might want to opt for a bronzer instead. You'll get more even coverage *and* hide the spots. My absolute favorite moisturizing body bronzer is Garnier Ambre Solaire No Streaks Bronzer Dry Body Mist, which has a faint shimmer and will make your legs look long and lean.
- Apply in thin, even layers and rub in well. If you just slop a bunch of self-tanner on your body, you'll be more likely to turn your skin orange

rather than bronze. Lotions and creams are better than sprays, which can streak. (Hint: If you use a tinted lotion, it'll be easier to see where and how much you're applying than if you use a clear liquid tanner.)

- Wash your palms and soles. The skin on the palms of your hands and the soles of your feet is thicker than the skin elsewhere on your body, so it will become darker than the rest of your skin—a total giveaway that you're faking it.
- A fake tan won't protect you from the sun. Even if your skin looks darker with a self-tanner, you still need just as much sunscreen as usual. And if your self-tanner contains SPF, that protection will last only 3 to 4 hours (even if the tan lasts 3 to 4 days).

DERMATOLOGY 911: HELP! MY FAKE TAN IS *ORANGE*, AND NOW I LOOK LIKE AN OOMPA-LOOMPA!

*D*on't panic. If your fake-'n'-bake tan has left you spotted, streaked, or an unsightly shade of orange, there is a way to reverse the damage. Get yourself to a chemist, girl! Acne treatment pads (with glycolic or salicylic acid) contain ingredients that actually "unglue" the top layer of the skin—the part that holds the fake tan. Wipe vigorously and you'll be back to your old, pale self in about a day (as opposed to three or four).

If you'd like to avoid this kind of problem in the future, you might want to look into professional spray-on tanning, which utilizes tanners with the same ingredients as the stuff you use at home but with slightly different formulas. The best method is airbrush tanning, where you stand stark naked in front of a technician while she sprays a fine, even mist over your body. The artist can even custom contour your body, giving the illusion of sculpted arms, rippling abs, and thinner thighs. A less pricey (and humiliating) option is to get sprayed at a salon with individual spray-tanning booths. (If you have asthma, allergies, breathing problems, or sensitive airways, the spray could aggravate your condition, so check with your doctor first. You might want to stick with at-home tanning.)

To make sure you get the best results, use a loofah or washcloth to exfoliate in the shower, preferably every day for a week before your appointment to avoid any dry spots that might soak up more color. Then apply a thin layer of Vaseline around your fingernails and cuticles to avoid staining. You'll also want to avoid the dreaded "butt crease." Many of us, when we stand up straight, have a little "overhang" in the rear—a crease of skin just under the cheeks. If you don't account for this, you'll end up with bright white crescents of skin on the backs of your upper thighs, totally visible if you bend over in your bathing suit. To make sure your crease is covered, bend over slightly when the spray is at your back. Just don't bend over too much, or your butt will catch all the pigment and your back will stay pale (and *that* wouldn't look good, either)

Phytophotodermatitis, the Other "Lime Disease"

For many people, squeezing a lime into a Corona bottle or making fresh lemonade just *feels* like summer. But, believe it or not, these simple pleasures could leave you with a nasty rash. Phytophotodermatitis (*phyto*—plant; *photo*—light; *dermatitis*—rash) is a common condition that may develop when you touch natural plant compounds called coumarins and then spend time in the sun.

Coumarins are found in a variety of foods we eat, including lemons, limes, celery, parsley, parsnips, fennel, dill, and figs. When these compounds are hit with UVA rays, a chemical reaction occurs that can damage your skin and your skin's DNA, leading to redness, swelling, and blistering that may sting or burn, almost like a sunburn. Unlike a sunburn, however, which typically covers a large area (your entire chest or back), phytophotodermatitis occurs only where the lime juice drips or splatters, or where you touch your face with the hand that was squeezing the fruit. So you might wind up with streaks, splotches, or drip marks rather than a rash covering your entire face. These spots may fade in a few days or, if severe, can take several months to heal. The good news is that this rash goes away on its own. Cool compresses with a damp washcloth can soothe the blisters, and avoiding the sun will help your skin heal faster. And the next time you're mixing cocktails or preparing a meal, remember these tips:

- Avoid handling fruits and vegetables containing high levels of coumarins right before spending time in the sun. If you do touch a lemon or lime, be sure to wash your hands thoroughly before going outside and be careful not to touch your face or another part of your skin (while rolling up your sleeves, for example) before you make it to the sink. Rolling lemons or limes in your hands before squeezing them is a common way to encourage the fruit to release more of its juice. But even that simple act will deposit the fruit's natural oils all over your fingers, even if you don't touch the juice itself.

- UVA-blocking sunscreen may help prevent phytophotodermatitis since it's mainly UVA rays that react with the plant compounds, but it won't prevent it completely. Washing your hands is still the easiest way to avoid it.

- For years women have squeezed lemon juice in their hair to get sun-kissed highlights without visiting a salon. Unfortunately, this can give you a horrific rash on your scalp and anywhere else the juice drips. Do yourself a favor and leave bleaching to the professionals.

FROM THE **(CELEBRITY)** FILES OF *Dr. Wu*

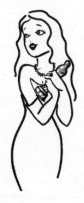

Patient: Kelly Meyer—Environmentalist, Hollywood Insider (her husband is Universal/NBC President Ron Meyer)

Skin Concern: Mysterious red and brown spots

Food Sensitivity: Limes

In Kelly's Words: I first came to Dr. Wu after developing a mystery rash on my face. Seemingly out of nowhere I had these red splotches that turned dark over the course of several days, then went away. I had already visited a few other dermatologists who told me it was probably allergies. But when new spots kept popping up above my upper lip and on my cheek, I figured something else must be going on. Within 30 seconds of meeting Dr. Wu she asked me a seemingly ridiculous question: "Have you been smelling limes?" The crazy thing was, I had! I live in Malibu, and I walk on the beach every day. That summer, every time I passed my lime tree, I'd pluck a piece of fruit, squeeze it, hold it up to my face, and smell the juice.

Dr. Wu's Diagnosis: Kelly's a natural beauty who doesn't wear much makeup, and she'd already told me she hadn't changed her skin care routine. But as soon as I saw Kelly's "mystery rash," I was sure I knew what it was. The odd red spots were characteristic of phytophotodermatitis. The good news is that this type of "lime disease" is super-easy to cure: I asked her to avoid squeezing limes and then touching her face. When I saw Kelly 2 weeks later, she hadn't touched another lime, and the rashes were gone.

Can *Eating* These Foods Cause a Rash?

Normally, eating foods that have high levels of coumarins won't cause a rash or skin reaction. It's touching the juice or the skin of the fruit that creates the problem. In fact, one study showed that volunteers who ate twenty stalks of celery, twenty-five figs, and 250g of parsley had no skin reaction when they were later exposed to sunlight (although I wonder how their stomachs felt, since figs have been known to cause gas and diarrhea—gross).

On the flip side, eating large amounts of celery—450g, which is like a pound of celery—and then going into a tanning bed (which emits UVA rays) has been shown to cause a severe widespread burn. Likewise, drinking 8 ounces of celery broth before hitting the tanning salon has been reported to cause a severe rash. The moral of the story? Just to be on the safe side, don't eat large quantities of foods that are high in coumarins before spending time in the sun, and stay away from tanning beds altogether. (Though who would eat a pound of celery?)

Recap of Chapter 6

Protecting Your Skin from the Sun

* Choose a sunscreen with UVA and UVB protection and a minimum SPF of 30. Reapply every few hours.
* Get a boost of carotenoids and polyphenols by eating lots of brightly colored fruits and vegetables, especially red and orange foods. Before you hit the beach, tennis courts, or neighborhood pool, eat a tomato-rich meal such as spaghetti with marinara sauce and a drizzle of olive oil, or pizza Margherita (which has very little cheese).
* To help prevent new and recurrent sun damage and skin cancers, limit the fats and dairy in your diet, and indulge in green tea, red wine, and dark chocolate (in moderation, of course).
* Add omega-3-rich fish to your diet to fight sun damage—even after the fact.
* Get your skin checked out regularly by a dermatologist. Yearly appointments can increase your chances of spotting suspicious growths before they turn cancerous.

7

Stop Wrinkles Before They Start

(How Food Can Help You Turn Back Time)

've always loved Los Angeles, but when I moved back to the West Coast after five years of living in Boston, I felt like a dumpy country mouse. I had gone to med school in the land of duck boots and Carhartt jackets. Most of my classmates didn't wear makeup; lots of them were still struggling with adolescent acne. And when I walked around campus in the dead of winter—when everyone was bundled up to their eyeballs to keep out the cold—it became damn near impossible to distinguish the men from the women. To say I had a bit of culture shock when I returned to Hollywood is the understatement of the century.

In Los Angeles, *everybody* cares about the way they look. Plus, the city is teeming with thousands of PYTs trying to break into "the industry." Restaurants, coffee shops, and supermarkets routinely hire wannabe actresses and models, so even grocery shopping can be intimidating. And if you're really looking for a confidence smasher, just try shopping for clothes.

I was having lunch recently with a friend who's a former model, when she told me that she wanted to stop by Maxfield, a high-end boutique in West Hollywood that caters to an impossibly posh celebrity clientele. My friend can wear the size 0 (and below) items they stock—*and* she can afford them— whereas I wouldn't be able to get the pants past my knees. Needless to say, I never shop there. My friend, however, is a regular.

When we got to the front door, my friend breezed right through. I, on the other hand, was stopped by a security guard who insisted on inspecting my purse. Then, as we walked among racks and racks of uber-expensive designer duds, not a single salesperson bothered to look my way. Since I wasn't "anybody," they completely ignored me, catering instead to the willowy 20-somethings who looked as if they had just stepped off a Paris runway (or the set of *Gossip Girl*). I thought I had gained a lot of confidence since my awkward days as a pimple-faced teen, but it's hard to be confident when you're a foot shorter than everyone in the room.

While my friend was in the dressing room, I browsed the sale rack (and actually found something I could afford). But when I tried it on, I realized it was too small. After some effort I managed to flag down a saleswoman to bring me a larger size. "Guess you had a little too much pumpkin pie over the holidays," she clucked as she handed me the larger dress. I froze. Was she trying to be funny? If so, it was the cruelest joke I'd ever heard.

I felt my face flush, got dressed as quickly as possible, and told my friend I'd wait for her outside. The whole episode brought back a rush of painful grade-school memories when I was triple-cursed with clumsiness, bad skin, and poor vision. It was like being picked last for games all over again. You *never* forget that feeling.

This is why I can relate to my patients and their various insecurities. I knew what it was like to have bad skin as a teen, and now I know what it's like to wake up and see wrinkles and crow's-feet where there weren't any before. Just as it's cruel to accuse someone of eating too much pie when they can't fit into a size 4, I can't imagine blaming anyone for what happens to her skin over time. After all, you can't fight gravity (unless you spend 8 hours a day on one of those upside-down tables they advertise at two o'clock in the morning). What you *can* do is make the best choices for your skin, three times a day, every time you sit down for a meal or reach for a snack.

In many ways being a dermatologist is a bit like being a therapist: It can be a very intimate relationship. People come to see me at their most vulnerable (either because they're self-conscious about some aspect of their appearance, or because they're naked on my exam table). And since I'm working *thisclose* to a person's face—as well as behind closed doors—lots of personal details and stories get shared. And you know what I hear more than anything else? Women often feel guilty (or embarrassed) about wanting to look their best.

One day I walked into my waiting room to introduce myself to a new patient, only to find the woman sobbing uncontrollably. It turns out that she'd caught her husband cheating with his much younger assistant (diddling the secretary, how original). And although she'd gathered the strength to leave him—and to start dating again for the first time in 20 years—she felt silly for getting caught up in worrying about her appearance. (By the way, I *never* hear this from men. They never feel bad about wanting to look their best.) My scorned patient wondered aloud (as do many of my patients) if she shouldn't just let herself "age gracefully." My response? I think aging gracefully means taking care of yourself, not giving up and letting yourself go.

The Best Place for Anti-Aging Products? Your Local Supermarket!

Most of my patients over the age of 20 eventually ask me what anti-aging products they should be using. It's no wonder: Cosmetics companies feed into our insecurities about getting older, and it seems as though we'll all turn into wrinkled old prunes without the latest (and often very expensive) miracle cream. While a few specific products can help your skin look healthier and more vibrant, skin-care products alone aren't enough to preserve or improve your looks over time. It's just as important to feed your skin what it needs to build healthy collagen and elastic tissue, and to fight the effects of falling estrogen that start to happen in our 30s.

When my patients make an appointment for an office consultation, in addition to asking them what their topical skin-care routine is, I ask them to bring in a food diary. (I also might ask them to bring in their makeup bag and dump the contents on my table.) You can tell a lot about a person by what, when, and where they eat. Still, most of my patients are surprised when I ask about their diets, typically because no doctor (let alone a dermatologist) has ever asked before. In fact, most are surprised that I don't automatically recommend some kind of injectable, a laser treatment, or something even more invasive.

Although I regularly conduct clinical research trials on the latest cosmetic procedures, and I teach these techniques at USC Medical School and to my colleagues nationwide, many of my patients don't necessarily want or need a laser treatment or a wrinkle filler. They just want my advice on how they can look their best. Actually, most celebrities (and noncelebrities) are somewhat fearful of cosmetic procedures, particularly Botox, because they equate them with the extreme examples we see in the tabloids. (I'm actually using lower doses of fillers and injectables and less invasive lasers—for a more natural look—than I did 10 years ago.) For that reason I spend much more time counseling patients on their diet and lifestyle choices. I know that those who eat the right foods and live a healthier lifestyle have more healthy, glowing skin (and cuter figures), while people who ignore their diet often have skin that's tired looking or broken out (and they're typically less happy with their bodies).

You don't have to resort to extreme measures to look younger, but you don't have to feel guilty about wanting to look your best, either. Whether you want to improve your skin or you're happy with what you've got and you want to keep it that way, you can look and feel your best by stocking your fridge with the right foods, making smart choices when you eat out, and choosing skin-friendly snacks in between meals. You have the power to feed your skin the foods that will help build collagen, preserve elastic tissue, and restore firmness. That, combined with using the right skin care, will help your skin look, feel, and *be* more healthy and glowing. But before we talk about how to turn back time with food, we need to understand what happens to the skin as time goes on.

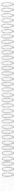

FROM THE (CELEBRITY) FILES OF *Dr. Wu*

Patient: Roma Downey—Actress (*Touched by an Angel*)

Skin Concerns: Dry skin, breakouts, sun damage

Food Sensitivity: Potatoes (particularly chips)

In Roma's Words: I'm Irish, and we are the original potato people, so I have a weakness for chips (especially Kettle Chips) as well as chips. But the closer I get to my 50th birthday, the more I realize that I can't eat the same quantity of food as before because I can't burn it off as easily. I can also pretty much guarantee that I'll have a breakout right after eating chips. So when

I'm thinking about indulging, I ask myself: Can you afford to have a pimple on your face next week? Usually I'll snack on almonds instead.

Back in Ireland (where I was born and raised), the sun didn't shine that often. Businesses would actually close on sunny days so people could spend time outdoors, and being tan was considered healthy, sexy, and attractive. That's probably why I sunbathed all the way up to my late 30s, but when I started to develop dark patches on my face (called melasma), I finally stopped sitting in the sun. Now, even though I travel to a lot of tropical locations with my husband [Mark Burnett, executive producer of *Survivor*], I'm very careful about my skin. I'm always the one in the big floppy hat.

At home I keep a very healthy pantry and fridge. However, it's easy to fall off your routine when you travel. So when I'm on the road, I try to be prepared. I pack my own snacks—typically a piece of fruit (like an apple or a banana), and a Ziploc bag of almonds. I also drink loads of water since plane traveling can really dehydrate you (and your skin). A typical day looks like this:

Breakfast: Cup of tea and a slice of whole-grain toast before driving my kids to school. Then I go to Pilates (5 days a week). Afterward I go home and have scrambled egg whites with chopped tomatoes.

Lunch: Slices of turkey breast wrapped around avocado.

Dinner: Chicken breast, Brussels sprouts, and green beans.

Dr. Wu's Diagnosis: Roma has glowing skin (and a great figure!) because she's usually very disciplined and aware of what she eats. She has some sun damage from previous years of sunbathing, however, so she needs to be extra careful to choose sun-protective foods. Since she often travels to exotic beach locations—or wherever *Survivor* is filming—she should pack tomato paste, sun-dried tomatoes, and green tea. That way, if she gets caught outside and feels a burn coming on, she can incorporate these foods in her next meal as well as apply green tea compresses to her skin. When it comes to snacking, Roma could try high-antioxidant berries (such as blueberries, blackberries, or strawberries) instead of an apple or banana, both of which are high in fructose, which can speed up aging in the skin. When traveling she can add dried, unsweetened cherries or cranberries to her bag of almonds.

What Happens to Your Skin Over Time

In Chapter 6, I explained the concept of extrinsic aging—how environmental factors such as smog, cigarette smoke, and especially sun exposure produce free radicals that can make your skin appear older, drier, and dull. But in this chapter I'd like to focus on *intrinsic* aging, which are the effects of hormones and heredity (the skin you inherited from your parents), combined with the passage of time.

When you're young, your skin cells are actively pumping out new collagen, so your skin is smooth, firm, and wrinkle-free. You could smile a hundred times and the skin would still spring right back into place. But somewhere around the age of 30, your skin's natural metabolism begins to slow; eventually we're no longer producing enough collagen to replace what's being broken down by extrinsic factors like free radicals and stress. As our collagen reserves are depleted, the skin begins to thin. (In fact, research tells us that the skin will get approximately 30 percent thinner between the ages of 20 and 80.) And thin skin wrinkles easily, which makes sense when you think about it. After all, thin silk and linen fabrics wrinkle much more easily than corduroy and velvet.

Aside from making wrinkles more obvious, thinner skin and less collagen also means there's less structure surrounding the pores, so they sag open. As a result, your pores can look larger as you age even if your skin isn't necessarily oilier. (Actually, the oil glands produce less oil over time, and water evaporates more quickly from the skin. Since these changes are most prominent after menopause, dry skin becomes a major concern for women over the age of 55.)

WHY "BLACK DON'T CRACK"

You may have heard the somewhat crude expression "black don't crack," which refers to the fact that people with darker skin tones appear to age slower than people with porcelain complexions. (Korean American comedienne Margaret Cho prefers the phrase "beige don't age.") The crazy thing is that the jokes are based in fact: African Americans and Asians don't tend to wrinkle as much or as early as fair-skinned individuals. Here's why:

Studies have shown that people with darker skin tones tend to have thicker skin (and thicker collagen bundles) than folks with lighter skin, which makes them less prone to wrinkling and creasing. People with darker complexions also tend to have more melanin in their skin, which acts as a sort of built-in SPF. This natural sun protection doesn't completely guard against skin cancer and sun damage, but it does help prevent the UV rays from attacking the collagen and elastic tissue in the skin. While people with fair skin may start to notice fine lines in their 30s and 40s, those with darker skin tones typically seek treatment for discoloration or sun spots long before they notice any wrinkles.

But before you get your panties in a bunch (or cheer with glee, depending on *your* complexion), people with darker skin do tend to experience sagging along the jaw and neck, and often have more pronounced nasolabial folds (the creases that run from the sides of the nose to the corners of the mouth) since their skin is thicker and "heavier."

In addition to collagen loss, your skin cells also slow down their production of healthy elastic tissue. Studies show that the elasticity in your skin will decrease by 1½ percent every year after menopause, which means that the skin gets looser and starts to sag. These changes are most prominent in the jawline (jowling) and the neck (looseness, crepeyness). Over time, not only will you produce less healthy elastic tissue, but the skin actually starts to make abnormal elastic material. This abnormal tissue sits under your skin and has no real elastic function. It can't help your skin "bounce back" when you frown, squint, or furrow your brow. And if you have a lot of sun damage, this process speeds up. The areas with the most sun damage (typically the chest and arms) can actually develop yellowish leathery patches where these blobs of faulty elastic tissue coalesce into large masses. (Ew.)

It's also normal for your complexion to show signs of change over time. In your 20s and 30s, your skin tends to have a rosy glow. But as your metabolism begins to slow in your 40s and 50s, the skin makes fewer new blood vessels, and the ones it does make can be abnormally dilated, causing

AGING BY THE NUMBERS

Now that you know what *kinds* of changes your skin will experience over time, it's important to determine *when* those changes will start to take place. Here's a quick look at what you can expect in your 30s, 50s, and beyond:

20s: In your 20s, the skin generally looks healthy and radiant. You may develop some freckles that appear in the summer and fade in the winter, but the most common concerns in this age group by far are acne, blackheads, and large pores.

30s: This is generally the time when mild sun damage starts to show up on the face and body. Freckles that used to fade in the winter may appear larger and darker or morph into larger sun spots. You may notice the beginnings of crow's-feet and lines between the eyebrows when you're squinting or frowning, but these generally go away when the face is relaxed.

40s: In your 40s, sun damage (like sun spots and blotchiness on the neck, chest, and face) may become even more prominent. Crow's-feet and smile lines now remain visible even when the face is relaxed, and as your body enters perimenopause, the skin may begin to appear dry and dull.

50s: In your 50s, you may notice deeper wrinkles on the forehead and around the mouth, as well as the appearance of new wrinkles on the cheeks and above the upper lip. With the onset of menopause, the skin may start to feel thinner. Sun spots get larger and may appear in new places such as the arms, legs, and the backs of the hands.

60s and beyond: With the continued loss of collagen, the skin may begin to sag, especially along the neck and jawline, as well as bruise more easily. The sebaceous glands will begin to grow larger (even though they'll be pumping out less oil); they may look like tiny flesh-colored bumps on the forehead and cheeks. Dry skin is also a major concern for women in their 60s and 70s.

irregular circulation. Some areas of the skin will have less circulation and look pale, while other areas will experience excess circulation and look flushed. This is the reason you may develop blotchy patches or "broken" capillary veins, which aren't actually broken but, rather, dilated (or stretched out) from excess blood flow. They then rise to the skin's surface where they become visible. The skin may also begin to lose its healthy glow and appear sallow. Weaker circulation also means that wounds heal slower.

Along with irregular blood circulation, the production of new skin cells begins to slow down. When the body is no longer creating enough new cells to "push off" or slough off the old skin of the epidermis, the dead cells hang around on the surface of your skin for a longer time, which causes brown spots and uneven pigmentation. Over time, these dead cells can accumulate and turn into rough, flaky patches that represent precancerous growths. If left untreated, a small percentage of these may develop into skin cancer. The melanocytes (pigment-making skin cells) also become affected: Instead of making smooth, even pigment (for an all-over tan), they begin making clumpy patches of pigment in the form of sun spots or melasma.

What Happens When You Hit Menopause

As teenagers, our hormones made us irritable and anxious with stubborn breakouts and oily skin. For some women, adolescent acne then becomes hormonal acne, which can drag on into your late 30s and 40s. Then, when you finally think you have things worked out, *wham,* menopause cuts off your estrogen, and you wind up with a whole new set of skin problems.

Menopause, which technically begins the year after your last menstrual period, is responsible for the majority of changes we see in aging skin. (The beginning stages of menopause, which include the onset of irregular periods, are referred to as "perimenopause.") As your ovaries begin to slow down their production of ripe eggs (and eventually stop producing ripe eggs altogether), the amount of estrogen in the body begins to plummet. The ovaries continue to produce some estrogen (and your body will begin to convert other sex hormones *into* estrogen), but you'll still have much less than when you were menstruating. It's this fluctuation in estrogen levels that causes the classic symptoms of menopause, particularly hot flashes and flushing. The drop in estrogen also contributes to a loss of collagen, at a rate of 2 percent per year after going through "the change" (although 30 percent of total collagen loss happens in the first 5 years after menopause). With all the changes going on in your body, you can expect major changes in your skin. Spider veins and "broken" capillaries, thinning or sagging skin, and thicker, darker hair growth on the upper lip and chin are all common when you enter this phase of your life.

While hormone replacement therapy (HRT) has been shown to increase collagen, elasticity, and skin hydration, it's still quite controversial among medical professionals, especially since it's been linked to such side effects as an increased risk of breast cancer and stroke in some women. You should talk to your doctor about HRT if you're experiencing menopausal symptoms like severe hot flashes or insomnia or if you have osteoporosis, but wrinkles shouldn't be the only reason to take hormones.

As a potential alternative to HRT, an increasing amount of evidence suggests that dietary antioxidants may be able to offset some of the symptoms of menopause. For example, it's estimated that as many as 75 to 85 percent of women in the U.K. and America experience hot flushes associated with menopause, but only 25 percent of Japanese women have them. Some researchers believe that's because Asian women eat roughly fifteen to twenty times more soy than British or American women (for a total of 40 to 80mg a day, which is equivalent to 1 cup of dried soybeans or 2 cups of fresh tofu).

Soy contains a type of phytoestrogen, or plant estrogen, that has a weak estrogen-like effect on the body. (The implication, of course, is that eating soy is a way to supplement the loss of estrogen that occurs at the onset of menopause.) There is no conclusive evidence, however, that supplementing your diet with soy-based foods (such as tofu, soy milk, or soy cheese) is a safe or effective treatment for everyone. In fact, a diet high in soy may have negative side effects for women with estrogen-receptor positive (ER-positive) breast cancer. If you're entering perimenopause and considering adding more soy to your diet, be sure to discuss it with your family doctor or gynecologist first, particularly if you have a family history of breast cancer; he or she can help you determine if adding soy is right for you.

Eat to Beat the Clock: Foods That Fight Wrinkles

When my dear friend Bari was in the fifth grade, she had to write a paper on Ponce de León, the Spanish explorer who supposedly discovered the Fountain of Youth in the early 1500s. While Bari was busy working away, her father arranged for one of his buddies to give her a call, claiming to be the man himself. Of course, Ponce de León would have been somewhere around 500 years old at the time, but Bari totally bought it. And even if he hadn't discovered the Fountain of Youth, she thought, he was clearly doing something right.

The idea of staying young forever (or at least looking that way) is an intoxicating one. It's why we spend hundreds of dollars on wrinkle creams, collagen injections, and those funny little eye masks that are supposed to make you look well rested. But what most women don't realize is that the real Fountain of Youth (or at least the most effective way to beat back wrinkles) might just be in your refrigerator. Here's how certain foods can help you turn back time:

Eat More Protein

Recent research from the University of Michigan shows that matrix metalloproteinases (MMPs), which are enzymes activated by free radicals and a diet high in sugar, not only devour healthy collagen, but they also leave collagen fragments floating around in the skin. When healthy fibroblasts (the skin's collagen-making cells) come into contact with these damaged fragments, they basically get confused; they shut down and stop making collagen. In aging skin these collapsed or "confused" fibroblasts make little collagen and *lots* of collagen-destroying MMPs, so the effect is exponential. One damaged cell leads to two damaged cells, two cells lead to four, and so on and so on.

By doing what you can to stimulate new collagen, however, the damaged or nonfunctioning cells can essentially be "woken up." In fact, researchers have been able to take skin cells from an 80-year-old woman (wimpy collapsed fibroblasts that were no longer making much collagen) and manipulate them in a lab to behave like the fibroblasts of a 20 year old. What does that mean? By stimulating new collagen, you can actually turn back the clock!

While there are cosmetic procedures that can stimulate collagen growth, the least invasive and less expensive course of action is to feed your body the building blocks of collagen. (Conversely, when you crash-diet or stop eating altogether, you deprive the body of the nutrients it needs to function properly, so collagen production drops quickly.)

Collagen itself is a protein, so all proteins (like chicken, lean meats, and soy) will help keep the skin strong and flexible, but the major components of collagen are the amino acids glycine and proline. Beef, lamb, and chicken breasts have high concentrations of both amino acids, so they're excellent staples in an anti-aging diet. You can also find glycine in pork, quail, bison, and such seafood as lobsters, crabs, scallops, and shrimp. Cottage cheese and cabbage are other good sources of proline. You'll also want to eat plenty of foods containing vitamin C, magnesium, and copper; these are called collagen cofactors because they're essential for collagen production.

The Problem with Sugar

At this point you already know that added sugars and refined grains can lead to dramatic spikes in your blood sugar (as well as increased oil production, elevated androgens in the bloodstream, and more frequent hot flashes and flushing). But if you're worried about wrinkles and fine lines, there's another reason you should refrain from eating lots of sugar: Glucose actually eats away at your skin's collagen and elastin in a process called "glycation."

When you eat sugar, the glucose molecules react with proteins in the body and produce compounds called Advanced Glycosylation End-products (AGEs). When these AGEs accumulate in the body (after you eat lots of sugar), they end up aging *you*. AGEs activate MMPs, the enzymes that digest and destroy healthy tissue. And in the skin AGEs interfere with your body's ability to make collagen and elastin, leaving your skin less supple and resilient. (AGEs may also explain why diabetics heal more slowly when they're injured and why they're at greater risk for skin infections.) Additionally, UV rays react with AGEs to produce harmful free radicals that further digest your skin's healthy collagen and elastin, leaving your skin thinner and weaker.

By following the *Feed Your Face* Diet, you'll already be cutting out added sugars and simple carbs (like white bread, white rice, and white flour). Since fructose speeds up the AGEing (and *aging*) process even faster than glucose, you'll also want to avoid high-fructose corn syrup (found in fizzy drinks, salad dressings, ketchup, and some cereals). But certain high-fructose fruits can make you AGE too, so if you want your skin to look younger, you'll want to eat the following fruits sparingly and *only* when paired with protein or healthy fats:

Apples (2 apples have the same amount of fructose as a can of Coke)
Apple juice and applesauce
Pears or pear juice
Canned fruit (these often use pear juice to make a heavy syrup with
    added sugars)
Watermelon
Grapes
Raisins and dates
Dried fruit

Dried fruit and nuts are actually one of my favorite snacks as well as a fairly large component of the *Feed Your Face* Diet. Luckily, dried fruits with *no* added sugars are fine if you eat them in moderation. (I like Crunchies all natural freeze-dried fruit snacks.)

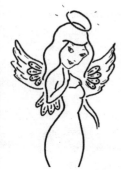

Anti-Aging Fruits

Not all fruits are "bad" for your skin. Fruits that are naturally low in fructose have less of an AGEing effect (as well as a powerful boost of antioxidants). Whether you're 15 or 50, you can eat the following fruits guilt-free:

Strawberries	Oranges
Blueberries	Lemons
Blackberries	Limes
Raspberries	

Eat Tomatoes

Tomatoes have been shown to help protect the skin from UV damage, but they also have powerful anti-aging effects. In a recent study, female volunteers who took tablets containing 60mg of lycopene (the super-powerful antioxidant found in tomatoes), 50mg of soy isoflavones, and 60mg of vitamin C showed significant improvement in fine lines, skin hydration, elasticity, and radiance after six months.

FROM THE **(CELEBRITY)** FILES OF $\mathcal{D}r. \mathcal{W}u$

Patient: Kat Von D—Tattoo Artist, Reality TV Star, Author
Skin Concerns: Dry skin, sun protection (for her tattoos!)
Food Sensitivity: No sensitivity per se, just a weakness for Mexican food
In Kat's Words: Even though skin "awareness" is part of my job, and there is a noticeable difference in my skin when I eat well, I have to admit I find it difficult to stick with a consistent diet.

When I'm busy filming or tattooing, it gets hard to carve out time to eat throughout the day. And when things are really crazy, the day is often over before I realize I haven't eaten at all. (Those are usually the days when late-night pizza sounds like a good idea, and it's a downward spiral from there.) For example, my last book tour [for *High Voltage Tattoo*] was a 3-month whirlwind of traveling from city to city. I would start my early mornings with nonstop press, then head into a 5-hour book signing almost every day. By the time I got back to the hotel, I'd had hardly anything to eat, drank probably three sugar-free Red Bulls, and had minimal water. Too drained to exercise, I'd order comfort food or dessert in the room, and then do it all over again the following day. So before long I definitely noticed more breakouts (which don't often happen for me) and dried-out skin.

Lately I've had a decent break from filming *LA Ink,* so I've been able to dive back into my healthy regimen, which includes a lot of training and, of course, a healthier diet. Usually this veers toward mainly raw foods. That's why my food diary might seem a bit "squeaky clean."

Dr. Wu's Diagnosis: To anyone who's looking, it's obvious that Kat cares about her skin. As the owner of more than fifty tattoos, it's the showcase for her incredible art. She does make good food choices (like chicken sandwiches and dried fruit) and stays hydrated with plenty of water. Like any other busy woman, however (whether you're a sought-after tattoo artist or a working mom), sometimes she skips meals. But it's important not only to eat the right *kinds* of foods; she also needs to eat enough of them. A diet too low in calories won't provide enough protein and nutrients to make healthy collagen and elastic tissue. Additionally, not eating all day and then ordering comfort food or dessert at night can cause blood sugar spikes that will further AGE your skin. Kat is young, so her skin still looks smooth and supple. She can get away with skipping meals *now,* but she should try to eat more regularly to keep it that way.

When Kat doesn't have time for a sit-down meal, she should find protein-rich grab-and-go snacks that she can eat in between tattoo clients. She could add almonds or walnuts to her dried strawberries for a more skin-friendly midday snack. Kat should also eat plenty of cooked tomatoes to protect her fair skin from UV rays, keep her tattoos from fading, and prevent future sun damage.

Watch Your Saturated Fat

Most people know that a diet high in saturated fat can increase your risk of heart attack and stroke, but three separate studies have shown that saturated fats can also jeopardize the health of your skin:

- In a Japanese study, volunteers who ate more saturated fat had significantly more facial wrinkles than those who ate less.
- In a study published by the *Journal of the American College of Nutrition,* people who ate lots of butter or margarine (both contain a large amount of saturated fat per serving) had more wrinkling than those who ate less.
- In a study published by the *American Journal of Clinical Nutrition,* researchers found that a diet high in total fat (including both saturated and unsaturated fats) leads to decreased skin hydration and, therefore, drier skin.

So how much saturated fat is too much? According to the American Heart Association, saturated fat should account for less than 7 percent of your daily calories, while the rest of your daily fat intake should come from *un*saturated fats (the kinds found in nuts, seeds, fish, and vegetable oils). For the average woman on a 2,000-calorie-a-day diet, that works out to about 16g (or less) of saturated fat per day. And since most of us have no idea how much saturated fat we're eating, I'll try to help you out.

Saturated fat is most commonly found in animal products; beef, veal, lamb, pork, butter, milk, cream, and cheese all contain saturated fat (as well as dietary cholesterol). Some plant-based foods, however, including coconut, coconut oil, palm oil, palm kernel oil (often referred to as tropical oils), and cocoa butter, also contain saturated fat. Margarine, which comes from a plant source, is also particularly high in saturated fat because it has been hydrogenated, which is a process that makes it melt more slowly. If a stick of margarine stays hard on your countertop, think about what it's doing inside your arteries.

While meat and other proteins can be good for your skin in other ways (beef, for example, is especially beneficial for people with acne due to its high zinc content), you'll want to choose the leanest cuts available. (Bison, by the way, has a rich, meaty flavor, but it is lower in fat than chicken breast.) Remember that prepared and takeout foods, as well as foods made with cream, sour cream, and butter, can also be high in saturated fat. (A grande Java Chip Frappuccino from Starbucks, for example, has 12g.) And if you're going to have margarine, choose the softer kind that comes in a tub. Better yet, opt for nonhydrogenated trans-fat-free margarine spread or, when possible, cook with healthier fats such as olive oil.

Saturated Fat by Serving

It's not always easy to know how much saturated fat you're really eating. Use the chart below to get an idea of how many grams of fat these common foods contain:*

Food	Saturated Fat
1 large egg yolk	2g
Chicken breast, roasted (7 ounces)	2g
Top sirloin (trimmed to 1/8-inch fat), grilled (7 ounces)	5g
Dark meat chicken, roasted (7 ounces)	6g
Flank steak (trimmed of all fat), grilled (7 ounces)	7g
1 tablespoon butter	7g
Pork chops, grilled (7 ounces)	10g
85% lean ground beef (7 ounces)	12g

*Nutritional information provided by the USDA.

Eat Green and Yellow Vegetables

Studies show that people who eat lots of green and yellow vegetables (such as peppers, squash, spinach, and green beans) tend to have fewer wrinkles—especially around the eyes—than those who don't. Why? Because just as carotenoids and other antioxidants can protect you from the sun, they also fight the free radicals that break down collagen over time. Even better, new research shows that people who eat a diet high in saturated fat *and* eat lots of green and yellow vegetables have fewer wrinkles than people who eat a high-fat diet and little or no greens. So here's a general rule of thumb: If you're going to eat a steak (or some other high-fat food), pair it with a side of brightly colored veggies.

FROM THE (CELEBRITY) FILES OF *Dr. Wu*

Patient: Christa Miller—Actress (*Cougartown, Scrubs, The Drew Carey Show*)

Skin Concern: Having glowing, radiant skin on camera

In Christa's Words: When I'm not working, I'm pretty lax about my diet. I like the way I look in real life. It's very easy to look bloated on camera, though, so when I am working, I'm more mindful of what I eat. (I have to be thinner so that I look like a normal size on TV!)

When I'm on the set of *Cougartown,* I'll start the day with egg whites, slices of tomato and avocado, and whole wheat toast. (Courteney Cox and I usually eat together, but she skips the toast. She's more disciplined than I am.) Then for lunch I'll have a salad. Snacking, however, is imperative; otherwise, I'll crave pizza around 1:30 PM. If I cave and end up eating the pizza, then at night I'll have a small snack (like popcorn) instead of dinner.

Things get a little tricky if I have an event in the evening. For example, my husband and I went to a charity dinner in Beverly Hills recently, and dinner wasn't served until 9 PM. By then I was starving, so I had the pasta. They also have this amazing butterscotch pudding with caramel, whipped cream, and sea salt, so I had that, too. I've got a weakness for sugar, especially when I'm tired or if I have to be on set really early (like before 6 AM). I also love to bake homemade chocolate chip cookies.

Dr. Wu's Diagnosis: Christa's a relatively new patient of mine, and she does what a lot of women do when they're watching their figures: She compensates for midday indulgences by skipping dinner. Not only is this counterproductive for looking svelte on camera (starving yourself can slow the metabolism, so your body starts holding on to fat), it causes your blood sugar to surge wildly—and that can affect your face. Even on the days when Christa has pizza for lunch, she should still eat a small, healthy snack in the late afternoon to modulate her blood sugar. Then for dinner she can have something light, such as a small leafy green salad with yellow and red veggies, chopped walnuts (for protein and a dose of omega-3s), and a drizzle of olive oil—much more satisfying (and face-friendly) than popcorn. When she goes out to eat, she should ask for a side of green beans, spinach, or squash to help keep her skin smooth and wrinkle-free.

Christa already makes a delicious homemade trail mix to snack on when she's filming *Cougartown*. (Read the recipe on page 237.) She should tuck an extra bag in her purse so she'll be prepared for any future late-night events. By "pregaming" with a snack before dinner, her blood sugar won't dip so low, and she won't crave sweets as much.

Eat More Omega-3s

Not all fats are bad for you. In fact, fat serves as a source of energy in cell metabolism, so your skin actually needs some fat to function properly. But whereas saturated fats can contribute to wrinkles, healthy omega-3s can keep your skin looking firmer and younger.

Back in Chapter 1, I explained that each skin cell is wrapped in a protective layer of fatty tissue. This helps seal in moisture and protects your skin from chemicals and toxins that may irritate your skin or cause an allergic reaction. If you don't eat enough healthy fats to replenish this fatty "bubble wrap," moisture will evaporate more quickly, and your skin will dry out. But if you add plant-based omega-3s to your diet (called alphalinolenic acid, or ALA), you can improve the dryness associated with aging. In addition, eating more omega-3s (especially those from fatty fish like salmon, sardines, and albacore tuna) can dramatically improve the skin's elasticity, which helps it bounce back into place after smiling or squinting.

You can increase the amount of omega-3s in your diet by eating plenty of fish, flaxseeds, walnuts, almonds, and olive oil.

Stop Smoking

You already know that cigarette smoke produces free radicals that eat away at your skin's collagen and elastin. But cigarettes also stimulate the skin cells to produce matrix metalloproteinases (MMPs), the enzymes that destroy healthy skin tissue. Remember that more cigarette smoke equals more collagen destruction, which equals weaker, thinner skin. Plus, sucking on cigarettes causes wrinkles in the upper lip, commonly referred to as smoker's lines.

CAN A RETINOID CREAM SMOOTH MY WRINKLES?

Patients often ask me if retinoid creams such as tretinoin (found in Retin-A) and retinol can really help their wrinkles. Here's what you need to know:

Retinoid creams work by helping to slough off dead skin, so they're most helpful for those with sun damage, blotchy pigmentation or dark patches, and fine lines and wrinkles. Retinoids also stimulate new collagen production as well as block the enzymes that break down collagen after UV exposure, thereby making wrinkles appear smoother. In fact, research shows that these vitamin A–derived creams are among the most effective topical anti-aging tools on the market, but retinoid creams can also irritate sensitive skin and leave your face a flaky mess if used incorrectly.

To minimize redness and flaking, I tell my patients to start slowly. Although prescription-strength retinoids like Retin-A will yield the fastest results, these can be more irritating. Instead, start with a mild, nonprescription cream like RoC Retin-Ox Wrinkle Correxion Regenerating Night Cream (especially if you have sensitive skin). Apply a thin layer before bedtime two to three times a week and gradually work up to four or five applications per week. Since retinoid creams can make your skin more sensitive to the sun, it's extra important to use a sunscreen with UVA and UVB protection and to avoid facial scrubs and waxing.

You may be slightly pink or flaky the first few weeks after starting a retinoid treatment, but that typically subsides. After the first month you'll notice an improvement in your overall skin texture because retinoids help increase cell turnover, leaving you with softer, smoother, "newer" skin. After three months you'll notice a softening of fine lines and wrinkles. And after four to six months dark patches may begin to fade.

Topical Treatments for Younger-Looking Eyes

Dark circles, puffiness, and fine lines can make you look tired and run-down even when you're not. Since the eyes are the windows to the soul, it's important to keep them looking fresh and clear. Here's how:

- Gently pull down on the skin beneath your eye. Do you see freckles or dark patches underneath your lower lashes? Skin-brightening creams can reduce this excess pigmentation that contributes to dark circles.
- Thin skin under the eyes can also contribute to dark circles because dark eyelid muscles become visible beneath the skin (the same way that black panties are visible through white pants). Studies show that eye gel with retinol can decrease dark circles after 4 weeks by thickening the skin of the lower eyelid. Try RoC Retin-Ox Wrinkle Correxion Eye Cream.
- Excess salt in your diet can make your body retain water, so when you lay down at night, some of that extra fluid redistributes to your face, causing puffy eyes and under-eye bags. Seasonal allergies and sinus problems can also contribute to swollen eyes, so ask your doctor about an antihistamine if you have either of these conditions.

The next time you wake up with puffy lids, try soaking a cotton ball in cold soy milk and holding it to your closed lids for a few minutes. The cold temperature and anti-inflammatory properties of soy can help shrink the swollen tissue. If your dark circles are caused by hollowness, an injectable filler such as Restylane or Juvéderm may help lessen the circles. You can read more about fillers in Chapter 12.

Don't Forget Your Hands!

Your hands can show the telltale signs of aging, so you'll want to give them just as much attention as you give your face. Here's what you can do to keep your hands looking their best for a lifetime:

Plump up thin skin. As time goes by, we lose collagen and fat in our hands, which can make them appear bony and have more pronounced veins. To keep them looking youthful, look for a hand cream with retinol to support collagen growth in the skin such as Chantecaille Retinol Hand Cream or Vaseline Healthy Hand & Nail Conditioning Hand Lotion. Because thin skin also bruises easily, be sure to eat plenty of fruits and vegetables with vitamin C, which helps strengthen blood vessels.

Remove rough patches. While a hand sanitizer kills germs, it also contains a high concentration of alcohol that can dry out your skin. Keep your hands soft and smooth by reapplying hand cream throughout the day. Choose a cream with glycerin (to soften) and urea (to remove dead skin)—I like Eucerin Dry Skin Intensive Handcream 5% Urea—and be on the lookout for scaly bumps that don't heal. They could be a type of precancerous growth called actinic keratosis (AK).

Banish brown spots. Chances are you have more freckles and spots on the backs of your hands than almost anywhere else on your body. That's because those spots are signs of sun damage, and your hands are almost always on display. Look for a product with soy (like Philosophy When Hope Is Not Enough) or arbutin, a natural extract found in bearberry, wheat, and certain types of pears (try Chantecaille Vital Essence with Arbutin), and be sure to wear sunscreen on your hands. UV rays can be strong on a clear day even when it's freezing outside. Stubborn brown spots can also be removed by a dermatologist with a laser treatment, chemical peel, or liquid nitrogen spray (which freezes them off).

FROM THE FILES OF *Dr. Wu*

Patient: Hilla

Skin Concerns: Dry skin, anti-aging

In Hilla's Words: I spent my childhood on three acres nestled in the German countryside, where we grew our own fruits and vegetables and got fresh eggs from the neighbor's chickens (in exchange for Grandma's homemade jam). The milkman came every morning with still-warm milk straight from the cow; it wasn't pasteurized or homogenized (and, of course, the cows weren't treated with antibiotics or hormones).

In 1986 I moved to Los Angeles. It was the first time I experienced McDonald's, "American" staples like hot dogs, and refined or processed food. (Honestly, I never understood the hype; I found most of it rather tasteless.) But you have to eat, and a few years later—at the age of 30—I found myself at the local spa, complaining about my dull complexion. On top of that, I started to get severe migraines and in general felt puffy and bloated. It wasn't until I got my diet back under control (and ate the way I used to) that the migraines went away.

I'm 52 now, and getting older ain't always pretty, but it sure beats the alternative, which would be not getting older at all! My skin has become drier, probably from the blazing Southern California sun, so I eat plenty of healthy fats (like organic olive oil) and drink lots of water.

Over the years I've learned not to fret too much. You have to love yourself and take care of yourself: eat well, sleep well, and spend your time doing things you truly enjoy (I love gardening). I also think it's important to pamper yourself more as you get older. You deserve it! Here's what I eat on a typical day:

7:30 AM: A glass of water with a splash of organic apple juice. (Then I walk the dogs for 45 minutes.)

8:30 AM: Smoothie (made with organic raspberries, pineapple, strawberries; organic yogurt; and apple juice), oat or rice cereal with almond milk, and espresso

11:00 AM: Slice of toasted spelt bread with butter and a soft-boiled egg

2:00 PM: Caesar salad with spelt croutons and roasted chicken

5:00 PM: Almonds, apple splices, olives, cherry tomatoes, a bit of cheese, and espresso

8:00 PM: Pan-roasted white King salmon, cauliflower and sweet potato mousse (prepared like mashed potatoes but with cauliflower and sweet potatoes instead of regular potatoes), small scoop of vanilla ice cream, and two glasses of Champagne

Before bed: Herbal tea with lemon and honey

Dr. Wu's Diagnosis: Hilla is someone who has eaten well for most of her life. Now, in her 50s, she has smooth glowing skin and a knockout body to show for it. She eats small, frequent meals to keep her blood sugar stable and to prevent AGEing. She also has protein with every meal to supply her body with the building blocks of collagen and elastic tissue. For an added antioxidant boost she could consider swapping Champagne for red wine, herbal tea for green tea, or indulging in a piece of dark chocolate for dessert. Check out Hilla's recipe for roast chicken in Chapter 9.

Recap of Chapter 7

Slowing the Signs of Aging

✳ Supplement the loss of collagen and elastin by eating the proper proteins. Starving yourself can actually make your skin age faster.

✳ Sugar makes you AGE (and *age*). Once you hit 50, it's particularly important to curb your intake of sugar and avoid fruits that are high in fructose.

* Studies show that people who eat lots of saturated fat (especially butter and margarine) have more wrinkles than those who don't. Choose lean or extra-lean meats and a nonhydrogenated trans-fat-free margarine spread. Avoid foods made with cream or sour cream and be wary of prepackaged and fast food.

* Fight dry skin and boost elasticity by adding omega-3s to your diet (such as fish, flaxseeds, walnuts, olives, and olive oil).

* For fewer wrinkles (especially around the eyes) eat lots of green and yellow veggies. If you eat a steak or a high-fat meal, pair it with spinach, squash, or green beans.

* Talk to your dermatologist *now.* Early action can keep your skin looking young and vibrant without the need for cosmetic procedures.

* Never feel bad about wanting to look your best.

8

Eating for Stronger, Healthier Hair and Nails

People often assume that Asians all have silky, glossy, gorgeous hair. But in its natural state mine is a frizzy, puffy mess that bends in all different directions, and it's especially unruly in humid weather. A few years ago when I was in Miami, it reached such epic proportions—we're talking Kramer hair, people—that my husband, who like many men normally wouldn't even notice if I dyed it pink, turned to me and said, "Uh, what's up with your hair? I don't think you can go back to the office like that." (Charming, isn't he?) But he was right. As soon as we landed in L.A. (thank God for the dry weather on the West Coast), I tamed the beast. I washed it, conditioned it, blow-dried it, and put in about a bottle of smoothing serum.

Despite the natural state of my hair, I learned at an early age that it could be beaten into submission. And over the years it has served as a kind of security blanket: Even if I was a chubby kid or an awkward, pimply-faced teenager, I could still have pretty hair. Which is why, when I was in the eighth grade, I fought with my mother for weeks to get this ridiculous haircut—layered "wings" on the top and long, straight layers on the bottom (proving that it is possible to have two different hairstyles at the same time; you saw the picture). But, hey, it was the era of Farrah Fawcett's feathers, and I was a tiny Asian girl living in Southern California. It was a last-ditch effort to fit in with the carefree surfer girls I'd always envied. (By the way, that totally backfired, but it did instigate a sort of hair obsession.)

When I was an undergrad, I spent time studying French at the Sorbonne in Paris. Although I loved spending afternoons at the Louvre and eating pastries at nearly every meal, I lived in a dark, tiny dorm room, not much larger than my twin mattress. The bathrooms were coed and communal, with no doors on the stalls or showers (how French!), and the hot water was unreliable (the showers were either ice cold or scalding hot). I'd jump in and out as quickly as possible, and I sure as hell wasn't going to wash my hair every day in those conditions. (That turned out to be a good thing since I nearly burned down the building the first time I plugged in my blow-dryer.) Luckily, I figured out how to use my curling iron, and I'd get up an hour early to tame my tresses before class.

The obsession only got worse in medical school. Even though most of my female classmates put their hair up in a ponytail, mine was always styled and sprayed. I'd even tape lecture notes on the walls of my bathroom so I could study for exams while blow-drying (which I *still* think was rather ingenious). And then when I finished my medical training and it was finally time to become a "real doctor," I decided it was also time to get "serious hair." So I chopped if off into a severe, straight, chin-length bob. (I have since burned all the pictures from this period.) Years later, around the time I ditched the white lab coat, I learned to embrace my natural waves. And these days when I get my hair cut, I tell the stylist I'm going for Victoria's Secret hair—full and flowing but still well groomed.

Like your skin, your hair (and nails) are accessories that you wear every day. They're always on display, so it's understandable that our identities are sometimes wrapped up in these visible parts of our anatomy. For example, some people chop off their hair or dye it crazy colors after a bad breakup; others cling to the same style for 20 or 30 years. And how many times have you seen an angst-ridden teen with jet-black nails or a woman sporting long acrylics decorated with decals and tiny rhinestones? But while the style of your hair and the state of your manicure can be reflections of your personality, the overall *condition* of your hair and nails says much more about you than what's in vogue at any given time. More than mere accessories, they're a barometer of how well you're feeding your body as well as an indication of your overall health.

Lots of people ask their hairstylists or manicurists for advice when they notice a problem with their hair, scalp, or nails. After all, you might get your nails done every week (or your hair trimmed every few months), whereas you may not see a doctor more than once or twice a year. Hairstylists and nail technicians certainly do have expertise in grooming and styling (and many of us couldn't live without them), but they work on your hair and nails *after* they've grown out of the skin. As a dermatologist I know that certain dietary deficiencies or imbalances can affect the health of your hair and nails *before* they grow out, and I can tell you which foods you need to eat to help them grow strong, shiny, and healthy. We'll get to the foods that can strengthen and protect your nails in a bit, but for now let's concentrate on your hair.

Hair: The Stuff on Your Head

If you're not eating the right foods, your hair can get dull, dry, and thin. In fact, thinning hair is one of the most distressing problems my patients ask me about. But before we can talk about how and what to feed your hair, we first need to understand what hair is and how it grows.

Why Do We Have Hair?

Great hair may be what separates mere mortals from perfectly coifed goddesses like Jennifer Aniston, but how the hair looks is really secondary to what it *does*. There are a number of biological reasons for having hair, including:

Insulation. The hair on our bodies, particularly on the scalp, helps trap heat and regulates body temperature.

Sensation. Since the hairs are attached to nerve endings, they can help with your sense of touch.

Sexual signaling. At puberty a rise in androgens (the male sex hormones) triggers the growth of armpit and pubic hair (and men, of course, develop facial and chest hair). Aside from protecting the delicate skin of the genitals, scientists believe that this "androgenic" hair is used to send signals about our sexual status and sexual maturity—to identify a woman as being fertile, for example. The relatively large amount of hair in the armpits and pubic region also provides a large surface area for sweat to evaporate and disperse pheromones, the natural odors our bodies secrete that may play a role in mating. In pop culture, pheromones are thought to serve as a kind of aphrodisiac, though that hasn't actually been scientifically proven. But as any woman who has ever lived with female roommates knows, it's common for our menstrual cycles to "sync up" over time. This is most likely due to how our bodies perceive these odors.

Display and identity. Close your eyes and imagine any kind of distinct social group—ballerinas, Rastafarians, punk rockers, or military men—and I bet you could also come up with a corresponding hairdo (such as buns, dreads, Mohawks, and buzz cuts). You see, it's not uncommon for members of the same group to have the same hairstyle—we use our hair to identify as members of the same social class or to stand out in a crowd. It's a part of who we are.

What Is Hair, Anyway?

You can think of your hair as a green onion: You might eat only the green stalk, the part that grows aboveground (likewise, you might only *care* about the strands that grow out of your head), but there's a lot going on below the surface.

Deep inside your skin (all the way down in the subcutaneous tissue or the "fat layer" of the skin) are little hair-making machines called hair *follicles*. These follicles are surrounded by blood vessels that bathe them in nutrients and help them produce keratin. Eventually, all that keratin gets pushed out of the follicle and out through an opening in the scalp, forming a strand of hair.

Your individual strands of hair are made of many, many layers of keratin stacked on top of one another, a bit like shingles on a roof or scales on a fish. The outermost layer is called the hair cuticle. When your hair is healthy and undamaged, the cuticle is smooth, shiny, and strong because the keratin layers lie flat against each other. But when the hair becomes damaged (from chemical processing or heat styling, for example), the cuticle gets ragged and peels away from the underlying keratin layers. When that happens, the individual hairs can't lie flat against each other, so your hair becomes frizzy and flyaway.

Why Is My Hair Curly, but My Sister's Hair Is Stick-Straight?

The shape and texture of your hair depend on the size and shape of your hair follicles. In that sense, the follicles are kind of like mini pasta makers: Different shapes make different kinds of pasta, from fettuccine to linguini to angel hair. Similarly, large, wide follicles make thick hair, while smaller follicles produce thinner, finer hair. If the opening of the follicle is round, the hair growing out of it will be straight like spaghetti (and round in cross-section). If the opening of the follicle is oval, the hair will be wavy (oval in cross-section). And if the follicle is flat (like linguine), the hair will be kinky or curly (flat in cross-section).

The shape of your hair follicles is determined by a number of factors, including genetics, hormones, and other chemical changes in your body, which means that the shape of the follicles—and therefore the texture of your hair—can change over time, at certain stages of your life (such as during puberty or pregnancy), as well as when taking certain medications (particularly chemotherapy drugs). In general, though, the shape of the follicle is fixed, as is the hair that comes out of it. The shape of the hair is held in place by very strong sulfur bonds, which can only be broken by chemical perms or relaxing solutions. The individual strands, however, also contain weaker hydrogen bonds that can temporarily be broken with heat. That's how blow-dryers, flat irons, and curling irons work: They break the hydrogen bonds, which then reform as soon as the hair gets wet.

$E = mc^2$ **Did You Know . . .**

The hair follicles contain two types of melanin pigment: a darker, brown-black pigment called *eumelanin,* and a lighter, reddish pigment called *pheomelanin.* Brunettes have much more eumelanin, while redheads have more pheomelanin. Blondes have small amounts of both pigments. Gray hair has only a small amount of pigment, and white hair has none at all.

The Many Ways Your Hair Changes Over Time

On average, people have about 100,000 hair follicles on their head. Not all of the follicles are actively growing hair at the same time, however. Your hair actually grows in cycles. Follicles typically remain active for several years; then the hair falls out, and the follicle "rests" for a while. Later, the follicle resumes growing hair.

At any given time you have a number of hairs that are ready to fall out and go into the resting stage. In fact, the normal range of hair loss is somewhere between 50 and 100 hairs a day. If you don't shampoo or brush every day, these loose hairs can accumulate, so you may lose more the next time you get around to taking a shower. (Don't worry if you see more hairs in the drain than normal; you're not actually going bald.)

Even though we all have about the same number of hair follicles, people can have fine or thick hair depending on how fine or coarse each individual strand is as well as how many hair follicles are actually active. Over time, the number of follicles that are actively producing hair decreases. (Men are at a real disadvantage here: By the time they hit 50, they may have only 250 to 300 active hair follicles.) This is why most of us notice that our hair gets thinner as we get older.

Hormones also play a major role in hair growth. Female hormones (estrogens) increase the growing phase in the hair cycle: The hair grows longer before the follicle goes into its resting phase. This is why many woman notice that their hair and nails seem to grow faster during pregnancy, when there's a surge in estrogen. It's also why thinning hair is a common concern during menopause (when the estrogen in our bodies starts to decline) as well as during other major hormonal changes, such as after a hysterectomy. On the other hand, the hair of the scalp is particularly sensitive to the effects of male hormones (androgens), which are present in both men and women but in different proportions. Androgens cause thinning of the hair and shrinkage of the follicles, which is why some men go bald, but, typically, women do not. Thyroid conditions can also affect hair growth all over the body: An overactive thyroid triggers more and faster hair growth, while a sluggish thyroid can cause thinning hair or hair loss. In fact, a telltale sign of low thyroid activity is thinning or loss of the outer half of the eyebrows.

MINOXIDIL, THE TOPICAL TREATMENT FOR THINNING HAIR

Minoxidil is a topical ingredient that grows scalp hair, and it's the only approved treatment for hair loss in women. (Men also have a prescription pill called Propecia, which blocks the effect of testosterone on the hair follicles, but it hasn't been shown to work for us ladies.)

Minoxidil, which is the active ingredient in brand name Regaine as well as in several generic products, is a liquid that you put on your scalp twice a day to stimulate hair growth.* (This can take 4 months or longer, so you'll have to be patient.) It's thought to work by increasing the hair's growth phase (or postponing the resting phase). Although it's available in two strengths (2 percent and 5 percent), I usually recommend the 5 percent solution since it's more effective in many patients. However, this stronger formula can sometimes trigger facial hair growth in women (which is reversible if you stop using it, so don't freak out, OK?). Some women who have hair follicles that are very sensitive to minoxidil may respond well to the weaker formula. Other side effects include scalp itching and irritation, and if you stop using it, the hair will eventually thin out again as if you'd never used it in the first place. Don't worry, though, it won't *all* fall out!

*Regaine cannot be prescribed by the NHS, so patients must either buy it over-the-counter or have a private prescription for it.

Aside from the normal thinning we see over time, certain health conditions (including thyroid disease and iron-deficiency anemia) and medications can also cause hair loss. Additionally, any extreme change in your health, like a severe illness, hospitalization, or surgery requiring general anesthesia, as well as significant emotional or psychological stress, can lead to *sudden* hair loss. This condition, called telogen effluvium, causes the hair follicles to suddenly shut down and go into their resting phase, as if your body had shut down all nonessential functions and preserved its energy to fight the particular stress or illness. The good news is that when you recover from your illness, the hair will grow back, although there can be a lag time of three to four months before you start to see new growth.

Nutrition plays a major role in the look and feel of your hair. If you don't feed your body the right nutrients (if you dine on, say, Oreos rather than fruits and veggies), the hair will begin to grow finer and lighter in color. Additionally, the cuticle will fray more easily and lift up, so the hair becomes rough in texture instead of silky smooth, and more prone to split ends. If you fully deprive your body of the nutrients it needs, your body will stop producing hair altogether in order to preserve its energy for more important functions, such as pumping blood and making brain cells. In extreme cases of poor diet or malnutrition, the hair can even fall out. In the office I see this in patients who have anemia (especially iron-deficiency anemia), those with eating disorders or who are crash dieters, and people who just have a really poor diet in general (like those who subsist on Cheerios and martinis—you know who you are!).

If you notice sudden severe hair loss, if your hair continues to fall out despite your best efforts to eat well, or if you notice areas of complete baldness (which can be a sign of an autoimmune condition called alopecia areata), make an appointment with a dermatologist. She can examine your scalp and perform further testing to rule out an underlying internal cause of hair loss.

What to Eat for Bouncy, Beautiful Hair

Although the hair that grows out of your head is dead, the living part of the hair—the follicle—is very much alive. If you're not eating a balanced diet (and therefore supplying the follicles with the nutrients they need), your hair will pay the price. While there are products that can help with limp, unruly hair as well as hair loss, adding the following foods to your diet can help you regain a more youthful, damage-free 'do.

For Stronger Hair . . .

Eat foods that are high in cysteine. Most proteins are made of many different amino acids. Keratin is unique, however, in that it's made largely of one amino acid in particular: cysteine. Cysteine molecules are linked together in a strong bond called a disulfide bond, which gives your hair its strength. So by eating cysteine, you can help make your hair stronger.

You can find large amounts of cysteine in the following foods:

pork	red peppers	Brussels sprouts	dairy products
poultry	garlic	oats	broccoli
egg yolks	onions	wheat germ	

$E=mc^2$ *Did You Know . . .*

Some people think cysteine might be a hangover remedy since it helps break down acetaldehyde, a by-product of alcohol metabolism. This may be the reason raw egg yolks are part of common hangover "cures." Unfortunately, scientists haven't gotten around to *proving* this one yet. (Hurry up!)

Eat Silicon. Silicon, a naturally occurring element that's found in the earth, has been shown to be essential for healthy bone formation. (That's silicon, not *silicone,* the stuff in breast implants and bad lip jobs.) Research shows us that people who take silicon supplements have stronger bone density and less osteoporosis as well as stronger nails and hair. In one study in particular, volunteers who took a silicon supplement had significantly stronger hair and nails after 20 weeks.

Although you can find silicon in a variety of foods, people who eat a diet rich in whole grains and cereals have higher silicon intakes than those who eat more dairy and animal products. In fact, studies have shown that those who eat a traditional Asian or Indian diet (which emphasizes grains and less dairy) have higher silicon intakes than Western populations. (Isn't it interesting, then, that Asians and Indians also have thicker hair and fewer hip fractures?)

While the EU has not established guideline daily amounts (GDAs) of silicon, studies show that 10mg/day is enough to help strengthen the hair and nails. The best sources of dietary silicon include the following:

• Green beans (one of the richest sources of silicon as well as one of the lowest calorie foods; if you can, choose organic green beans, which retain more silicon from the soil)

- Whole grains and cereals (oats, barley, brown rice)
- Spinach
- Lentils
- Mineral water (especially from volcanic areas; try Volvic, which contains 14.5mg/liter)
- Coffee (made with mineral water)
- Perrier mineral water (5mg/liter)
- Beer (one of the reasons that men often have higher silicon intake than women)

FYI: Bananas have a high concentration of silicon, but only a very small fraction is absorbed into the GI tract (and therefore by your hair and nails).

FROM THE (CELEBRITY) FILES OF *Dr. Wu*

Patient: Nicole Sullivan—Actress, Comedienne
(*Rita Rocks, MADtv, The King of Queens*)
Skin Concern: Cystic acne

In Nicole's Words: I really wanted to lose weight before my wedding [to actor Jason Packham in 2006], so I tried all kinds of crazy diets—cleanses, fasts, no carb, low carb. You name it, I tried it. Sometimes I'd break down and have a slice of pizza for lunch, but then I wouldn't eat again for the rest of the day, just so I could lose the weight. Several months went by when I didn't so much as look at a vegetable (because veggies, of course, have carbs). The thing is that all those crazy diets really messed up my face. I'd always had pretty decent skin, so when I started getting cystic acne, I was crushed. It wasn't until after the wedding, when I started eating like a normal person again, that I was able to get my skin back under control.

A few months after I gave birth to my second child (in August 2009), I was ready to slim down again. But this time I wanted to do it right, so I signed up to be a spokesperson for Jenny Craig. I liked the program (I lost 15kg in 4 months!), and I learned some tricks: 28g of meat is the size of a tube of lipstick, 85g is the size of your palm. Now I'm on the "maintenance" plan.

As a mom your kids are your number-one priority, but priority number two needs to be yourself. I don't touch the stuff my kids sometimes snack on, like graham crackers and macaroni cheese—but we eat dinner together as a family, and I make a healthy meal. I've also given myself permission to go out and buy *good* food (like organic meats and produce) even if it's a little more expensive. My favorite snacks are raw almonds and green beans. (I eat them just about every day.) And before I go on camera, I drink double the amount of water.

Dr. Wu's Diagnosis: One of the reasons Nicole has such beautiful blond hair could be that she eats so many green beans, which are one of the richest dietary sources of silicon, a natural element that gives you shinier, healthier tresses. (Find out how she gives green beans a kick of flavor on page 242) It's great that she snacks on almonds, which are a good source of protein and may help keep the grays away. And now that she's eating more sensibly, her acne has calmed down and her skin looks clearer. It's also good that she's willing to buy the best-quality food she can afford (especially since organic green beans have more silicon than nonorganic). The sad truth is that cheaper food is often less healthy. If your food budget is already tight, I'll give you some tips in Chapter 9 for getting fresher food without breaking the bank.

For Thicker Hair . . .

Eat iron and zinc. Since red meat is such an excellent source of both zinc and iron, it's not uncommon for vegetarians (or people who eat disproportionately large amounts of legumes and whole grains) to have low levels of these important minerals in their bodies. In fact, such foods as unfermented soy (soy milk, tofu), brown rice, corn, and wheat bran contain a compound called phytate, which interferes with your body's ability to absorb iron and zinc into the bloodstream, further depleting mineral reserves. So what does that have to do with your 'do? Low levels of iron and zinc have been linked to thinning hair, especially in women.

Zinc is essential for producing keratin (the basic component of hair), so people with low levels of zinc may produce finer, sparser hair (read "weak hair") or even begin to lose their hair altogether. Meanwhile, anemia from iron deficiency is one of the most common causes of thinning hair in otherwise

STYLING TRICKS FOR HAIR LOSS SUFFERERS

air loss is a common problem, and not just among men. Many of my female patients are concerned about thinning hair, too. In some people the condition is hereditary, but in others it can be the result of a hormonal imbalance, nutritional deficiency, illness, severe stress, or a side effect of certain medications.

Unfortunately, there's no miracle cure for hair loss. The best thing you can do is practice good grooming and learn how to make the most of the hair you have. If your locks are a little thinner than they used to be, try these tricks:

Get the right hairstyle. A straight-across-the-bottom cut can actually make your hair hang heavy, so it looks thin and straggly. Be sure to trim split ends regularly and have your stylist layer your hair for added volume.

Avoid tight ponytails and headbands. Hair accessories that constantly tug on your hair can end up pulling it out at the roots.

Limit heat styling. Blow-drying can literally boil the water in your hair, causing "bubbles" to form inside the hair. This weakens your hair and makes it break easily. To minimize hair breakage, gently towel-dry first and then use the lowest setting on your hair dryer that still gets the job done. And since coloring and chemical processing can also weaken the hair, stretch out your salon appointments as much as possible.

Use styling products sparingly. Gels, mousses, and leave-in conditioners coat the individual strands, which *can* make your hair appear thicker. But use too much, and the goop will make your hair fall flat. Experiment to see which products you can do without (maybe stick with the mousse but toss the smoothing cream, for example) or switch to lighter formulas, such as an aerosol over a liquid pump hairspray. Personally, I couldn't live without my Bumble & Bumble Classic Hairspray.

healthy adult women. Additionally, women with hereditary hair loss (androgenetic alopecia), as well as alopecia areata (an autoimmune condition that attacks the hair follicles), have significantly lower levels of iron in their blood compared to those without hair loss.

It's estimated that 25 percent of premenopausal women (meaning women who are still menstruating, not women entering perimenopause) are iron deficient. For healthier, thicker hair, increase the amount of iron and zinc in your diet by making lean red meat (like beef or lamb) your main course as often as twice a week and incorporating other zinc- or iron-rich foods (such as lentils, kidney beans, raw oysters, pork, turkey, and spinach) in your diet, too. (If you're a vegan or vegetarian, you can get plenty of zinc and iron from the plant sources listed above, as well as from zinc- and iron-fortified foods, such as enriched cereals and pastas.) For maximum mineral absorption try to avoid eating foods that are high in iron or zinc alongside foods containing phytate (like rice and corn). And avoid zinc supplements—*excessive* zinc intake can actually be toxic; if you're eating zinc-rich foods, you won't need help from a pill.

Avoid fish with high levels of mercury. Fish is an important part of the *Feed Your Face* Diet because it's a good source of protein and omega-3 fatty acids, and it's naturally low in saturated fat. Some fish, however, contain high levels of mercury, which can accumulate in the bloodstream and, in high enough concentrations, can actually lead to mercury poisoning. Aside from being hazardous to your health (in *extreme* cases mercury poisoning can actually be fatal), too much mercury can lead to hair loss.

Although mercury poisoning is rare, I do see it from time to time. Some of the trendiest restaurants in L.A. are sushi bars; in fact, there are eight sushi restaurants within a mile of my office. While sushi and sashimi are great sources of protein for those who are watching their waistlines (or who need to look thin on camera), over the last few years I've discovered that it's not uncommon to meet people who eat it as often as five or six times a week. And there *is* such a thing as too much. So whenever a patient comes to the office complaining of thinning hair, I ask about her diet—in particular how much and what type of fish she eats.

Since mercury accumulates in the tissue of fish over time, large species that are higher in the food chain naturally contain higher levels of mercury. To reduce your risk of mercury poisoning (and thinning hair or hair loss), avoid eating these larger fish, including swordfish, shark, and King mackerel.

If you're a tuna fan, limit your intake of albacore, ahi (yellowfin), and hamachi (yellowtail) to no more than once a week. These are all larger species of tuna (and likely to have higher levels of mercury) and are commonly served in restaurants as sushi (raw fish and rice), sashimi (slices of raw fish), as well as steaks or fillets. (Albacore is also found in canned tuna, where it's labeled "solid white.") "Light" tuna comes from a smaller species and therefore has less mercury; it can be eaten up to twice a week. Low-mercury seafood, including salmon, catfish, shrimp, clams, scallops, squid, eel, octopus, and sea urchin, can be enjoyed more often.

If you have thinning hair *and* you eat a lot of fish (more than once or twice a week, especially tuna or other large fish), ask your doctor if you should be tested for mercury. A blood test can indicate acute exposure, while a hair test is better suited to detect chronic mercury exposure. (Your hair contains a high concentration of sulfur, which binds with mercury over time.)

Exposure to other heavy metals—including lead (from water traveling through old lead pipes) and arsenic (from well water in areas with high levels of arsenic in the soil)—has also been linked to hair loss, but it's much less common than mercury poisoning.

Hey, Dr. Wu

Q: When I was in college, I wanted super skinny eyebrows, just like a Vargas pinup girl. But the fashion fetish led me to overpluck, and now they won't grow back. What can I do to get back my thick natural brows?

A: Sometimes you have to be careful what you wish for—the damage to your eyebrows could be permanent. Repeated plucking can inflame the hair follicles, causing them to grow finer, shorter hairs than usual. Over time, the hair follicles become scarred and eventually stop sprouting hairs altogether. There is a chance you can get your brows back, but it'll take some dedication.

Hide your tweezers and let your eyebrows grow in even if they're sparse and uneven for a while. This helps allow the follicle to heal. When you do start plucking again, choose tweezers that don't break off your hairs (I like Tweezerman) and only tweeze stray hairs below—not above—your natural arch.

If you've lost so many hairs that you don't know what your natural brow shape is, try using an eyebrow stencil. Hold the stencil up to your brow and fill in with short strokes of an eyebrow pencil. For a soft, natural look, choose a pencil color that's a little lighter than your hair.

Beware of tattooed eyebrows! Permanent makeup tattoos might be tempting, but my mother got them several years ago, and now her brows are purple. That's right, *purple*. Tattoo ink (even on your face) can fade and change color over time.

To Prevent Gray Hair . . .

Eat almonds. When I was in medical school, we were taught that our hair turns gray because the hair follicles eventually stop producing melanin, the pigment that gives hair its color (as well as our skin its tan). But new research shows that that's not entirely true: Our hair follicles don't stop producing pigment once you reach a certain age. They do, however, lose their ability to *keep* the pigment they make. Here's why:

Everybody knows that the fastest way to go from mousy brunette to white-hot blond is to bleach your hair with hydrogen peroxide. Well, it turns out that our hair follicles actually make their own peroxide. When you're young, the hair follicles also produce a large amount of an enzyme called catalase, which neutralizes this "natural" peroxide as soon as it accumulates. But as time goes by, our bodies make less and less catalase, so this balance is disrupted. As a result, peroxide builds up, leaving us with an ever-increasing amount of grays. What's worse, once that balance shifts, the peroxide that builds up actually inhibits your body's ability to make more catalase, so it becomes a vicious cycle: Once you start seeing your first grays, the process speeds up, and you get even more. You know that old wives' tale that plucking one gray hair leads to two growing in its place? While it's not actually true (one hair follicle can't multiply and start producing two hairs), it is common to start seeing more and more gray hairs because of this snowball effect. Scientists have also found that this spiral starts before you even see the signs of aging (meaning before you actually see your first gray hair).

At the moment, researchers are busy searching for ways to prevent gray hair (i.e., to stop the bleaching process before it starts). If they can discover a way to restart your scalp's ability to make catalase again, it would even be possible for people who have already turned gray to revert to their natural darker color. Until then, one way to prevent grays *may* be to eat foods that will boost your body's ability to generate its own catalase.

Almonds are one food that has been shown to increase the levels of catalase in the body. In a Chinese study, men added 84g (3 ounces) of almonds per day to their diet. After four weeks there was nearly 10 percent more catalase in their bloodstreams compared to those who didn't eat the almonds. This particular study included male smokers, so more research needs to be done to confirm that the results would be the same in women and nonsmokers. I can assure you, however, that I eat almonds almost every day since I'm getting tired of plucking my gray hairs.

While you can eat almonds any time of the day (because you can easily carry them around in your purse or pocket), some brands are heavily salted, so choose dry-roasted, unsalted nuts. Avoid smokehouse or honey-roasted flavors, which tend to be high in salt, sugar, and artificial flavors. I also like to use almonds in different ways:

- Toss whole or sliced almonds into a veggie stir-fry or side dish (like green beans)
- Sprinkle sliced almonds on a salad
- Stir chopped almonds into oatmeal
- Make homemade trail mix with roasted almonds and dried cherries or cranberries

Eat fruits and veggies. Hydrogen peroxide (which is produced in the hair follicles and is responsible for "bleaching" our hairs gray) is actually a type of free radical—that means it's a by-product of the body's natural metabolism as well as a product of such environmental stress as UV rays, secondhand smoke, and pollution. And new studies show that the hair follicles in particular generate a high level of free radicals, which damage the melanocytes (the pigment-producing cells) as well as the stem cells that maintain the melanocytes. So in the simplest possible terms, gray hair is caused by free radicals. And how do you fight free radicals? Eat more antioxidants. For the biggest boost choose brightly colored fruits and vegetables, especially berries, tomatoes, asparagus, spinach, squash, and peppers.

Stop smoking. Smoking cuts circulation to the hair follicles, so they don't get the oxygen and nutrients they need to make healthy hair. Cigarette smoke also triggers inflammation and scar tissue formation in the hair follicle, which interferes with hair growth. This is one reason why smokers have a particularly tough time healing after hair transplant surgery. Studies have also shown that men who smoke more than ten cigarettes (or half a pack) a week are nearly twice as likely to go bald as nonsmokers.

For an Itchy, Dry Scalp or Dandruff . . .

Eat yogurt. I've often noticed that people with itchy, flaky scalps are reluctant to wash their hair for fear of aggravating "dry" scalp. A flaky scalp, however, isn't typically caused by lack of oil or moisture but rather an overgrowth of yeast.

At any given time there's a small amount of yeast that lives on your scalp and feeds on dead skin cells and oil. Normally your skin's "good" bacteria keep this yeast in check. Hormonal fluctuations, stress, overactive oil glands, and spikes in blood sugar, however, can all trigger an overgrowth of yeast, leading to flaking, itching, and red patches—all signs of a common condition known as seborrheic dermatitis, or dandruff (which you can read more about in Chapter 5). Since the yeast is concentrated in hairy areas of the body (the scalp, eyebrows, behind the ears, and, on men, in the center of the chest), it's not uncommon for someone with dandruff to also have flaking on the eyebrows or behind the ears. And because yeast feeds on oil, it's actually a good idea to wash your hair daily if you're dealing with dandruff. This will help remove excess oil and dead skin as well as control the growth of yeast.

For additional relief from dandruff and flaking, new research suggests that taking an oral probiotic may help. Probiotics are dietary supplements that contain live organisms (like the "good" bacteria found in yogurt) that help your body maintain its balance of "good" and "bad" organisms. They're typically used to treat an overgrowth of yeast (as in women who are susceptible to vaginal yeast infections). But since many cases of dandruff are also associated with yeast, yogurt could help an itchy scalp, too.

In a recent French study, men with dandruff took powdered probiotics (in this case a type of bacteria called *Lactobacillus paracasei*) every day for several months. Within 4 weeks the volunteers had noticeably less dandruff.

After 2 months nearly two-thirds reported good improvement or total healing of their symptoms, including flaking, itching, redness, and greasiness. The volunteers also had significantly less dandruff-causing yeast on their scalps.

While more research is needed to determine the ideal dose and exact type of probiotic that will treat dandruff most effectively (the effects also need to be studied in women), I encourage my patients with dandruff to supplement their diets with yogurt or probiotics. Just stick with low-sugar, low-fat brands and avoid fruit-on-the-bottom yogurt, which is packed with added sugars and sometimes high-fructose corn syrup.

Eat more snacks. This isn't the first time we've discussed the benefits of eating every few hours (and it probably won't be the last), but maintaining a steady blood sugar with face-friendly snacks is particularly important for people struggling with dandruff since yeast tends to grow out of control when your blood sugar gets too high. For steady blood sugar (and less yeast) choose foods that are low on the glycemic index, and pair your carbohydrates with proteins and healthy fats to further slow the absorption of sugar into the body. (If you pair a whole wheat bagel with peanut butter, for example, the resulting blood sugar spike will be less dramatic than if you eat the bagel by itself.)

Hey, Dr. Wu

Q: Look, no one told me my pubic hair was going to turn gray. I'm not even married yet. How can I get serious with anybody when my hoo-ha makes me look like a grandma?

A: There are lots of annoying things about getting older, but going gray "down there" has to be one of the worst. You do have options, though. Here are a few ways to make sure the carpet matches the drapes no matter what your age.

Color it. Believe it or not, there's a specially formulated, nonirritating dye especially for use in the pubic area. The dyes from BettyBeauty don't contain ammonia or parabens (a type of chemical preservative commonly used in hair products and cosmetics), and they're not tested on animals, so you can finally become a "true blonde" without fear. Choose from "natural" colors like blond, brown, or auburn, or "fun" colors like hot pink. But if you're looking for a more dramatic change—going from black to, say, platinum—consider getting it done professionally. Some salons actually specialize in bikini waxing and dyeing.

Camouflage it. If you're looking for a more low-maintenance alternative to dyeing, you can temporarily cover gray pubic hair with a touch-up pen or even mascara. Just remember that the skin in your pubic region is thinner and more delicate than the skin on your scalp, so avoid products that contain peroxide, and try not to get the color on your skin. You should also avoid coloring right after you wax or shave, when the skin is most sensitive. And color only the pubic hair that's visible when your legs are closed—not the hair that grows on your labia.

Coif it. If coloring or camouflaging gray pubic hair isn't your style, you can always use electric hair clippers to trim the hair short enough to make the grays less noticeable. You may also consider waxing your entire bikini area (known as the Brazilian) or having your pubic hair removed with laser treatments or electrolysis.

Regardless of the method you choose, I recommend doing a patch test (or, in this case, perhaps a strand test) before any big event—like a romantic getaway with a new man.

Taking Care of the Hair You Have

Now that you know what to eat to promote healthy hair *growth,* it's important to discuss how to care for the hair you have now (so you can make bad hair days a thing of the past).

Imagine a brand-new leather handbag—soft and buttery, chic and stylish. But leave it out in the sun, carry it in the rain, or drag it around town for too long, and pretty soon it looks beat-up. The same goes for your hair. Although hair is technically "dead" (which is a good thing; otherwise, haircuts would be pretty excruciating), it can look healthy, lustrous, and bouncy if you take care of it. On the other hand, if you don't protect it from such environmental stress as UV rays and chlorine, or you abuse it by overdoing the brushing, blow-drying, coloring, and processing, it will look dull, damaged, and dry.

The first step to hair care is pretty basic: It's knowing how and when to wash it, and when to give your hair a break. As with skin care, everyone's hair routine may be a little different depending on the kind of hair you have, whether you process it, and how you style it. Here are some common hair conditions and how to make your hair look its best:

Greasy hair. The hairs on our head are lubricated by sebum (the same oil that lubricates our skin). The oil travels down the hair shaft to lubricate your hair and keep it soft, shiny, and healthy looking. Oil doesn't flow as easily down the hair shaft, however, if it's very kinky or curly, which is one reason that curly hair tends to be more dry and fragile than straight or fine hair. How much oil your glands produce is mostly determined by heredity, but just as your skin can get oilier during puberty (which is one reason teenagers struggle so much with acne), your hair can become oilier during similar hormonal shifts (like the week before your period).

Greasy hair is caused by a buildup of your skin's natural oils; the more oil you have, the greasier your hair. Additionally, if you use a lot of product in your hair (like gel or mousse) and don't wash it out thoroughly, your scalp oils combine with the product residue and weigh your hair down even more. That's why washing your hair regularly is so important: It removes the buildup of dirt, natural scalp oils, and hair care products, not to mention pollution, secondhand smoke, and anything else that may have fallen onto your hair during the course of the day. Yet many stylists recommend not washing your hair daily since shampoo can also strip the hair of its natural oils too much. So what's a girl to do?

You'll want to strike a balance between overwashing and looking like you've got an oil slick on your head. People with naturally oily hair should consider washing it at least every other day. The same goes for those who notice that their hair gets oilier when they're PMSing or when they're taking certain hormones (which can both cause increases in your body's oil production). Likewise, people who use lots of hair products every day are more likely to have product buildup, and they tend to accumulate a larger amount of dirt, dust, and pollution (which can stick to the product). They should also wash every day. People with dry hair, on the other hand, should wash less often. They should also look for shampoos specially formulated for dry or damaged hair, which strip less of the hair's natural oils. (Try Garnier Fructis Fortifying Shampoo.) Since curly or coarse hair is more likely to be dry, people with very wavy hair may have to shampoo only once or twice a week.

$E = mc^2$ *Did You Know . . .*

Have you ever heard that rotating among several different brands of shampoo can keep your hair from falling flat (or that you shouldn't stick with the same brand for too long because your hair will just "get used to it")? It's true that sometimes your shampoo can "stop working" and may not clean as well as when you first started to use it. This is because it leaves behind a residue that can build up and make your hair look dull and limp. Changing brands can help remove that residue, so your hair will regain its bounce and shine.

Dry hair. Like dry skin, dry hair doesn't have enough moisture—either because the scalp isn't producing enough oil or because the hair itself has been damaged, so water evaporates quickly, leaving the hair brittle. Since long hair has been around longer and therefore has had more exposure to UV rays, shampoo buildup, and heat-styling and processing, it's more likely than short hair to be dry and to feel coarse. Dry hair can also be difficult to style.

Conditioners are basically like moisturizers for the hair—they make dry hair softer, smoother, and more manageable. For the best results look for these ingredients:

• Panthenol, a form of vitamin B_5 that helps moisturize as well as makes the individual strands thicker and fuller, so your hair is more flexible and less prone to frizzies and flyaways.

- Dimethicone, which coats and seals the keratin layers so the hair is smoother and shinier. Dimethicone also helps detangle hair, so not only will it be easier to brush, but you'll also have less breakage from tangles and knots.
- Natural oils, like almond and coconut oil, which help coat and seal the strands and supplement your scalp's own natural oil, increasing hair flexibility.
- Wheat and rice proteins. Think about the old-school magnets you used to play with as a kid, when you learned that opposites attract and like charges repel. (Remember?) Your hair is kind of like a magnet, too. In damaged hair the keratin layers have negative charges, so the individual strands repel each other, making the hair flyaway and unmanageable. Wheat and rice proteins, however, have large positive charges that are attracted to the negative charges in the hair. They coat the hair and help it lie flat. Additionally, the proteins concentrate in the most damaged parts of the hair, making it stronger and smoother.

Overprocessed hair. Chemical hair processing works by opening the hair cuticle (the outermost layer of keratin), allowing the chemicals to get into the hair and react with the proteins, either to straighten your hair or make it curly, depending on what you're going for. After treatment, the cuticle closes again, so the keratin layers lie flat against each other and your hair looks shiny and healthy. Repeated processing (as well as excessive heat styling and exposure to UV rays), however, can damage the hair. The keratin layers don't reseal and the hair develops tiny holes, allowing water to evaporate more easily and leaving the hair very dry, fragile, and frizzy. It's a vicious cycle: The more porous the hair gets, the more water enters when it's washed, and the more water evaporates when it dries. Eventually overprocessed hair will break off.

The best treatment for overprocessed hair is pretty obvious: Cut back on the processing. It may be hard to quit cold turkey, but you can at least reduce the amount of processing; for example, if you color your hair *and* chemically perm or straighten it, choose one or the other but not both, at least until the damaged part grows out. Minimize the amount of heat styling and ask your hairstylist to give you a cut that will make the most of your hair as it's growing out. And since repeated washing and drying can make things worse, try not to shampoo more than once every other day.

PROTECTING YOUR HAIR AT THE POOL OR BEACH

*Y*ou know that you have to protect your skin with sunscreen, but UV rays can do a number on your hair, too. In fact, a recent study showed that exposure to ultraviolet light actually slows hair growth. The sun's UVA and UVB rays also break down hair proteins (as well as damage the color), making your hair look dull and brittle. The next time you're headed outdoors or taking a dip in the pool, protect your hair with these tips:

- Use a leave-in product with UV filters to protect your hair color. I like Aveda Sun Care Protective Hair Veil, which protects against UVA *and* UVB rays.
- Rinse your hair with tap water *before* getting in the pool. Nonchlorinated (i.e., tap) water binds to your hair, making it less likely to absorb copper from pool water. It's the copper—not the chlorine—that turns your hair green.
- After swimming, rinse and shampoo as soon as possible. Boots Sun, Swim & Gym Shampoo helps remove chlorine and copper deposits from the hair.
- Apply a deep conditioner or hair mask once a week to restore moisture to damaged hair. Try Toni & Guy Nourish Reconstruction Mask.

Choosing the Right Hair Care: Which Products Really Work?

I normally get my hair cut every 2 months at a relatively inexpensive salon located not far from my office, so I can run in after work. But every now and then, for a big event, I'll book an appointment at one of the really fancy celebrity spots in Beverly Hills—the kind of place where you might find paparazzi camped outside the entrance (even on an otherwise uneventful Wednesday afternoon). Not long ago I decided to splurge and scheduled a blowdry at just such a place. When the woman washing my hair asked if I wanted a Kérastase "mask" to make my hair shinier, I said sure (because I figured she was merely offering me a choice in conditioners). Little did

I know that that 5-minute treatment added 60 dollars to the bill. (My hair *did* feel softer and shinier, but not $60 worth.)

When it comes to hair care, the difference between chemist and salon- or professional-grade products is not nearly as dramatic as the difference between, say, on-the-shelf and prescription-strength skin care. High-end and low-end hair care products often contain the same ingredients. In fact, many companies make lines of inexpensive products in addition to their more expensive professional brands. L'Oreal, for example, makes Elvive shampoo and conditioner, sold in chemists, professional products, *and* the more expensive Kérastase range. But you know what? Kérastase dandruff shampoo contains zinc pyrithione, the same active ingredient found in Head & Shoulders.

What you pay for with salon products is the formula (professional products often have a nicer smell and a more luxurious lather) as well as the packaging. Salon products tend to look nicer on your countertop than store brands (and it might be less embarrassing to keep Kérastase in your shower than Head & Shoulders, especially if you've got a new man spending the night). Also, larger companies can invest in extensive research and product testing, an undertaking that a smaller company might not have the funding to support. I would know—I served as a consultant for the Aveeno Nourish Plus hair care line, so I've seen firsthand how much work it takes to make sure a shampoo gives you a consistent, creamy lather, rinses out well, and leaves your hair soft, smooth, and easy to style.

There's a whole science behind the formulation of hair care products, and the Aveeno lab in New Jersey is absolutely *huge*—they even have a whole section devoted just to lather. (Who knew?) For days during product development, scientists watched as a giant device mixed water and shampoo round and round. Then they measured the size of the bubbles, the thickness of the lather, and how long the lather lasted (so you don't have to keep adding more product mid-shampoo). They tested the products on lengths of human hair. And finally, in an actual hair salon located right inside the laboratory, they gave the products to stylists to try out on volunteers. *So* much work. But, hey, our hair is worth it!

At some point in the testing phase I gave some hairstylist friends of

SHOULD I BE AFRAID OF SULFATES?

*M*ost shampoos contain sulfates, which break up grease and produce a rich lather when mixed with water. (One of the most common ones is sodium lauryl sulfate, or SLS.) Many of my patients tell me, however, that they're avoiding products that contain sulfates because they've heard that these ingredients can be harmful to their health. While there is no published medical research linking sodium lauryl sulfate to cancer or other diseases in humans, sulfates, especially SLS, can irritate your skin and sting your eyes, particularly if you have allergies or sensitive skin. They can also strip your hair color.

If you have sensitive skin or just want to avoid sulfates in your hair care products, try such brands as Avalon Organics, L'Oreal EverPure, Naked or Origins, which use ingredients like coconut oil and palm kernel extract instead of SLS as a cleansing agent. Just be aware that these products may not lather or clean as well as "regular" shampoos.

mine unmarked samples of Aveeno shampoo and asked for their professional opinions. I picked women whom I knew were loyal to Kérastase (one of the most expensive and most well regarded product lines), but they were all impressed by the Aveeno stuff—proof that you don't have to spend a fortune to have luxurious locks. Choosing hair care products really comes down to what's most important to you. If you're happy to spend the money for prettier packaging and prefer the aroma, then go ahead and enjoy the expensive stuff.

The one instance where pricier hair products really can make a difference is in women who color their hair. Some less expensive products may use harsher chemicals that can strip the color. I always tell my patients to try new products (regardless of the cost) right before you're due at the salon. If you don't like the results, you'll be getting your color redone anyway. The same goes for medicated shampoos or prescription scalp products that your doctor recommends.

If you buy products in a salon, you have the benefit of asking your stylist for her opinion based on her experience and knowledge of your hair in particular. But beware: Stylists often get a percentage of the sales, which is why some more aggressive stylists may push certain brands harder than others. If you're interested in a pricier product, have your stylist use it on your hair (for free) during your appointment to figure out if you like it. If it's an expensive department store brand you're interested in, ask for a sample. And if you're contemplating a cheaper product from the chemist, ask about the return policy, just in case it doesn't agree with your hair.

Get Longer, Stronger Nails

I don't get manicures very often since I'm really hard on my nails. I wash my hands about a million times a day, and when I'm not seeing patients, I'm typing on a laptop or lifting weights at the gym. Plus, I have to keep them short so I can work with needles and other sharp instruments near people's faces. Likewise, the color's got to stay sheer or nude. (Can you imagine getting Botox injections from someone with claw-like, fire-engine-red nails? Yikes!) But even though I have somewhat limited freedom with the shape and color of my manicure, it's still distressing when a nail chips or cracks. (Actually, it might even be more depressing because I can't run to a salon and slap on a set of acrylics to cover stubby nails or sudden breaks.)

As we discussed earlier in the chapter, people often wait weeks or even months before seeing a doctor about a problem with their nails. They most often head to the manicurist first for advice. While nail technicians have expertise in grooming, and many of the more experienced pros have even learned how to recognize nail infections, they don't have the medical training or equipment to test for different types of infections, such as yeast, fungus, and bacteria, all of which must be treated differently. Manicurists are also not trained to diagnose other medical conditions, such as eczema and psoriasis, that can affect the nails as well as the fingertips. Nor are they able to treat severe ingrown nails (which may need to be surgically removed). It never hurts to ask your manicurist, but if you notice pain, tenderness, or pus on or around the nails, or if the nails are thickened or discolored, you'll want to visit a dermatologist, who can diagnose and treat the problem before it spreads to all your fingers (or toes).

Why Do We Have Fingernails and Toenails?

As with hair, your nails can be a fashion accessory, but they do much more than make a style statement. Your fingernails and toenails, not surprisingly, protect the ends of your fingers and toes. They increase your sense of touch, help you pick up small objects, and let you scratch (either an itch or in self-defense). They're also useful for opening packages, packs of gum, and pop-top cans of tomato paste. They're not, however, indestructible; they need to be nourished from the inside and cared for on the outside.

$E=mc^2$ **Did You Know . . .**

Fingernails grow faster than toenails—3.5mm per month (about the thickness of a graham cracker) versus 1.5mm per month (the thickness of a stick of Wrigley's gum) for toenails. Of all the fingernails, the pinky nail grows the slowest; of the toes, the big toenail grows the fastest.

Like hair, the nails are made of many layers of keratin, a protein produced by the "living" part of the nail, which sits just under the cuticle. Both the nail itself and the skin around the nails are affected by changes in your health. Certain illnesses, including heart, lung, kidney, and liver disease, can cause changes in nail color and their rate of growth. Nutritional deficiencies (such as iron-deficiency anemia) can also affect the shape and condition of the nails. Poorly "fed" nails get thinner and often curl up on the sides. Thin, weak nails are more likely to split, peel, and break off, in addition to being more vulnerable to bacterial and fungus infections. And, like your hair, our nails lose their luster with age.

As we get older, our nails also begin to grow more slowly and typically become thicker and yellowish, especially the toenails. They lose their water content, so instead of looking smooth and shiny, they can look dull and dried out. The surface may also become uneven and develop vertical ridges that run from the cuticle to the tip of the nail. Despite all these changes, feeding your nails the right foods can prevent chipping, cracking, and breaking.

Foods to Maintain Your Manicure

Since your nails are made of the protein keratin, it's important to include an adequate amount of protein in your diet to keep them strong and free of flakes and splits. In fact, patients of mine who crash-diet—either to lose weight for a photo shoot or before filming a swimsuit scene in a movie—often notice that their nails become thin and brittle, too. That's why when patients come to see me for help with their thin or weak nails, I always ask them about their diet. It can take 6 months or more for a nail to grow out, so there may be a lag time of a few months before you see the effects of crash dieting. Likewise, once you get on the right track and feed your nails what they need, it can take another couple of months to see stronger, thicker nails.

There's no shortage of products on the market—from powdered drinks to "strengthening" polishes—that claim to give you a healthier, stronger manicure. While a polish may help prevent cracking and splitting, it won't have any effect on the way your nails actually *grow*. (Remember, the nails are dead, so nothing you do to them on the outside will make them grow any thicker, longer, or stronger.) Research shows that only two food-based ingredients have actually been proven to strengthen the nails before they grow out from your skin: biotin and silicon.

Biotin

Biotin is a form of vitamin B that has been shown to heal brittle nails. (One study in particular found that taking 2.5mg per day of biotin for 2 months helped heal dry, splitting nails in two-thirds of the participants.) While biotin is available in various dietary supplements, studies have shown that it's best absorbed when included in a well-balanced diet. (In other words, if your nails are brittle due to crash dieting, they won't grow back as strong if you just pop a supplement. You also need to eat the right foods.)

For strong nails make sure these rich sources of biotin are in your diet:

Salmon

Organ meats (liver and kidney)

Broccoli

Peanuts, almonds, walnuts

Egg yolks

Whole grains

Cabbage, swiss chard

Yeast (whole wheat bread and pizza dough)

Stop Smoking to Preserve Biotin

I know, I've been harping on smokers. However, studies have shown that women who smoke have significantly less biotin in their systems compared to nonsmokers, which means they have less biotin available to make healthy nails. It's also especially important to avoid smoking during pregnancy—not just because it has been linked to low birth weight, cleft palate, and other defects, but because biotin is broken down even more quickly during pregnancy, which can cause a deficiency even in women who don't smoke. Researchers even think that some of the birth defects linked to smoking may be caused by a smoking-related biotin deficiency at conception or in early pregnancy.

$E=mc^2$ *Did You Know . . .*

While egg whites are a great source of protein (and my go-to breakfast), raw egg whites contain a protein called avidin, which binds biotin and prevents your body from absorbing it. Heating the egg whites, however, destroys the avidin, allowing the biotin to be absorbed. It's a good idea, of course, to avoid eating raw eggs and foods containing raw eggs anyway, to reduce your risk of salmonella infection.

Silicon

If you read through the section on the foods that promote healthy hair growth, you'll remember that silicon is an element that's been linked to stronger bone density as well as stronger hair and nails. (In one study in particular, volunteers who took a silicon supplement had significantly stronger hair and nails after 20 weeks.)

While biotin supplements are widely available and show no evidence of toxicity, there are fewer studies on the safety of silicon supplements. Some reports even link silicon supplements with a greater risk of kidney stones. That's why the best way to supply your nails (and hair) with the silicon they need is to eat silicon-rich foods. For your convenience I've repeated the best sources of dietary silicon below:

- Green beans (one of the richest sources of silicon as well as one of the lowest calorie foods; if you can, choose organic green beans, which retain more silicon from the soil)
- Whole grains and cereals (oats, barley, brown rice)
- Spinach
- Lentils
- Mineral water (especially from volcanic areas; try Volvic, which contains 14.5mg/liter)
- Coffee (made with mineral water)
- Perrier mineral water (5mg/liter)
- Beer (one of the reasons that men often have higher silicon intake than women)

FYI: Bananas have a high concentration of silicon, but only a very small fraction is absorbed into the GI tract and, therefore, by your nails.

Correcting Common Nail Problems

Even when you're eating the right foods, there are a number of additional reasons that the nails may change in appearance; for example, onychoschizia—or brittle nails—is a common concern in my office. (Actually, it's estimated that as many as 20 percent of people have brittle nails, and they're more common in women than in men.) Many of my patients with nails that peel and split assume they have some type of fungus infection. Fungus infections tend to make nails thick and crumbly, however, rather than thin and flaky. Most of the time thin or brittle nails are caused by some kind of trauma, such as slamming your hand in the car door or using your nails to open soda cans, or from repeated exposure to moisture, like frequent or excessive hand washing. (The nails absorb a lot of water—up to ten times as much as the outer layers of the skin—so repeated wetting and the subsequent evaporation of moisture can dry out the nails and make them weaker.) Research shows that brittle nails are also associated with professional manicures and the frequent use of nail polish remover. In fact, people who get professional manicures are three times more likely to have brittle nails than people who use nail polish remover once a month. Why? The nails split and peel when the chemical bonds that hold the keratin layers tightly together become loose. The keratin layers lift off one by one, kind of like paint cracking and peeling over time. It is thought that repeated exposure to nail polish remover and other harsh chemicals weakens the bonds that hold the layers of keratin together, making them more likely to flake, peel, and eventually break.

Brittle nails can also be hereditary. If someone in your family has brittle nails, your risk of developing onychoschizia increases by 600 percent. (Rarely, an underlying illness or nutritional deficiency—such as anemia—can be the primary cause of brittle nails.) A general rule of thumb: If your fingernails split easily but your toenails are strong, then an external factor (like trauma) is likely to blame. Here are some other common conditions that may affect your nails:

White spots on the nail. Contrary to popular opinion, white spots on the nail are not calcium deposits or signs of a fungal infection. They're caused by trauma. Since the nail itself is technically "dead," any injury or damage to the surface of the nail can't be repaired. It has to grow out, and it usually will within six months. On the other hand, yellow-brown spots can be signs of psoriasis, even if you don't have psoriasis elsewhere on the body. A dermatologist can tell you if your yellow-brown spots are something to worry about.

Yellow discoloration. Thick yellow nails *can* be a sign of something contagious, such as a fungal infection, but the nails can also turn yellow for other, relatively harmless reasons, like poor circulation or walking around barefoot.

In some cases, yellow discoloration is caused by dark nail polish that has stained the nail bed. You'll know polish is the culprit if the nail surface is smooth and the discoloration affects all the nails equally. You can prevent future discoloration by using a base coat, by periodically removing polish and going au naturel for a while, or by switching to a lighter color. It's a good idea to remove polish once a month anyway, just so you can check to make sure the nails look healthy.

If you do have some kind of fungus, it's most likely the same as the one that causes athlete's foot. Fungal infections can make the nails appear discolored (usually yellow or brown rather than black) as well as thick and crumbly, and the skin between the toes and on the bottoms of the feet can be scaly and itchy. But the only way to know exactly what's going on with your nails is to have them tested; your doctor can take a tissue sample and send it to a lab for culture. If it's a fungus, he'll likely recommend a topical treatment such as Clotrimazole 1% cream or Lamisil (both available at chemists) or prescribe Lamisil pills. If you have nail psoriasis, which can look exactly like a fungus infection, your doctor may suggest cortisone injections around the nail or a systemic treatment if psoriasis also affects other parts of the body.

It's also possible for the nails to become infected with *Pseudomonas* bacteria, which live in moist dirt and hot tubs. Bacterial infections can turn your nails dark green or black, while the affected toe may become tender, red, and swollen—you might also notice some pus draining under the cuticle. If your toes are sore and you see drainage, see a doctor right away since the infection can spread to the rest of your foot.

Hey, Dr. Wu

Q: I've been trying to grow out my nails, but they keep splitting and cracking. I've even tried those "nail-grow" polishes, but nothing seems to work. What can I do?

A: Your nails are already dead by the time they grow out, so applying polish won't make them grow any faster. You can prevent chips, cracks and splits, however, by following these tips:

- To prevent splitting, try to be gentle on your nails. Avoid using them to open packages or pop the tops of soda cans, and if you do see a split or crack, resist the urge to peel the nail off. Instead, immediately file the ragged edges with a nail file or emery board. This will prevent the split from getting longer. Also avoid buffing the entire nail since that can lead to thinning. Apply a clear polish once a week to strengthen the nails and lock in moisture, and remove it no more than every other week to minimize your exposure to the harsh chemicals in polish remover.

- Filing your nails into a soft rounded shape (rather than straight across) will make them stronger and less likely to split. I call this the "squoval," square with rounded edges.

- Since frequent hand washing can dehydrate the nails (and predispose them to splitting), be sure to moisturize the nails after they've been in water. You can use hand cream or cuticle oil, but my favorite topical product for nails and cuticles is food-grade sweet almond oil, which is nontoxic, nonirritating, and contains natural vitamin E. (And it smells like almond cookies. Yum!) For added protection, wear gloves when you're doing the dishes, gardening, or working with chemicals or solvents.

- If you wear nail polish, avoid polish removers with acetone, which can dry out the nail. (Look for "acetone-free" products instead.)

- Many of my patients have had success with topical products that contain acetyl mandelic acid. They won't make your nails grow faster, but the alpha-hydroxy acid can smooth out splits. Try NeoStrata or Neo-Ceuticals Nail Conditioning Solution.

Melanonychia striata. Dark stripes on the nails, or melanonychia striata, are caused by increased or excess pigment, and it's more common in people with darker skin tones. Although it's a harmless condition, if you notice any new discoloration, rapid growth, or sudden darkening of the toenails, be sure to show a dermatologist, who may need to do a nail biopsy to make sure it's not melanoma.

Subungual hematoma. One of my patients, a busy mother of two, went to a manicurist the morning before she was to attend a big event (in sexy strappy sandals she'd bought for the occasion). During her pedicure, however, she felt that the woman was a little rough on the toenails, and when she looked down, she was a little nervous to see her wielding a seriously sharp instrument. The manicurist warned her that she had a lot of dead skin that needed to be removed. Afterward, her toes were a little sore, but everything seemed fine. Later that night, though, her nails became more tender and red, and she hobbled around all night in her new shoes. By the next day her nails were dark purple and turning darker by the hour. When she finally came to see me a week later, the nails on her big toes (and several other nails) were completely black. I took one look and knew what had happened: The manicurist was overzealous and punctured the veins beneath the toenails, causing bleeding under the nail, a condition known as subungual hematoma. When that happens, the nails typically fall off and it can take 6 months or longer for them to grow back.

I've had my own experience with subungual hematomas—every year I come back from my annual ski trip with bruised toes. (Maybe I need new ski boots?) But in the winter of 2009 things looked particularly bad. After 3 days of skiing, my big toenails were dark red, and by the last day of my trip, it had become painful to walk, though I managed to get my shoes on. Unfortunately, I made the mistake of taking off my shoes on the plane, and by the time we landed, I couldn't get them back on, so I had to walk around LAX barefoot. (Note to self: Always travel with flip-flops in your carry-on.) The next day my toes were throbbing so badly that I had to trade my pumps for Dr. Scholls' open-toed sandals, making it necessary to explain my extra-casual footwear to every patient who walked through the door. (Um, embarrassing.) Over the following week my toenails turned black and eventually fell off. It took 9 long months for them to grow back.

Subungual hematomas are common in runners, hikers, and skiers who tend to hit their toenails against the inside of their shoes or boots. If enough blood collects under the nail, the condition can be extremely painful. A doctor can drain the blood, providing instant relief. If you don't seek treatment, the blood will dry into a scab (which turns the nail black), and you'll have to wait for the nail to grow out. To help prevent hematomas, make sure your athletic shoes and boots are properly fitted and always keep your toenails trimmed short.

SEE YOUR DOCTOR IF . . . YOUR NAILS ARE PAINFUL, RED, OR SWOLLEN

The majority of changes in your nails (from white spots to vertical ridges) are completely harmless. Sometimes, however, changes in surface texture or discoloration can indicate a more serious problem. If you notice any of the following, it's time to seek medical attention:

- Pain, swelling, redness, or pus around the nail (which can be signs of a bacterial or yeast infection)
- Thickened or crumbly toenails (fungal infection)
- Bleeding under the nail; if severe, subungual hematomas can cause permanent damage to the nail.
- Yellow, green, or brown discoloration (fungus or bacterial infection)
- Changes in nail shape or surface texture (can be a sign of anemia)
- Brown or black discoloration of the nail or cuticle (can indicate melanoma)
- Pits or divots on the surface of the nail (can indicate psoriasis)

A Word About Your Cuticles

The cuticle—the thin strip of skin that surrounds the nail—is meant to protect your skin and keep out harmful bacteria, fungus, and viruses. So it pains me, literally, when a manicurist whips out a sharp pair of scissors and starts snipping away. The first time this happened—years ago, before I knew better—I didn't say anything because I figured the woman knew what she was doing. But before long there was a pile of skin on the table. At one point she even drew blood, which is when I told her to stop. It's *never* normal to bleed when you're having a manicure. Plus, cutting the cuticles makes them fray and split, which can be really painful, as well as allows bacteria to enter the nail bed. If your cuticles are growing like weeds, you can gently push them back, but not too far. Over time they can become thick and callused, and you can develop a gap between your nail and the skin big enough for germs to enter and cause an infection.

There's also a thin layer of tissue along the underside of your nail; this is

KEEPING YOUR NAILS HEALTHY
WHEN WEARING ACRYLICS

A patient of mine (who happens to be a manicurist) was once called to a photo shoot when a certain pop princess showed up with all ten fingernails bitten off to the quick. Since no amount of polish can disguise stubby nails, my patient saved the day by applying semipermanent acrylics. I've always envied women with perfectly groomed and polished nails, and I have to admit that the idea of getting acrylics—that is, a perfect chip-resistant manicure that lasts for several weeks—*is* pretty appealing.

Studies have shown, however, that health care workers who wear artificial nails carry more germs (including Staph bacteria and yeast) on their nails than those who don't, and I can't risk spreading infection to my patients just to have a nice manicure. I've also treated many patients who have lost their own nails or developed allergic reactions to the acrylate chemicals, so I've seen firsthand the damage that acrylics can do. If you have acrylics or are thinking about getting them, here are some things to keep in mind:

- Acrylic nails should be removed every 6 to 8 weeks—leaving them on too long can cause the fake nail to separate from the natural nail. When water gets trapped underneath, you've got a breeding ground for germs. It's better to let your own nails "breathe" for a few weeks between applications.
- For a more natural look, ask your manicurist to go light on the acrylic glue and request a shape that mimics the shape of your cuticle. (A more natural shape also makes typing, texting, and counting change easier.)
- If the cuticles become red, flaky, or swollen, remove the acrylics and see a dermatologist. These symptoms can be signs of a candida yeast infection or an allergic reaction even if you've used acrylics for years.
- If the nail under the acrylic becomes thick, crumbly, or discolored, see your doctor—these may be signs of a bacterial or fungal infection.

your skin's barrier to infection and water. Don't clean too hard under the nails, and don't let anyone stick a sharp instrument under there. The same goes for hangnails; trim only the ones that are actually hanging. If you pick and cut too much, the cuticles along the sides of the nail can't adhere as well, and you'll be even more likely to develop an infection (called paronychia).

Recap of Chapter 8

Keeping Your Hair and Nails Strong and Healthy

* Nutrition plays a major role in the look and feel of your hair and nails—keep them looking their best by feeding them healthy proteins. Never crash-diet.

* Eat plenty of foods containing silicon, iron, and zinc; mineral deficiency is a major cause of hair loss.

* Going gray? Eat more almonds and stock up on antioxidant-rich fruits and veggies.

* Hair getting thinner? Avoid mercury, which is found in large fish like tuna and swordfish.

* Remember that most shampoos contain similar ingredients; more expensive doesn't necessarily mean better.

* To reduce flyaways, choose a conditioner with wheat or rice proteins and rich emollients, like panthenol or natural oils.

* Most nail-growth products, such as drink mixes and strengthening polishes, won't do much to improve the condition of your nails. (A polish may help prevent splitting and cracking, but it won't make your nails actually grow any faster.) For a prettier manicure, stick with foods containing biotin, silicon, and protein.

Part III

Feed Your Face in *Action*

9

. . . .

The *Feed Your Face* Diet

Not long ago, during a routine checkup, one of my regular patients marveled at the fact that I basically wear fitted skirts and sky-high stilettos day in and day out. It's not that she's *not* into fashion—Maggie has a closet full of designer duds and a truckload of Manolos and Jimmy Choos. She's even hired a stylist to help her navigate the trendy boutiques of Beverly Hills—she just can't pull an outfit together on her own. Her unorganized and overflowing closet had become overwhelming, so every day (and I do mean *every* day) she reaches for the exact same thing: jeans and a plain white tee. (Luckily, she lives in Malibu, a place so casual that people wear jeans even to church.) The thing is, I totally get Maggie's predicament, because the way she feels about her closet is the way I used to feel about my pantry.

I've never been much of a cook (much to my mother's disappointment), and 12-hour days at the office leave little time to prepare gourmet meals. Before, I'd do my grocery shopping at the end of a hectic workday, with a growling stomach and dwindling patience. I'd rush in, grab whatever was on sale, and get out as quickly as possible. And when I was *really* busy (like during awards show season, when I'm on every actress's speed dial), the groceries would get shoved into the pantry according to the way they were bagged at the store—randomly. Food got lost in the back of the cupboard.

I always managed to forget what I'd bought. And I'd end up reaching for my favorite (and sometimes least healthy) snacks—my old standbys, the jeans and T-shirts of my pantry. What I've learned is that when I *do* take the time to shop and can come home and put everything away properly, I end up eating better. No desperate handfuls of crisps to satisfy a midday craving, no cold cereal for dinner because there's just nothing else to eat. (I also discovered that if you plan your meals ahead of time, you can make the best use of what's already in the cupboard *and* waste less food—which means more money left over for shoes or whatever you'd rather be shopping for!)

The *Feed Your Face* Diet is the culmination of everything we've talked about in the previous eight chapters—how to minimize fine lines and wrinkles, boost UV protection, fuel collagen production, heal acne, reduce inflammation, and soothe rashes—organized into a month-long meal plan that takes the fear and stress out of eating for healthier, more beautiful skin.

Starting on page 255 you'll find 28 days' worth of breakfast, lunch, dinner, and snack suggestions. Every meal is easy to prepare and has been designed to provide a balance of antioxidants (to fight free radicals), protein (to fuel collagen production), omega-3s (to soothe inflammation), and lycopene (for UV protection). While the *Feed Your Face* Diet will benefit all skin types, I've gone ahead and made some necessary adjustments for certain skin conditions in particular, such as reminding you to avoid dairy if you're pimple-prone, adding more soy if you're worried about fine lines and wrinkles, or avoiding gluten if you suffer from stubborn rashes.

The meal plan, however, is merely a way to put the *Feed Your Face* philosophy into practice—it's designed to take the guesswork out of deciding what to eat, not to tell you what you *have* to eat. (After all, you'll eventually graduate to preparing your own face-friendly meals.) If you don't like, say, tofu, swap it out for another lean protein such as chicken. Likewise, if you don't care for broccoli, choose a different green veggie instead. And if you love the chocolate smoothie (on page 261), feel free to make it your new go-to breakfast. Don't be afraid to be flexible. Just make sure that you replace any foods you don't like with other healthy proteins, whole grains, and vegetables. (So swap brown rice for quinoa or couscous, not white rice.) Otherwise you might not be getting enough calories, and you'll wind up rummaging through your cupboards at two in the morning. Never a good idea.

And here's the best part of the *Feed Your Face* Diet (if I do say so myself): You don't actually have to cook anything if you don't feel like it or if you just don't have the time. Believe me, I've had nights when the idea of preparing dinner made me break into a cold sweat. That's why the majority of these meals can be assembled from items you can pick up at your local supermarket or favourite takeaway establishment. For the days when even *that's* too much work, I've also included the *Feed Your Face* Guide to Eating Out, a listing of the healthiest options available at popular restaurants. (Besides, you shouldn't have to sacrifice your social life to maintain great skin.)

While you can continue to use the meal ideas in the *Feed Your Face* Diet long after the initial 28 days, at some point you'll be ready to graduate to making your own meals. That's why I've given you loads of help stocking your pantry, fridge, and spice rack. We'll go over the ingredients you need to whip up the meals in the *Feed Your Face* Meal Plan, but keep these essential items on hand and you'll be able to create your own face-friendly dishes, too. I've also listed some of my favorite snacks and food brands (where-to-buy information for these as well as all the products mentioned in *Feed Your Face* is located in the Resource Guide) as well as tips from some of my celebrity patients (so you'll know what the stars *really* snack on when they're killing time in their trailers).

For smooth, clear skin and a healthy, sexy body, here's what you should *Feed Your Face*.

Stocking Your Cupboards

Your kitchen cupboard is where you'll find the core ingredients of any healthy meal, but it's also the place where half-eaten boxes of stale cereal and mystery canned goods go to die. Start by cleaning yours out. Toss (or donate) all that processed, sugar-filled, nutrient-free junk (like crisps, biscuits, and ready meals) and anything else that's been in there longer than you can remember. Then stock your pantry with these face-friendly staples:

Cooked and Canned Tomatoes

Tomatoes are packed with the antioxidant lycopene (for extra UV protection), and I keep every variety in my pantry. Sun-dried tomatoes are great in omelets or pasta, while jarred, low-sodium salsa gives baked chicken a kick. In fact, when I'm headed on vacation, the two most important things in my suitcase are a bathing suit and tomato paste. Three tablespoons every day at lunch—mixed into marinara sauce or on top of a pizza, not smeared on your face—helps protect against sunburn, so I come home to L.A. with a golden glow rather than looking like a lobster. Aim to incorporate tomatoes in at least one meal a day (it's surprisingly easy when you think about it), and you'll help protect your skin from sun spots, freckles, and premature wrinkling.

CELEBRITY SKIN SECRETS—
Marina Sirtis's Kokkinisto

OK, I'll admit it. I am a total *Star Trek* nerd. So when I first met Marina Sirtis (a.k.a. Deanna Troi), I kind of geeked out. Born in London to Greek parents, Marina grew up eating a mostly Mediterranean diet and tons of tomatoes—which is probably why she looks 15 years younger than her actual age. She was kind enough to share her family's recipe for Kokkinisto, a traditional Greek dish made with tomatoes and meat. Try it!

INGREDIENTS:

1½ to 2 pounds leg of
  lamb or lamb shank
1 yellow onion, chopped
½ cup olive oil
1 cup dry red wine
1 can stewed tomatoes
1 tablespoon tomato paste

2 bay leaves
1 cup water
Salt and pepper to taste
2 or 3 russet potatoes,
  peeled and chopped
½ cup peas
2 cups spinach, cleaned and dried

Kokkinisto is traditionally prepared with lamb (shoulder chops or cutlets), but you can substitute beef or chicken. Cut the meat into individual portions (larger than bite-size).

In a stockpot, sauté the onion in 2–3 tablespoons of olive oil until tender. Add the remaining oil and brown the meat on both sides. Add wine and stir. Add the tomatoes, tomato paste, bay leaves, salt, and pepper. Cover and let simmer until the meat begins to soften, 30–45 minutes. (Add water as needed if the sauce begins to dry.) Add the remaining vegetables and simmer until the meat is tender and the sauce is reduced and thickened.

Serves 2–3

Grains, Nuts, and Seeds

Whole grains, which are lower on the glycemic index than refined grains and contain loads of essential nutrients, are an important staple in any diet. Serve a small scoop of brown or wild rice (instead of white rice) alongside fish and veggies or try quinoa, a protein-packed grain that's similar to couscous. For a quick and easy breakfast, keep plenty of slow-cooking or rolled porridge oats on hand (rather than instant porridge). Don't worry—despite their name, slow-cooking porridge oats can actually be prepared in a jiff. That's key—I know, because I don't have time to stir a pot of porridge for thirty minutes while I'm trying to get ready for work. And when it comes to snacking, you can't beat whole-grain crackers and hummus. I especially like Ryvita crackers, which are ridiculously crunchy and absolutely packed with fiber.

For sandwiches and wraps you can go with 100 percent whole-grain bread or check out sprouted grain bread. Unlike foods made with refined flour, sprouted grains are allowed to sprout (that is, germinate) before being turned into bread. Sprouted grain products are flourless (though not gluten-free), low-carb, and low on the glycemic index.

If you suffer from rashes (especially eczema or psoriasis), you'll want to avoid gluten, a protein found in such grains as wheat, barley, and rye, which may contribute to inflammation and aggravate itchy, flaky skin. You still need plenty of whole grains in your diet, however, so get to know the gluten-free aisle in your grocery store. You'll find gluten-free bread, waffle and pancake mixes, granola, and cereal, as well as gluten-free soy sauce. You should also aim to incorporate more naturally gluten-free grains in your diet such as corn, flax, brown rice, millet, and quinoa.

Nuts like almonds, walnuts, and pecans are loaded with omega-3s, magnesium, vitamin E, and other nutrients, but they're also full of fiber so they'll keep you feeling fuller longer, which is one of the many reasons that nuts—paired with dried fruit for a burst of sweetness—are one of my favorite snacks. Nuts are high in fat, so you do want to limit yourself to a small handful. (If you're eating nuts with dried fruit, that's a small handful total, not a handful of each.) I'm also addicted to roasted cashews (sea salt flavor is my favorite). They have less sodium per serving than most chocolate bars and contain only three ingredients: dry-roasted cashews (no oil!), sea salt, and gum acacia (a natural tree resin for texture). Natural nut butters make an equally excellent snack when spread on whole-grain or sprouted grain bread or alongside a piece of fruit, but stay away from Jif, Skippy, and other brands that contain added sugar, high-fructose corn syrup, salt, and other additives. Instead, try Fairtrade Organic Unsalted Crunchy Peanut Butter, which is made entirely from peanuts and contains no added sugars, salt, or oil.

If you're concerned about the appearance of fine lines and wrinkles, add Brazil nuts to your diet. They're one of the richest dietary sources of the antioxidant selenium (1 ounce, or about a handful of nuts, provides about 1000 percent of your Daily Value), which is essential to preventing the breakdown of collagen. (There is such a thing as too much selenium, though, so you don't want to overeat Brazil nuts.) You might also try soy nuts, which are roasted soybeans; they have a taste and texture similar to peanuts.

Seeds, including sunflower and flaxseeds, also provide a range of nutrients. Flaxseeds in particular (also known as linseeds) are an excellent source of omega-3s, but they must be finely ground for your body to absorb the nutritional benefits. Buy it premilled or use a coffee grinder to do the milling yourself. Sprinkle flaxseeds in smoothies, oatmeal, or yogurt for an omega-3 boost.

Christa Miller's Homemade Trail Mix

In between takes on the set of *Cougartown*, Christa Miller snacks on homemade trail mix. Combine pumpkin seeds, sunflower seeds, and pistachios with a splash of maple syrup and a pinch of sea salt. Roast at 300° for 20 minutes. Add dried cherries (with no added sugars).

Whole-Grain Pasta

Switching white pasta for whole wheat pasta doesn't have to affect your taste buds, but it will affect your blood sugar—for the better. Until recently whole-grain pastas were mostly grainy, gummy, and unappetizing. But these days, delicious good-quality whole wheat pastas are widely available. Don't be fooled by multigrain or fortified varieties, however, which are just mixtures of refined grains with added vitamins and minerals. Whole-grain is still the best. Remember that all pastas should be cooked *al dente,* or slightly firm—overcooked pasta breaks down more quickly in the body, causing your blood sugar to spike more rapidly. If you prepare your pasta the night before (for pasta salad, for example), be sure to rinse in cold water to stop the cooking process; otherwise, the pasta will continue to cook even after you've placed it in the refrigerator. And remember that pairing your pasta with a protein (such as lean chicken) will curb blood sugar spikes even more.

Tofu

Made from soy milk with added coagulants (such as calcium and various enzymes), tofu is an excellent low-calorie source of protein. Tofu is rather bland on its own, but it adopts the flavors of the foods with which it is cooked, so it can easily be added to both sweet and savory dishes. While tofu is most commonly found packed in water in the refrigerated aisle, you can also look for silken tofu, so named for its silky smooth texture.

It's sold in aseptic packaging (similar to juice boxes) so it won't spoil, and you can stock up if there's a sale. Soft silken tofu is great for smoothies and desserts. It also comes in a firm variety, which you can use in stir-fries or as a substitute for meat in baked dishes or casseroles. An added benefit: Firm tofu is higher in protein and calcium than the soft variety. Just keep in mind that tofu is a fermented food, so you'll want to avoid it if you have hives or eczema since fermented foods can trigger your body to release histamine.

Hey, Dr. Wu

Q: Should I be choosing foods that are fortified with nutrients and omega-3s?

A: "Whole" foods (meaning natural, unprocessed foods) are generally better for your skin and your body, but if you're a picky eater, you may want to consider choosing fortified foods to help you get the nutrients you need. For example, if you hate fish, flax, and walnuts, you can choose pastas, orange juice, or cereals that contain added omega-3s. Read the labels carefully, however. The pasta may not be whole grain, the orange juice is likely to be high in sugar and calories (with no fiber), and the cereal may list sugar and corn syrup much higher on the ingredient list than the omega-3. When it comes to fortified foods, you're getting only what the manufacturer adds; you're not getting the full benefit of the whole food (such as fiber, natural antioxidants, protein, and other nutrients). The bottom line: Whenever possible, it's best to get your nutrients from natural sources.

Sugar Substitutes

It's hard to quit eating sugar cold turkey, especially if a daily Starbucks with two sachets is what gets you going in the morning. While you're weaning yourself off the sweet stuff, it's OK to *occasionally* use a sugar substitute. Although there has been much concern about the potential dangers of such artificial sweeteners as sucralose (Splenda), aspartame (Candarel), and saccharine (Sweet 'N Low), so far scientists and the FDA have concluded that they are safe when consumed in reasonable quantities. The real problem with artificial sweeteners, I think, is that they perpetuate your craving for sweet-tasting treats, so they should always be used sparingly, if at all.

Just can't quit the sugar habit? At least try switching to an unrefined sugar (such as brown sugar, honey, molasses, or agave nectar) when possible. Agave, which has become all the rage among raw foodies and vegans, comes from a cactus-like desert plant, and though it contains fructose and glucose, it has a lower glycemic load than white sugar. While unrefined sugars will still spike your blood sugar, they also contain disease- and age-fighting antioxidants. You can think about it like this: Much like refined grains lack the nutrients found in whole grains, refined sugar lacks the antioxidant benefit of *un*refined sugar. If you've gotta have it, you might as well go with the best quality you can find.

Shopping List: Keep These Items in Your Cupboard

Sun-dried tomatoes

Canned tomatoes

Low-sugar pasta sauce

Tomato paste

Whole wheat pasta

Canned tuna in water

Dried fruit (cranberries, cherries, apricots)

Nuts (almonds, walnuts, pecans, soy nuts)

Silken tofu

Natural nut butter (peanut, almond, or cashew)

Lentils

Capers

Whole-grain crackers

Canned beans (black, kidney)

Onions and garlic

Whole grains (oats, quinoa, brown or wild rice)

Flaxseeds

Whole wheat or sprouted grain bread

Filling Your Fridge

If your fridge drawer is filled with beer (you know who you are), I'm talking to you. Toss the fizzy drinks, fruity beverages, fruit-on-the-bottom yogurt (which usually contains corn syrup and several teaspoons of sugar), and chili-cheese dip, and load your refrigerator with fresh fruits and veggies. The little bit of room you have left over? That's for reduced-fat dairy and lots of lean proteins. Trust me—your face will thank you.

In the Produce Section

OK, I'll admit it. If given the choice between an apple and a chocolate bar, I'd be seriously tempted by the chocolate bar. But fruits and vegetables don't have to be boring! Stone or pitted fruits, such as plums and peaches, make an easy grab-and-go snack, but throw them on the grill (and top with a drizzle of balsamic vinegar) and they make an elegant dessert. Berries, especially blueberries and raspberries, are packed with free radical–fighting antioxidants, and they're easy to work into your main meals. Toss them in smoothies, layer them in low-sugar yogurt, or serve them on top of whole wheat pancakes (instead of syrup) for an indulgent weekend brunch. And a toasted cheese made with pesto, fresh mozzarella, and thick tomato slices beats a take-away burger any day.

When you're shopping for fresh produce, be sure to choose fruits that are just underripe. A slightly underripe banana, for example, is firm in texture and filled with fiber—you have to chew it more, which slows down the absorption of sugar in the body. An overripe banana, on the other hand, is brown and mushy—you could practically swallow it without chewing because most of the starch has already been converted to sugar and will start to get absorbed into your bloodstream as soon as it hits your tongue. Overripe fruit has essentially been predigested; it will taste sweeter, but it will also have a more dramatic effect on your blood sugar—and your skin!

$E=mc^2$ *Did You Know . . .*

Love fresh berries but hate their short shelf life? Submerging berries in hot water kills mold spores, which helps them stay fresher longer. In fact, the heat will actually stimulate the formation of active antioxidants, so your body can absorb more nutrients. As soon as you bring them home from the supermarket, run berries under hot tap water (about 125°, which is the upper limit on most residential water heaters), for 30 seconds or so.

When it comes to veggies, load up on green, yellow, and red varieties, which contain the most anti-aging and sun-protective antioxidants. And be sure to keep green beans (also known as string beans or snap beans) in your salad drawer since these have a high silicon content for smooth skin and strong, healthy hair and nails. (They're also one of the lowest calorie foods!) You can toss green beans in salads or bake or stir-fry them, but my favorite treat is Simply Green Beans, which are crunchy freeze-dried green beans (no salt or sugar added) that make a satisfying on-the-go snack.

Just as it's important to steer clear of overripe fruit, it's also important not to overcook your vegetables. In some cases boiled or steamed vegetables may deliver more antioxidants than raw veggies (for example, lycopene is more *bioavailable* in cooked tomatoes, meaning it's easier for your body to absorb), but overcooking can break down starchy vegetables (such as potatoes and squash), sending your blood sugar higher faster. Additionally, some vitamins (such as vitamin C, which is essential for collagen production) are water soluble, so they can be leached out during the cooking process.

CELEBRITY SKIN SECRETS—

Nicole Sullivan's Jazzed-Up Green Beans

To give ordinary green beans a kick of flavor, Nicole Sullivan stir-fries them in 1 tablespoon of olive oil and sprinkles in sesame seeds, sweet peppers, and a bit of chopped onion.

Dairy Alternatives: Soy Milk, Soy Yogurt, and Soy Cheese

While dairy foods aren't completely forbidden for followers of the *Feed Your Face* Diet (unless you're suffering from breakouts, in which case they are), you should be limiting your intake of dairy as much as possible. Choose only reduced-fat or skim milk, yogurt, and cheese or go completely dairy-free and opt for soy-based products. (An added bonus: Soy is loaded with a type of plant estrogen called isoflavone, which has been shown to improve fine lines and skin elasticity.) These days you won't have any trouble finding dairy alternatives: Soy milk is available in virtually any supermarket and comes in a variety of flavors and brands. Soy cheese (which is a bit like tofu but firmer) is less ubiquitous, but you can find it in some specialist shops. I personally don't think it has much flavor on its own—it's certainly no match for fresh Brie—but it *does* add a rich, creamy texture to sandwiches, wraps, and salads. As an alternative, try cashew cheese, a spreadable "cheese" made from whole cashews; it is delicious on whole-grain crackers or paired with veggies. It isn't very widely available but you can easily make your own.

Before you load your fridge with soy products, it's important to remember that a diet high in soy may potentially have negative side effects for boys and men in general and for women with estrogen-receptor positive (ER-positive) breast cancer. Soy contains plant estrogens that may interfere with the male hormone, testosterone. Women with a personal or family history of breast cancer should consult their doctor, who may recommend limiting their intake of soy products, including tofu, soy milk, edamame, and soy nuts. Try swapping soy milk for almond or coconut milk, and soy yogurt for dairy-free coconut yogurt. You might also try Greek yogurt. It's not dairy-free, but authentic Greek yogurt is thick, tart, and contains no added sweeteners, thickeners, or preservatives. It also has about twice the protein as regular yogurt, so it's infinitely better for you than the super-sweet sugary stuff that most of us are used to. One of my favorites is Total 0% Greek Yogurt. Look for the plain fat-free versions, which are just as thick, creamy, and satisfying and have about half the calories. Sprinkle a few berries on top, and it tastes just like cheesecake. (Really!)

Choosing Lean Meats

Red meat can be high in saturated fat and cholesterol, but it's also an excellent source of zinc, a natural anti-inflammatory as well as an inhibitor of *P. acnes* bacteria (which is great if you're struggling with breakouts). Get the benefit of red meat without all the fat by limiting your intake to twice a week and choosing lean cuts; sirloin, shoulder steak, flank steak, top loin, tenderloin, and filet mignon are your best bets. Avoid fattier rib cuts, such as rib eye and prime rib, and opt for extra-lean ground beef, which contains no more than 15 percent fat, as opposed to regular ground beef, which may contain as much as 30 percent fat.

As an alternative to beef, try bison. A bison burger tastes just like the real thing, but it's leaner and lower in cholesterol than most other proteins, including beef and chicken. When it comes to making sandwiches, avoid processed luncheon meats at all costs; they're often a source of hidden sugars, starches, and—get this—*dairy products*. (Many deli meats, including ham, sausage, and hot dogs, use lactose, a sugar found in milk, as a flavor enhancer. Some meat also contains casein, a milk protein.) Instead, choose fresh roasted turkey, fresh roast beef, rotisserie or grilled chicken, and meats labeled "dairy-free" or "kosher." Ham is fine, too, provided you choose a low-sodium variety and stay away from honey-glazed ham, which is full of added sugars.

Shopping List: Keep Your Fridge Full
of These Healthy Foods

Fresh fruits
  (especially berries)
Fresh veggies (especially
  green, yellow, or red)
Kalamata olives
Hummus

Low-fat, low-sugar yogurt or
  soy yogurt
Low-fat or soy cheese
Low-fat milk or soy milk
Lean proteins (ground beef,
  white fish, poultry)
Eggs

Herbs, Spices, and Condiments

While you may think of condiments as relatively guilt-free, ketchup, barbecue sauce, salad dressing, and pasta sauce are all loaded with hidden
sugars and high-fructose corn syrup. Look for low-sugar or sugar-free versions, as well as alternative ways to flavor your food. A drizzle of olive oil
and a splash of balsamic vinegar is better than commercial salad dressing
(if you've got rosacea, skip the vinegar and choose an olive oil that's been
infused with fresh garlic and herbs). Swap jams for sugar-free preserves (or
better yet, choose fresh berries). And if you're acne-prone, use kosher salt
rather than table or sea salt, both of which contain iodine, a possible acne
irritant.

Shopping List: Face-Friendly Spices and Condiments

Fresh herbs
Kosher salt
Balsamic vinegar
Olive oil (extra virgin
  and infused)

Low-sodium soy sauce
Dijon mustard
Low-sugar ketchup
Low-fat mayonnaise made with
  olive oil

Are Organic Foods Worth the Cost?

When I was 10, my grandpa dug up our well-manicured Southern California lawn to grow a vegetable garden. The neighbors couldn't understand why anyone would rip out beautiful Kentucky bluegrass, but back then no one had even heard of organic gardening. (I guess Grandpa was just ahead of his time.) He planted all kinds of foods—tomatoes, squash, Chinese leafy greens, zucchini—and it was my after-school job to wash the vegetables after they'd been harvested. I enjoyed working alongside my grandpa until one day I found—horror of horrors—a *worm,* which sent me into a fit of hysterics. I tossed my basketful of vegetables sky-high, sending squash and zucchini flying across the yard. That was the end of my work in the garden.

These days you're not likely to find a worm in any of *your* produce because the majority of conventionally grown fruits and vegetables at the store have been treated with a range of pesticides. Ironically, you'd be better off eating a worm. (Hey, it's a great source of protein!) Organic produce, on the other hand, is grown without the use of most chemical pesticides and herbicides, while organic livestock are reared without the use of antibiotics and growth hormones, and generally are fed an organic diet of grass or grain (as opposed to animal by-products, manure, fats, oils, and grease).

Eating organic is generally healthier (by reducing your exposure to chemical pesticides and antibiotics), more humane for the animals, and better for the environment. While buying organic foods can be more expensive, there are ways to keep the cost in check, including choosing supermarket brands or shopping at the local farmers market. (Regular customers can almost always score a discount.)

Here's what you should know about when to go organic:

Understanding the Terms

Organic standards in the U.K. are enforced by certification authorities, such as the Soil Association and the Organic Food Federation who inspect each stage of the organic food chain.

An organic product is classified according to the percentage of organic ingredients it contains. If a product contains 95 percent or more organic ingredients, it may be called 'organic' in the product title. If it contains between 70 percent and 90 percent organic ingredients, the term 'organic' may be used in the list of ingredients, and if a product contains less than 70 percent organic ingredients, the term 'organic' may not be used anywhere on the product packaging, Consequently, if a product is labeled 'organic', you can be confident that almost all of the ingredients it contains have also been certified as organic.

Fruits and Vegetables

If you can afford to buy only *some* organic foods, the produce section is a good place to start, especially since fruits and vegetables should make up the bulk of your diet (rather than, say, meat and poultry). Nonorganic fruits and vegetables are routinely sprayed with pesticides. Even if you wash your produce at home (which you should *always* do), those chemicals have had weeks to sink deep into your food.

Choose organic fruits and vegetables when you plan to eat the skin or peel (as with apples, berries, green beans, and lettuce) or when buying produce that's especially vulnerable to insect attack (such as tomatoes, cabbage, and cauliflower) since these items are more likely to have pesticide residue. Fruits that you have to peel, such as oranges, bananas, and pineapples, tend to have a tough skin that isn't as easily penetrated by pesticides, so it's not as important that they be organic.

Dairy Products

Organic milk and dairy products come from cows that are allowed to free range on pastures which are not sprayed with synthetic chemical pesticides. Unlike many non-organic cows, they are not fed on genetically modified cattle feed and are not given routine antibiotics to prevent the spread of disease and infection. When cows are treated with a steady stream of antibiotics, trace amounts of the drugs wind up in the milk supply (and, eventually, in *you*).

Research has also established that organic milk contains higher levels of Vitamin E, Vitamin A and antioxidants than non-organic milk.

You can avoid added hormones and antibiotics by choosing organic milk and dairy products. Imported cheese is fine, however, since the hormone is banned in European countries.

Meat and Poultry

Like dairy cows, non-organic cattle and poultry are also treated with antibiotics to prevent the spread of infection. For this and other reasons, organic meat and poultry may be healthier for you, too. For example grass-fed cattle have five times the omega-3 content as those fed on grain (although it is worth bearing in mind that "grass-fed" does not necessarily mean "organic" and vice versa). When it comes to poultry, many nonorganic chickens are injected with a saltwater solution in order to increase the weight (and therefore the price) of the chicken by as much as 15 percent.

Go Ahead, Try It

My fabulous patient Hilla (you'll remember her from Chapter 7) agreed to share this excellent recipe for Roast Chicken in a Clay Pot—her go-to meal for flawless, wrinkle-free skin. Here's what you'll need:

Clay pot (Roemertopf)	1 cup celery, chopped
1 Organic Chicken	1 cup carrots, chopped
Olive oil	1 cup leeks, chopped
Salt	2 bay leaves
Pepper	5 juniper berries
1 apple, chopped	1 cup chicken broth
1 lemon with peel, chopped	1 cup dry white wine
¼ cup parsley, chopped	Sour cream
½ cup raisins	Organic chicken base
Paprika to taste	seasoning

You can find a good-quality clay pot (also called a Roemertopf) at stores like Williams-Sonoma. Soak in cold water before use (about 15 minutes) and always put the pot in a cold—not preheated—oven; otherwise, it might crack.

Wash the chicken. Rub the inside with olive oil and sprinkle with salt and pepper. Fill with the chopped apple, lemon, parsley, and raisins. Close with kitchen twine or toothpicks.

Make a marinade with olive oil, salt, pepper, and paprika. Brush the marinade on the outside of the chicken. Place the chicken in the pot, breast side down, and add the celery, carrots, leeks, bay leaves, juniper berries, chicken broth, and white wine. Put the cover on the pot and cook at 350° for 1½ hours.

Remove the chicken and place it in an open baking dish. Brush again with olive oil. Raise the heat to 400°, place the chicken in the oven, and brown until crispy (15–20 minutes). The meat will be very tender, and the skin should be crisp.

Discard the bay leaves and put the remaining vegetables from the clay pot in a blender. Blend with a dollop of sour cream and organic chicken base seasonings, and you'll have the perfect gravy without adding flour. Serve with veggies and brown rice.

Serves 4–5

Eggs

One of my patients, Sarah, lives in an incredible modern estate in Malibu, a home so beautiful that it has been featured in a number of architectural and home décor magazines. She also raises chickens in her backyard. (Malibu is packed with well-to-do hippies, people who do a lot of yoga and communing with nature.) Sarah feeds her chickens—which she refers to as her "girls"— every day, and every time she comes to the office, she brings me a dozen hand-fed, hormone- and antibiotic-free, pastel-hued eggs. The flavor is rich, and the yolks are intensely orange—they're like no other eggs I've ever eaten.

Organic eggs come from chickens that are fed on a diet rich in organic cereals and are not treated with routine antibiotics. They are raised in free-range systems in which they are encouraged to roam outdoors and express their natural behaviour. Organic egg standards go further than the requirements for 'free-range' eggs. Chickens who produce free-range eggs can live in very large flocks with limited access to outdoor space and can be fed on genetically modified crops, so this is worth bearing in mind when you are choosing your eggs at the supermarket.

A Word About Calcium . . .

It's my belief that most people eat too much dairy, because even organic milk and dairy products can affect the condition of your skin. (For example, the naturally occurring cow hormone bovine IGF-1 has been linked to increased oil production, elevated insulin production, and heightened androgen levels *in humans.* You can read more about the relationship between dairy products and the skin in Chapter 4.) Despite this, dairy products *are* an excellent source of calcium, which is why everyone on the *Feed Your Face* Diet should take a calcium supplement—and a multivitamin isn't enough.

Multivitamins typically contain iron, which (along with some other vitamins and minerals) will interfere with your body's natural ability to absorb calcium. This means that even if your multi contains calcium, your body won't be able to use it. For that reason, calcium supplements should be taken alone, not alongside other vitamins (including prenatals) and not with an iron-rich meal such as a steak dinner. (You can still take a multivitamin if you like; just take it in the morning and save the calcium pill for later in the day, about an hour or so before lunch *and* dinner. Most calcium supplements are two-a-day doses.) As for what to look for, choose a calcium supplement with vitamin D (because vitamin D actually helps the body absorb the calcium) and aim for 1,000mg to 1,500mg of calcium per day.

Now here's the downside: If you've ever taken a calcium supplement, you know they're horse pills—they're absolutely *huge*. And if you're like me and have a problem swallowing pills, that's not good news. In fact, I once went to brunch with my husband and two friends and decided to take my calcium pill halfway through the meal. Well, it got stuck, right in the middle of my throat. I discreetly took a sip of water and then a bite of omelet in an effort to force it down. When that didn't work, I started gasping for air and finally coughed up the pill—along with a mouthful of water—directly onto the pretty white tablecloth. Conversation halted, and my husband looked over at me, eyebrows raised. "Are you *OK?*" he asked. I was practically on the floor, dying of embarrassment.

Luckily, there are other non-pill forms of calcium that are, in my opinion, much, much easier to take, such as Ellactive Chocolate Calcium Chews. Just know that many calcium chews and gummies *are* sweetened with sugar, so you can't eat them like sweets.

Washing It All Down: What to Drink for Healthy, Hydrated Skin

When it comes to keeping your skin healthy and hydrated, the best thing to drink is, of course, water—and plenty of it. (Dehydrated skin tends to look dry and wrinkly, while rashes and other imperfections can become more pronounced.) But with the insane amount of sodas, sports drinks, and juice cocktails available these days, ordinary tap water can seem, well, boring.

The problem with designer drinks is that the majority of them are loaded with sugar, which can wreak as much havoc on your blood sugar (and your skin) as a giant jam doughnut. A 354ml bottle of Coca-Cola, for example, packs 39g of sugar—that's 10 teaspoons of the sweet stuff *per can*. (Soda can also leach essential vitamins and nutrients—including calcium—from the body.) But even the stuff that *seems* healthy often isn't. For example, Drench Blackcurrant and Apple flavour drink has more than 40g of sugar per 440ml bottle—that's as much as five Krispy Kreme doughnuts. If you're inclined to try some fancy new beverage, don't be fooled by sleek packaging and savvy marketing. Read the label, and if there's any added sugar, put that drink back on the shelf.

What about drinks that promise to give you healthy, glowing skin? I've actually been invited to sit on advisory panels for some of these so-called beauty beverages (manufacturers sometimes ask doctors to provide expert opinions and give feedback on their data before launching a product), and so far I haven't been impressed. Most of the beverages I've reviewed boast a "special" blend of antioxidants that's been formulated (supposedly) to benefit the skin, but the research I've seen is generally weak, unconvincing, or proprietary (meaning the exact blend of ingredients is a closely guarded trade secret, so you don't really know what's in the bottle). Another problem? Some of these drinks are loaded with calories while others contain artificial sweeteners that can cause diarrhea and bloating (I know firsthand). As with all foods, it's imperative to read the label carefully. And don't believe the hype.

Now that we've ruled out all the stuff you shouldn't have, let's talk about what you can drink:

Water. The old "eight glasses a day" adage may be overstating things but we could all use a little more water and a little less coffee and soda in our diets. If plain tap water is too boring, try sparkling water with fresh-squeezed lemon or lime. But try not to reach for Vitamin Water (unless it's the low-sugar, calorie-free version), Antioxidant Water, or any other form of designer H_2O that's high in calories and added sugars.

Green tea is packed with antioxidants called catechins, and it has an anti-inflammatory effect, so it can help soothe conditions such as acne and eczema. Plus, as I mentioned before, green tea has been shown to protect against free radicals from UV rays, giving you added protection against sunburn and sun damage, including roughness, sun spots, and skin cancer. Be sure to drink green tea before, during, and after spending time in the sun. Iced green tea is delicious and refreshing.

Red wine, especially cabernet sauvignon, pinot noir, and merlot, is loaded with antioxidants called flavonoids, and moderate consumption has been shown to reduce sunburn and sun damage. As if that weren't enough, research shows that a daily glass of red can increase your good cholesterol (HDL) by up to 16 percent, as well as lower your bad cholesterol (LDL). Just remember that red wine, like white wine and Champagne, is a fermented beverage that contains histamine, so you'll actually want to avoid it if you have eczema, hives, or psoriasis because histamine can contribute to flare-ups and inflammation. Red wine also contains alcohol by-products, including acetaldehyde, which can cause flushing if you have rosacea.

Fresh-squeezed juice. The first time I had *real* juice, other than the fresh lemonade my mother sometimes made when I was a child, was a few years ago at my friend Scott Barnes's apartment in New York. Scott is an incredible makeup artist to the stars (he counts Jennifer Lopez and Kim Kardashian as clients) as well as a hip New Yorker. He had just visited the famous Union Square farmers' market, and I watched with eager anticipation as he piled leafy green veggies, carrots, apples, and pears high atop his kitchen counters and then ran them all through his juicer. Let me tell you: What came out was incredible. One sip and I couldn't understand why anyone would ever settle for V8. (By the way, one can of regular V8 has 480mg of sodium—that's almost twice the amount of sodium in a single serving bag of Chili Cheese Fritos. If you like V8 and don't have the time or inclination to juice, switch to low-sodium V8, which has only 140mg. It also makes a great low-sodium Bloody Mary mix!)

When you eat fruits and vegetables, you're getting an antioxidant boost plus a ton of fiber—the "pulp" left over that your body can't fully digest. Fiber is great for you, of course—it's like Roto-Rooter for your colon—but you can only have so much in a sitting. Drinking the juice of fruits and vegetables, however, allows you to get a dose of antioxidants without filling up too much. It's also a way to get several servings of fruits and veggies on the go, which is perfect for when you need your hands free to drive or text. (Just keep in mind that fresh juice isn't always low in calories, so one glass a day is all you need.)

Since that day in Scott's kitchen, I decided to make juicing a personal goal of mine, and I've been meaning to buy a juicer . . . for the last few years. (I just haven't quite worked up the energy.) See, I love the *idea* of juicing, but, frankly, it seems like kind of a pain in the ass. All that shopping and chopping. I haven't yet found the time. That's why I haven't officially included juicing in the *Feed Your Face* Diet. (Besides, I promised that no special equipment was required.) Still, I wanted you to be aware of the benefits. If you're at all inclined, I say go for it!

Hey, Dr. Wu

Q: You don't expect me to skip cocktail hour, right? Can I still have alcohol on the Feed Your Face Diet?

A: Absolutely. In fact, dry red wine—cabernet sauvignon, pinot noir, and merlot, in particular—is loaded with antioxidant-rich flavonoids, and research shows that moderate alcohol intake (about a glass of wine a day for women) has proven health benefits. (Chardonnay has the most antioxidants among white wines.) Besides, only a tiny amount of the alcohol you drink gets converted into sugar in the bloodstream. (Drinking on an empty stomach can actually *lower* your blood sugar.) The real health problems with alcohol are its effects on your metabolism:

- Having a drink or two before a meal will decrease insulin and blood sugar levels. That's why you're likely to feel famished after a night of drinking (and why pizza at 3 AM tastes sooo good).
- Alcohol is absorbed into your GI tract and travels to your liver, where it's converted to acetate, which your body uses as fuel. Your body will burn all the acetate before it begins to burn fat, which is why heavy drinkers wind up with a "beer belly."
- Mixed drinks and sweet cocktails provide empty calories with no nutritional value.

To maintain your skin's clarity you'll want to avoid mixed drinks and cocktails with added sugar, such as margaritas and daiquiris. Instead, choose dry red wine, white wine or Champagne, dry sake, or distilled spirits (vodka, rum, whiskey, brandy) served on the rocks or mixed with club soda (not tonic water, which contains high-fructose corn syrup and/or sugar). For a low-sugar mojito, ask the bartender to skip the simple syrup and use club soda instead of Sprite or 7Up. You can also try Shochu, a Japanese spirit that's similar to vodka but has fewer calories. Ask for Shochu at a sushi restaurant or look for it in Asian food markets. Try it the way they drink it in Japan: mixed with cold water, green tea, or grapefruit juice.

What to avoid: Margaritas, daiquiris, cosmos, drinks made with simple syrup (sugar water), dessert wines, liqueurs (Kahlua, Amaretto, Triple Sec), Bailey's Irish Cream, Schnapps, frozen or creamy drinks, tonic water, sugar- and salt-rimmed glasses.

More Tips, Tricks, and Pointers

The *Feed Your Face* Diet isn't just about *what* you eat. When it comes to regulating your blood sugar and controlling flare-ups and breakouts, *when* and *how much* you eat is just as important. Don't forget to do the following:

Watch your portions. I'm not one for weighing your food or obsessively counting calories, but you should always be mindful of how much you're eating—even when the food is *Feed Your Face* friendly. (Having one slice of sprouted grain bread is fine, but *five* slices is not.) Always read the nutrition labels to get a sense of the proper serving size. Serve your meals on smaller dishes (so it *looks* as if you're eating a heaping plateful), and never eat foods—including takeout—straight from the container. Here are some additional guidelines:

A serving of protein (such as chicken, beef, or fish) should be about 3 to 4 ounces, the size of a deck of playing cards or the palm of your hand.

A serving of cooked pasta, lentils, or beans should be somewhere between half a cup and a cup, about the size of your fist.

A serving of nuts should fit in your palm, like a small handful.

A serving of whole wheat crackers is about six crackers.

A smoothie should be somewhere between 12 and 16 ounces or 1½ to 2 cups. Use as much fruit as you like but go easy on the milk and yogurt.

Plan ahead. I attend a lot of evening events, from charity fund-raisers to medical conferences, and they don't often have dinner on the table before 8 or 9 PM. By then I'm ravenously hungry, and it's not hard to work my way through the entire bread basket. That's why I like to "pregame": I'll have a snack while I'm getting ready or in the car on the ride over so that I can control myself until the actual meal is served. Consider having an advance snack the next time you're dining out, and skip the bread basket entirely—reaching for the bread (whether you're hungry or not) is another example of eating on autopilot.

Snack regularly. To keep your blood sugar steady and your insulin in check, eat something small every 3 to 4 hours. The *Feed Your Face* Diet assumes a fairly regular dining schedule: breakfast at 8 AM, a mid-morning snack, lunch at noon, a 3 PM snack, and dinner by 6 or 7 PM. But if you don't eat dinner until much, much later or never have time for a proper lunch, feel free to fill in the gaps with additional snacks and downsize your main meals accordingly.

CELEBRITY SKIN SECRETS—

Kelly Hu's Favorite Snack

Kelly Hu's favorite snack is wheat-free, dairy-free dry roasted almonds which gives her a protein and fiber boost. Plus, almonds can help prevent gray hair!

THE *FEED YOUR FACE* MEAL PLAN

The time has come. By following the 28-day *Feed Your Face* Meal Plan, you'll get a jump on the path to clearer, younger-looking, more radiant skin. It's the no-muss, no-fuss guide to eating foods that will help make wrinkles, sun spots, and blotches a thing of the past. And by incorporating more tomatoes in your diet, you'll get built-in sun protection, too.

When it comes to preparing these meals, the recipes are super-easy to follow. You don't have to stress about exactly how much garlic to use in stuffed bell peppers or how much mayo to mix into your turkey salad; it's all to taste. And remember, don't be afraid to be flexible. If you don't like tofu, swap it for chicken. If you're not near an oven, choose a snack you can grab on the go (like dried fruit and nuts) rather than something you have to heat up (like tomato bruschetta).

You *do* have the power to change your skin. *The Feed Your Face* Meal Plan will get you started.

WEEK ONE

MONDAY

Breakfast: Flax-spiked fruit smoothie (for an omega-3 boost). In a blender, combine frozen blueberries, low-sugar vanilla yogurt or silken tofu, ground flaxseed, and ice. Blend until creamy and smooth. If you have acne, you'll want to avoid dairy. Stick with the silken tofu or use soy yogurt.

Snack: Whole-grain crackers with hummus. If you have rashes (like eczema or psoriasis), you'll want to avoid gluten. Choose gluten-free crackers or swap for veggie dippers. For added sun protection add a cup of green tea.

Lunch: Curried turkey salad—a great alternative to chicken salad! Combine deli-sliced turkey with reduced-fat mayonnaise, curry powder, celery, and red grapes, halved. Serve over crisp romaine lettuce with a whole wheat roll (or gluten-free bread) and a side of baby carrots.

Snack: Piece of fruit (your choice) with natural nut butter.

Dinner: Stuffed bell peppers. Fill red, yellow, and/or orange peppers with a mixture of sautéed extra-lean ground beef, red kidney beans, onion, garlic, tomato sauce (with no added sugars), fresh parsley, red pepper flakes, and cooked brown rice. Bake at 375° for 45 minutes or until peppers are tender and brown at the edges. Serve with a small side salad of mixed greens and light vinaigrette. Get an antioxidant boost (and fight aging) by enjoying a glass of red wine with dinner.

TUESDAY

Breakfast: Slow-cooking porridge oats. Sweeten with a sugar substitute and cinnamon or, for savory oats, a pinch of salt and a nondairy, trans-fat-free margarine spread. Add fresh fruit, such as raspberries or blueberries, and a small handful of nuts. (Try almonds or walnuts.) Avoid instant oatmeal; it's higher on the glycemic index because it's been processed to reduce cooking time.

Snack: Low-fat, low-sugar yogurt and fruit salad made with strawberries, cantaloupe, honeydew melon, and kiwi. If you have acne, skip the yogurt and eat a small handful of walnuts instead.

Lunch: Vegetarian wrap. Spread hummus on a whole wheat (or gluten-free) tortilla and fill with grilled vegetables (such as peppers, zucchini, squash, and onions) or fresh veggies (lettuce, tomatoes, carrots, peppers).

Snack: Whole wheat or gluten-free crackers and grape or cherry tomatoes.

Dinner: Salsa chicken (for a healthy helping of lycopene). Top boneless, skinless chicken breasts with low-sodium salsa (mild, medium, or hot, depending on your preference) and bake until the chicken juices run clear, about 30 minutes at 350°. Top with reduced-fat cheddar cheese and continue baking until the cheese melts. Serve with guacamole or sliced avocados. If you have acne, use a soy cheese or skip it altogether.

WEDNESDAY

Breakfast: Cantaloupe and low-fat cottage cheese (a great lean protein). Add some chopped walnuts or almonds and ground flaxseed for added omega-3s. (If you have acne, replace the cottage cheese with turkey sausage or a vegetarian sausage.)

Snack: Veggie dippers (such as green beans, baby carrots, celery sticks, and sliced red peppers) with hummus.

Lunch: Lentil soup. Find it at your local lunch spot, or try a canned soup (like Amy's Organic, the "light in sodium" variety). Boost the flavor with some fresh parsley and red pepper flakes. Serve with a slice of sprouted grain or gluten-free bread, carrots, snow peas, peppers, or another veggie of your choice.

Snack: Strawberries drizzled with 1 tablespoon of dark chocolate sauce. Melt dark chocolate chips or dark baking chocolate in a double boiler or on *low* in the microwave. Dark chocolate has more antioxidant-rich flavonoids, so choose one with at least 60 percent cocoa—the higher the percentage, the less added sugar.

Dinner: Tofu stir-fry. For an Asian-inspired dish, season cubed extra-firm tofu with low-sodium soy sauce. Cook with sliced peppers, water chestnuts, broccoli, cauliflower, sliced carrots, and peanuts. Serve with a small scoop of brown rice. If you have acne or rosacea, swap the soy sauce for a splash of sesame oil and fresh ginger. If you have hives or eczema, swap the tofu for chicken (tofu is fermented and can sometimes trigger a reaction) and leave out the peanuts.

THURSDAY

Breakfast: PB&J smoothie. (Pour in a traveling mug for an easy grab-and-go breakfast.) In a blender, mix strawberries, plain nonfat yogurt, fat-free or low-fat milk, ice, and a small amount of natural, trans-fat-free peanut butter. If you have acne, use soy milk instead of skim, and silken tofu instead of yogurt.

Snack: Whole wheat or gluten-free crackers and reduced-fat spreadable cheese (such as Laughing Cow) or soy cheese.

Lunch: Chicken Waldorf salad. Combine chopped apples, rotisserie chicken breast, and grape halves with reduced-fat mayonnaise and a splash of fresh lemon juice. Serve over a bed of greens and top with toasted walnuts and a whole wheat or gluten-free roll.

Snack: Edamame or Simply Green Beans.

Dinner: Whole wheat pasta with fresh tomato basil sauce, grilled shrimp, mushrooms, and cherry or grape tomatoes. If you have rashes, choose gluten-free pasta.

FRIDAY

Breakfast: Low-sugar granola and dried cranberries with nonfat milk or low-sugar yogurt. If you have acne, use soy milk instead of skim.

Snack: Choose an orange, tangerine, clementine, or grapefruit and a small handful of unsalted sunflower seeds.

Lunch: Make-your-own salad. Choose leafy greens (such as romaine, baby spinach, or mixed baby greens) and veggies of your choice. Add zinc-rich kidney or garbanzo beans, a lean protein such as grilled chicken, tuna (without mayo), roasted turkey or beef, and unsalted nuts, like pistachios, almonds, or walnuts (all of which are rich in zinc and healthy fats). Dress with a dash of balsamic vinegar and olive oil. If you have rosacea, avoid vinegar and dress with an infused or flavored olive oil.

Snack: Green tea and a small handful of soy nuts.

Dinner: Veggie pizza. Top a whole wheat pizza with a low-sugar tomato sauce, thick tomato slices, roasted peppers, spinach, and broccoli. If you have rashes, check your local health food store for a gluten-free crust or pita. Sprinkle with a *pinch* of reduced-fat or soy cheese.

SATURDAY

Breakfast: Mini whole wheat bagel. Spread with natural unsalted peanut butter or another nut butter (like almond or cashew). Enjoy with a piece of fresh fruit (your choice) and Greek or low-sugar yogurt. If you have rashes, have some gluten-free granola and apple slices with low-sugar yogurt (instead of peanut butter).

Snack: Fruit salad, made with strawberries, cantaloupe, honeydew melon, and kiwi.

Lunch: Turkey burger. Order yours with a whole wheat bun (or go bunless and serve over a green salad). Top with roasted red peppers, lettuce, tomato, and avocado.

Snack: Skim-milk latte with a dash of cinnamon (but skip syrup or flavor "shots," which are loaded with sugar). If you have acne, have a soy latte. To fight aging, have a cup of green tea and a piece of fruit.

Dinner: Zucchini boats—a meal dazzling enough for guests! Halve a zucchini lengthwise and scoop out the center. Stuff with sautéed extra-lean ground beef, onions, garlic, green bell pepper, tomato sauce, and cooked brown rice. Bake at 375° until zucchini is tender, about 15 minutes.

SUNDAY

Breakfast: Egg and tomato stack. Top a whole wheat or gluten-free English muffin with two scrambled eggs and sliced tomatoes. (Or, if you prefer, skip the muffin and use thick tomato slices to sandwich the eggs.) If you have ezcema, you'll want to skip the eggs. Instead, enjoy a smoothie of your choice and a piece of turkey sausage or a vegetarian sausage.

Snack: Sliced pear with natural peanut butter (or another nut butter such as almond or cashew).

Lunch: Spinach salad with baby spinach, grilled or rotisserie chicken, sliced apples, red onions, a small sprinkle of feta or goat cheese, toasted walnuts or almonds, and a low-sugar vinaigrette. If you have acne, skip the cheese. If you have rosacea, dress with olive oil (skip the vinegar).

Snack: Whole wheat or gluten-free crackers and grape or cherry tomatoes.

Dinner: Fish tacos. Marinate a mild white fish (such as halibut) in extra-virgin olive oil, salt, pepper, and lemon juice. Grill. Serve with whole wheat or gluten-free tortillas, shredded lettuce, chopped tomatoes, low-sodium salsa, and guacamole.

WEEK TWO

MONDAY

Breakfast: Whole-grain, low-sugar cereal. Choose one with less than 9g of sugar and more than 3g of fiber. Serve with fresh berries and soy milk. If you have rashes, choose a gluten-free cereal.

Snack: Piece of fruit (your choice).

Lunch: Chicken Caesar wrap. Fill a whole wheat or gluten-free tortilla with crisp romaine, chicken, a low-sugar dressing or vinaigrette, and a sprinkle of Parmesan cheese. Add a side of baby carrots or sliced peppers. If you have acne, skip the cheese.

Snack: Grape or cherry tomatoes with a part-skim or soy string cheese.

Dinner: Shrimp scampi. Sauté the shrimp (which is rich in protein but low in mercury) in extra-virgin olive oil. Add mushrooms, grape or cherry tomatoes (halved), lemon juice, garlic, a splash of white wine, a pat of butter, seasoning, and red pepper flakes. Meanwhile, cook whole wheat or gluten-free linguini. Top it with the cooked shrimp. If you have acne, leave out the butter.

TUESDAY

Breakfast: Orange soy smoothie. In a blender combine silken tofu, vanilla soy milk, a banana, ice, and a splash of orange juice. Sweeten with honey if desired.

Snack: A small handful of dried fruit and nuts. Try dried cherries and almonds. To fight aging, swap the almonds for selenium-rich Brazil nuts.

Lunch: Minestrone or gazpacho with a slice of sprouted grain or gluten-free toast and a few slices of deli turkey.

Snack: Veggie dippers and hummus.

Dinner: Pesto chicken and stuffed tomatoes. Brush store-bought pesto (made with olive oil) on top of skinless, boneless chicken breasts. Bake until the juices run clear, about 30 minutes at 350°. Slice large beefsteak tomatoes in half and scoop out the inside, discarding the seeds and reserving the pulp. Combine garlic, onion, fresh parsley, Parmesan cheese, cooked brown rice, olive oil, salt, pepper, and tomato pulp. Stuff the tomatoes with the mixture and bake for 20–25 minutes. If you have acne, skip the cheese.

WEDNESDAY

Breakfast: Scrambled eggs and smoked salmon (rich in omega-3s). Fold sliced smoked salmon, reduced-fat cream cheese, and chopped chives or scallions into scrambled eggs and warm. Serve with fresh berries. If you have acne, skip the cream cheese. For eczema, have rolled oats with some flaxseed and a piece of fruit instead of eggs.

Snack: Choose an orange, tangerine, clementine, or grapefruit and a small handful of unsalted sunflower seeds.

Lunch: Deli sandwich. Order yours on whole wheat bread or pita, and add fresh fillings such as roasted turkey, grilled or rotisserie chicken, or lean roast beef. Add lettuce, tomato, and mustard. If you have rashes, choose a gluten-free wrap or enjoy a chef's salad with turkey instead of a sandwich.

Snack: Tomato bruschetta. Top a slice of sprouted grain or gluten-free bread with a mixture of chopped tomatoes, garlic, fresh basil, salt, pepper, and olive oil. Warm under the broiler for 3–4 minutes.

Dinner: Sliced sirloin with black beans and rice. Top quinoa or brown rice with shredded carrots, zucchini, squash, peas, red onion, red peppers, black beans, and sliced sirloin.

THURSDAY

Breakfast: Ruby red grapefruit (another excellent source of lycopene). Sprinkle with a sugar substitute or try roasting in the toaster oven. Pair with nonfat Greek yogurt or low-fat cottage cheese. If you have acne, choose nondairy yogurt or a veggie sausage link instead of Greek yogurt or cottage cheese.

Snack: Whole wheat or gluten-free crackers and spreadable reduced-fat cheese (such as Laughing Cow) or soy cheese.

Lunch: Pasta salad. (Make a big batch, and you can enjoy it for several days.) Start with cooked whole-grain, spiral-shaped pasta. Add grilled chicken, steamed broccoli, red peppers, and grape tomatoes. Season with low-sugar vinaigrette or a splash of balsamic vinegar and extra-virgin olive oil. If you have rashes, choose gluten-free pasta. If you have rosacea, avoid the vinegar.

Snack: Veggie dippers with hummus.

Dinner: Fish with tomatoes, olives, and capers. This easy-to-prepare dish is a great source of vitamin C and lycopene. Sauté any white fish of your choice (such as halibut, sole, or tilapia). While cooking, mix store-bought low-sodium salsa with chopped kalamata olives and capers. When the fish is almost done, pour sauce over it and warm. Serve with a mixed green salad.

FRIDAY

Breakfast: Chocolate smoothie—sure to become an instant classic! In a blender combine silken tofu, vanilla soy milk, banana, ice, and unsweetened cocoa powder. Add a pinch of artificial sweetener if desired.

Snack: Low-sugar or nondairy yogurt (such as coconut yogurt).

Lunch: Greek salad made with romaine lettuce, kalamata olives (use what's left over from last night's dinner), feta cheese, red peppers, tomatoes, and red onion.

Snack: A small handful of dried fruit and nuts. Try dried apricots and walnuts.

Dinner: Beef and bean chili. Make a big batch of this skin-soothing chili and freeze it in smaller containers to eat later in the week. Sauté extra-lean ground beef with chopped onions, red and green peppers, and garlic. Add crushed tomatoes (choose a can with only tomatoes listed in the ingredients to avoid added sugars and sodium), red kidney beans, black beans, cumin, paprika, chili powder, and low-sodium beef broth (or water). Let the mixture simmer until the flavors combine, about 30 minutes. Fight aging with a glass of red wine at dinner.

SATURDAY

Breakfast: Yogurt parfait. Layer low-fat or nonfat Greek yogurt with fresh berries. Sprinkle with flaxseed to nourish your skin with essential minerals. If you have acne, swap regular yogurt for nondairy yogurt.

Snack: Piece of fruit (your choice).

Lunch: Tuna Niçoise salad. This Mediterranean salad contains a host of anti-aging ingredients, and it's an ideal choice when ordering from a menu. To make a simple version at home, combine light tuna canned in water, one hard-boiled egg, steamed green beans (fresh or frozen), cherry tomatoes, Niçoise or kalamata olives, sliced red onions, roasted new potatoes, and romaine or Bibb lettuce. Add low-sugar vinaigrette. If you have acne, leave out the potatoes. If you have rosacea, dress with olive oil (skip the vinegar).

Snack: Vegetable juice cocktail (choose low-sodium V8 or juice your own veggies) and soy nuts.

Dinner: Pasta with walnuts. Toss cooked whole wheat pasta with toasted walnuts, prosciutto or deli ham, chopped baby spinach, roasted garlic, and extra-virgin olive oil. Sprinkle with a pinch of Parmesan cheese. If you have rashes, choose gluten-free pasta.

SUNDAY

Brunch: Vegetable frittata. Frittatas are easier to prepare than omelets but just as tasty. Serve this with a green salad for a light but delicious protein-rich meal. Sauté chopped peppers and onions in a small ovenproof frying pan. Beat the eggs and then pour into the vegetable mixture. Let the eggs set on the sides; the middle will remain uncooked. Sprinkle with a small amount of sharp cheese and heat under a grill until the middle is cooked. Serve with a piece of fresh fruit or some berries. If you have acne, use soy cheese or skip it altogether. If you have rashes, opt for gluten-free pancakes (available at most health-food stores), fresh fruit, and Greek yogurt.

Snack: Spread one slice of toasted whole wheat or gluten-free bread with natural peanut butter.

Lunch: Tomato soup and toasted cheese. When it comes to lycopene, this rich soup is a superstar. Look for one that doesn't have high-fructose corn syrup, cream, or lots of sodium. Enjoy with an open-faced toasted cheese: Using an olive oil cooking spray, toast a slice of sprouted grain or gluten-free bread and top with one slice of low-sodium mozzarella. If you have acne, use soy cheese.

Snack: Piece of fruit and small handful of almonds.

Dinner: Orange pork tenderloin. This vitamin C-rich dinner is great for soothing dry skin. Combine 1 cup of orange juice, ¼ cup of low-sodium soy sauce, garlic, and a dash of honey. Pan-sear pork tenderloin cutlets to brown both sides, then add the orange juice mixture to the pan and cook for another two minutes. Transfer pork to a roasting dish and cook at 400° until the internal temperature of the pork reaches 155°. Serve with a side of steamed green beans. If you have acne or rosacea, swap the soy sauce for 2 tablespoons of spicy mustard and a splash of wheat-free Worcestershire sauce.

WEEK THREE

MONDAY

Breakfast: Strawberry smoothie. In a blender, add frozen strawberries (be sure to choose a package with no added sugars), soy milk, ground flaxseed, and ice. Blend until creamy and frothy.

Snack: Whole wheat or gluten-free crackers and hummus.

Lunch: Make-your-own salad. Choose leafy greens (such as romaine, baby spinach, or mixed baby greens) and green, red, or yellow vegetables of your choice. (Try green beans!) Add zinc-rich kidney beans, a lean protein such as grilled chicken, grilled turkey, grilled tofu, or beef. Also add a small handful of unsalted nuts (rich in zinc and healthy fats). Dress with a dash of balsamic vinegar and olive oil. If you have rosacea, dress with olive oil (skip the vinegar).

Snack: Piece of fruit (your choice).

Dinner: Nut-crusted halibut. Halibut is another omega-3-rich fish, so it's something to try in lieu of salmon. Dredge halibut fillets in whole wheat flour and egg wash (use just the whites), then coat with finely chopped walnuts, pecans, or pistachios, pressing to adhere. Bake or grill. If you have acne or rashes, dredge the halibut in a *small* amount of whole wheat flour or skip this step altogether. Serve over brown rice with a side of steamed veggies, such as broccoli.

TUESDAY

Breakfast: Slow-cooking porridge oats with blueberries and a sprinkle of flaxseed or a small handful of nuts, such as almonds or walnuts.

Snack: Yogurt parfait. Layer low-fat or nonfat Greek yogurt with fresh berries.

Lunch: Japanese lunch. Try sashimi instead of sushi rolls, which are typically made with white rice. While sushi rolls made with brown rice are fine, be careful about spicy rolls, which are often made with mayonnaise, and dragon rolls with tempura, which are rolls that have been deep-fried. Your best bets are salmon, tuna, and white fish. Enjoy with a side of edamame and a green salad with a splash of ginger dressing. If you have acne, avoid sushi rolls—the seaweed contains iodine, a common acne irritant. If you're pregnant, you'll want to avoid raw fish. Most Japanese restaurants have a baked fish option (such as cod or salmon), or go with the Kobe beef.

Snack: Veggie dippers with baba ghanoush (Middle Eastern eggplant dip).

Dinner: Chicken pasta. Top whole wheat rigatoni with a mixture of sautéed sliced portobello mushrooms, garlic, fresh parsley, rosemary, sun-dried tomatoes, green onions, and grilled or baked chicken. Dress with balsamic vinaigrette. If you have rashes, choose gluten-free pasta. If you have rosacea, toss with an infused olive oil (skip the vinegar).

WEDNESDAY

Breakfast: Whole-grain, low-sugar cereal with fresh berries and soy milk.

Snack: Choose an orange, tangerine, clementine, tangelo, or grapefruit and a small handful of sunflower seeds.

Lunch: Healthy BLT made with sprouted grain or gluten-free bread, low-fat mayonnaise or mustard, and low-sodium turkey bacon.

Snack: Cottage cheese or soy yogurt and an apple.

Dinner: Vegetable and beef kebabs. Thread cubed beef tenderloin on a skewer, alternating with zucchini, button mushrooms, quartered red onions, and grape tomatoes. Fire up the barbecue or use an indoor grill pan. Serve over brown rice, quinoa, or couscous.

THURSDAY

Breakfast: Low-sugar granola and dried cranberries with nonfat milk or Greek yogurt. If you have acne, choose soy milk.

Snack: Whole-grain or gluten-free crackers and hummus.

Lunch: Chinese chicken salad. Top shredded red and green cabbage with shredded chicken, carrots, bean sprouts, peanuts, and green onion. Toss with a peanut vinaigrette or a splash of sesame oil and low-sodium soy sauce. If you have eczema, skip the peanuts and opt for sesame oil and gluten-free soy sauce over peanut vinaigrette.

Snack: A small handful of dried fruit and nuts. Try dried apples and pecans.

Dinner: Turkey meatballs and marinara. Combine lean ground turkey, grated onion, minced garlic, egg whites (to combine), whole wheat bread crumbs, fresh parsley, and Parmesan cheese. Roll into meatballs. Sauté until browned on all sides and then simmer in store-bought, low-sodium marinara sauce (with no added sugars) for 20–25 minutes. Serve with a small mixed green salad. Fight aging with a glass of red wine at dinner.

FRIDAY

Breakfast: Flax-spiked smoothie. In a blender combine frozen blueberries, vanilla yogurt or silken tofu, ground flaxseed, and ice. Blend until creamy and smooth. If you have acne, swap the yogurt for soy yogurt or stick with the silken tofu.

Snack: Baby carrots or Simply Green Beans.

Lunch: Chicken Caesar salad. Toss crisp romaine and grilled or rotisserie chicken with a low-sugar dressing or vinaigrette. Add a sprinkle of Parmesan cheese. If you have acne, skip the cheese.

Snack: Tomato bruschetta. Top a slice of sprouted grain or gluten-free bread with a mixture of chopped tomatoes, garlic, basil, salt, pepper, and olive oil. Warm under the grill for 3–4 minutes. Spending some time in the sun? Get extra UV protection by spreading a bit of cooked tomato paste on your bread.

Dinner: Flank steak fajitas. Marinate flank steak with orange juice, garlic, coriander, cumin, orange zest, fresh lime juice, and two chipotle chilies (in adobo sauce). Grill and then serve with black beans, low-sodium salsa, and sautéed onions and peppers.

SATURDAY

Breakfast: Baked apples. Core large apples and fill with a mixture of chopped pecans or walnuts, lemon zest, a splash of fresh lemon juice, cinnamon, and a dollop of honey. Place apples in a baking dish and add ½ to 1 cup of water or apple cider. Bake at 400° for about 30 minutes, until tender but not mushy.

Snack: Piece of fruit (your choice).

Lunch: Portobello mushroom burger. Thick and meaty portobellos are a great alternative to beef. Grill or roast mushroom caps and top with grilled onions and roasted red peppers, a slice of Swiss cheese, and rocket. Serve on a whole wheat bun. If you have acne, skip the cheese. If you have rashes, go bunless and serve over a green salad.

Snack: A small handful of dried fruits and seeds or nuts. Try dried cranberries and pumpkin seeds.

Dinner: Salmon-in-a-pouch. In the center of a single piece of parchment paper, make a small bed of green beans or asparagus. Season a salmon fillet with salt and pepper and nestle in the greens. Top with lemon slices, diced tomato, basil leaves, and olive oil. Gather up the ends of the parchment paper to make a "pouch" and secure with kitchen twine. Place the pouch on a baking sheet and cook at 375° for 15–20 minutes. Serve with a small side of brown rice.

SUNDAY

Breakfast: Veggie omelet (use one whole egg and two egg whites) with mushrooms, peppers, and onions. If you have eczema, enjoy a smoothie of your choice and a piece of turkey sausage or a veggie sausage link.

Snack: Grape or cherry tomatoes with a part-skim or soy string cheese.

Lunch: Spinach-avocado-orange salad. Start with baby spinach and add sliced avocado, orange sections, red pepper, and roasted or grilled chicken or turkey. Drizzle with a low-sugar vinaigrette or a dash of balsamic vinegar and extra-virgin olive oil. If you have rosacea, dress with olive oil (skip the vinegar).

Dinner: "Fried" chicken with Southwestern salad. This meal will give you the sensation of a fried dish, but it's actually baked and therefore perfectly healthy. Combine salt, pepper, almond slivers, and whole wheat bread crumbs. Dredge boneless, skinless chicken breasts in whole wheat flour, egg wash (use only the whites), and the bread crumb mixture, coating all sides. Bake at 350° until the juices run clear, about 30 minutes. For the salad, combine black beans, grilled corn, diced tomato, onion, garlic, and diced jalapeño. Dress with a mix of olive oil, fresh lime juice, salt, pepper, cumin, and coriander. If you have rashes, use gluten-free bread crumbs or crushed rice crackers.

Snack (or Dessert!): Grilled peaches. Cut peaches in half, remove pits, and brush with olive oil. Grill the peaches cut-side down. Meanwhile, simmer ½ cup of balsamic vinegar in a saucepan until thick. Drizzle over the peaches. Serve with Greek yogurt. If you have rosacea, skip the balsamic vinegar glaze.

WEEK FOUR

MONDAY

Breakfast: Whole-grain (or gluten-free) waffle with natural peanut butter and fresh berries.

Snack: Veggie dippers and hummus.

Lunch: Tuna Niçoise salad. Combine light tuna canned in water, one hard-boiled egg, steamed green beans (fresh or frozen), cherry tomatoes, Niçoise or kalamata olives, sliced red onions, roasted new potatoes, and romaine lettuce. Add low-sugar vinaigrette. If you have acne, leave out the potatoes. If you have rosacea, dress with olive oil (skip the vinegar).

Snack: Hot chocolate and strawberries. Make hot chocolate with unsweetened cocoa powder and light vanilla soy milk.

Dinner: Pizza Margherita. Top a whole-wheat pizza crust with a low-sugar tomato sauce, thick tomato slices, chopped fresh basil, and a pinch of shredded mozzarella or soy cheese. Top with a drizzle of olive oil. If you have rashes, choose a premade, gluten-free crust.

TUESDAY

Breakfast: Mix low-fat cottage cheese with cinnamon. Top with berries and a low-sugar, high-fiber cereal. If you have acne or rashes, have a smoothie of your choice and a piece of turkey sausage or a vegetarian sausage.

Snack: Small handful of dried fruit and seeds or nuts. Get a flavonoid boost (and fight aging) by adding a few squares of extra-dark chocolate (at least 60 percent cocoa) to your snack.

Lunch: Greek salad wrap. Fill a whole-wheat tortilla with romaine lettuce, kalamata olives, feta cheese, red peppers, tomatoes, and red onion. If you have acne, replace the feta with chicken. If you have rashes, choose a gluten-free wrap or enjoy a Greek salad rather than a sandwich.

Snack: Low-sugar or soy yogurt and fruit salad made with strawberries, cantaloupe, honeydew melon, and kiwi.

Dinner: Pork tenderloin with apples and onions. Season the tenderloin with salt and pepper and pan-sear until brown on all sides. Transfer the pork to a roasting dish and rub with 2 tablespoons of Dijon mustard. Chop the apples and onions, sauté them, and then place around the pork. Roast at 400° until the internal temperature of the pork reaches 155°. Serve with steamed green beans.

WEDNESDAY

Breakfast: Sun-dried tomato scramble. Sauté sliced mushrooms, sun-dried tomatoes, and baby spinach. Add the mixture to eggs (one whole and two whites) and scramble. If you have eczema, enjoy porridge oats with fresh berries and flaxseed instead of eggs.

Snack: One slice of reduced-fat string cheese with a piece of fruit. If you have acne, swap the string cheese for a small handful of dried nuts.

Lunch: Minestrone or gazpacho with sprouted grain or gluten-free toast and a few slices of deli turkey.

Snack: Whole wheat or gluten-free crackers and hummus.

Dinner: Pesto chicken. Brush store-bought pesto (made with olive oil) on top of skinless, boneless chicken breasts. Bake at 350° until juices run clear, about 30 minutes. Serve with a medley of sautéed vegetables such as zucchini, squash, onions, and sweet potatoes.

THURSDAY

Breakfast: Chocolate smoothie. In a blender combine silken tofu, vanilla soy milk, banana, ice, and unsweetened cocoa powder. Add a pinch of artificial sweetener if desired.

Snack: Piece of fruit (your choice).

Lunch: Spinach salad with baby spinach, grilled or rotisserie chicken, sliced apples, red onions, a small sprinkle of feta or goat cheese, toasted walnuts, and a low-sugar vinaigrette. If you have rosacea, dress with olive oil (skip the vinegar).

Snack: Vegetable juice cocktail (choose low-sodium V8 or juice your own veggies) and soy nuts.

Dinner: Grilled, poached, or baked salmon. Serve on a bed of lentils with green beans or some other green, yellow, and/or red vegetable of your choice.

FRIDAY

Breakfast: Slow-cooking porridge oats. Sweeten with a sugar substitute and cinnamon or a pinch of salt and a nondairy, trans-fat-free margarine spread. Top with fresh berries and a sprinkle of flaxseed.

Snack: Green tea and a small handful of soy nuts.

Lunch: Chef's salad with sliced turkey, one hard-boiled egg, tomato, cucumbers, and soy cheese. If you have eczema, omit the hard-boiled egg.

Snack: Edamame.

Dinner: Dine out! Splurge on a restaurant meal or enjoy takeout in the comfort of your living room. Just make sure you're getting a balanced meal with vegetables, lean protein, and a side of whole grains. For help choosing the healthiest option, turn to the *Feed Your Face* Guide to Eating Out on page 275.

SATURDAY

Breakfast: Whole wheat pancakes. Choose a whole wheat (or gluten-free) pancake mix and top with wild blueberries and Greek yogurt.

Snack: Choose an orange, tangerine, clementine, or grapefruit and pair with a small handful of unsalted sunflower seeds.

Lunch: Make-your-own salad. Choose leafy greens (such as romaine, baby spinach, or mixed baby greens) and any green, yellow, or red veggies of your choice. Add zinc-rich kidney or garbanzo beans, a lean protein such as grilled chicken, roasted turkey, grilled tofu, or beef, and unsalted nuts (rich in zinc and healthy fats). Dress with a dash of balsamic vinegar and olive oil. If you have rosacea, dress with an infused or flavored olive oil (skip the vinegar).

Snack: Veggie dippers and hummus.

Dinner: Grilled lamb chops and stuffed tomatoes. Brush a little extra-virgin olive oil on lamb chops and season with kosher salt, pepper, and crushed garlic. Grill the lamb chops. Slice large beefsteak tomatoes in half and scoop out the inside, discarding seeds and reserving pulp. Combine garlic, fresh parsley, Parmesan cheese, cooked brown rice, olive oil, salt, pepper, and tomato pulp. Stuff tomatoes with the mixture and bake for 20–25 minutes. To fight aging, have a glass of antioxidant-rich red wine with dinner.

SUNDAY

Breakfast: Breakfast burrito. Fill a warmed 8-inch whole wheat or gluten-free tortilla with a scrambled egg, sliced avocado, and salsa. (Hint: The lycopene is best absorbed when paired with a little fat, making avocado a vital part of this dish.) If you have eczema, skip the eggs. Enjoy a smoothie of your choice and a piece of turkey sausage or a veggie sausage link instead.

Snack: A small handful of dried fruit and seeds or nuts.

Lunch: Tomato soup and toasted cheese, with sprouted grain or gluten-free bread and low-sodium mozzarella. If you have acne, choose soy cheese.

Snack: Piece of fruit (your choice).

Dinner: Beef and turkey meatloaf. Combine ground beef and ground turkey, Italian-style (or gluten-free) bread crumbs, onion, garlic, tomato paste, Worcestershire sauce, parsley, one egg white, salt, and pepper. Form into a loaf. Baste with ½ cup low-sugar ketchup (with no added sugar). Bake at 350° for approximately 1 hour. Serve with steamed asparagus.

The *Feed Your Face* Diet—at a Glance

	Monday	Tuesday	Wednesday	Thursday	Friday	Saturday	Sunday
Week 1	BREAKFAST: Flax-spiked smoothie	BREAKFAST: Porridge	BREAKFAST: Cantaloupe and cottage cheese	BREAKFAST: PB&J smoothie	BREAKFAST: Granola and dried cranberries	BREAKFAST: Mini-bagel and peanut butter	BREAKFAST: Egg and tomato stack
	SNACK: Crackers with hummus	SNACK: Fruit salad and yogurt	SNACK: Veggie dippers and hummus	SNACK: Crackers and cheese	SNACK: Citrus fruit and sunflower seeds	SNACK: Fruit salad	SNACK: Pear with peanut butter
	LUNCH: Curried turkey salad	LUNCH: Veggie wrap	LUNCH: Lentil soup	LUNCH: Chicken Waldorf salad	LUNCH: Make-your-own salad	LUNCH: Turkey burger	LUNCH: Spinach salad
	SNACK: Fruit (your choice)	SNACK: Crackers and cherry tomatoes	SNACK: Chocolate and strawberries	SNACK: Edamame	SNACK: Green tea and soy nuts	SNACK: Skim-milk latte	SNACK: Crackers and cherry tomatoes
	DINNER: Stuffed peppers with side salad	DINNER: Salsa chicken and avocado	DINNER: Tofu stir-fry	DINNER: Whole wheat pasta and tomato basil sauce	DINNER: Veggie pizza	DINNER: Zucchini boats	DINNER: Fish tacos

The *Feed Your Face* Diet—at a Glance *(continued)*

	Monday	Tuesday	Wednesday	Thursday	Friday	Saturday	Sunday
Week 2	BREAKFAST: Low-sugar cereal and berries	BREAKFAST: Orange-soy smoothie	BREAKFAST: Eggs and lox	BREAKFAST: Red grapefruit and yogurt	BREAKFAST: Chocolate smoothie	BREAKFAST: Yogurt parfait	BREAKFAST: Veggie frittata
	SNACK: Fruit (your choice)	SNACK: Dried cherries and almonds	SNACK: Citrus fruit and sunflower seeds	SNACK: Crackers and soy cheese	SNACK: Yogurt	SNACK: Fruit (your choice)	SNACK: Peanut butter on toast
	LUNCH: Chicken Caesar wrap	LUNCH: Minestrone or gazpacho	LUNCH: Deli sandwich	LUNCH: Pasta salad	LUNCH: Greek salad	LUNCH: Tuna Niçoise salad	LUNCH: Tomato soup and toasted cheese
	SNACK: Grape tomatoes and cheese	SNACK: Veggie dippers and hummus	SNACK: Tomato bruschetta	SNACK: Veggie dippers and hummus	SNACK: Dried apricots and walnuts	SNACK: Vegetable juice and soy nuts	SNACK: Fruit and nuts
	DINNER: Shrimp scampi	DINNER: Pesto chicken and stuffed tomatoes	DINNER: Sirloin with black beans and rice	DINNER: Fish with tomatoes and capers	DINNER: Beef and bean chili	DINNER: Pasta with walnuts	DINNER: Orange pork and green beans

The *Feed Your Face* Diet—at a Glance *(continued)*

	Monday	Tuesday	Wednesday	Thursday	Friday	Saturday	Sunday
Week 3	BREAKFAST: Strawberry smoothie	BREAKFAST: Porridge and blueberries	BREAKFAST: Low-sugar cereal	BREAKFAST: Granola and cranberries	BREAKFAST: Flax-spiked smoothie	BREAKFAST: Baked apples	BREAKFAST: Veggie omelet
	SNACK: Crackers and hummus	SNACK: Yogurt parfait	SNACK: Citrus fruit and sunflower seeds	SNACK: Crackers and hummus	SNACK: Baby carrots	SNACK: Fruit (your choice)	SNACK: Cheese and cherry tomatoes
	LUNCH: Make-your-own salad	LUNCH: Sushi	LUNCH: Healthy BLT	LUNCH: Chinese chicken salad	LUNCH: Chicken Caesar salad	LUNCH: Portobello burger	LUNCH: Spinach-avocado-orange salad
	SNACK: Piece of fruit (your choice)	SNACK: Veggies and baba ganoush	SNACK: Yogurt and apple slices	SNACK: Dried apples and pecans	SNACK: Tomato bruschetta	SNACK: Dried cranberries and pumpkin seeds	DINNER: "Fried" chicken
	DINNER: Nut-crusted halibut	DINNER: Rigatoni with chicken and mushrooms	DINNER: Veggie and beef kebabs	DINNER: Turkey meatballs	DINNER: Flank steak fajitas	DINNER: Salmon-in-a pouch with rice	SNACK: Grilled peaches

The *Feed Your Face* Diet—at a Glance *(continued)*

	Monday	Tuesday	Wednesday	Thursday	Friday	Saturday	Sunday
Week 4	BREAKFAST: Waffles with peanut butter and berries	BREAKFAST: Cereal and cottage cheese	BREAKFAST: Sun-dried tomato scramble	BREAKFAST: Chocolate smoothie	BREAKFAST: Porridge	BREAKFAST: Whole wheat pancakes	BREAKFAST: Burrito
	SNACK: Veggie dippers and hummus	SNACK: Dried fruit and nuts or seeds	SNACK: Reduced-fat string cheese	SNACK: Fruit (your choice)	SNACK: Green tea and soy nuts	SNACK: Citrus fruit and sun-flower seeds	SNACK: Dried fruit and nuts
	LUNCH: Tuna Niçoise salad	LUNCH: Greek salad wrap	LUNCH: Minestrone or gazpacho	LUNCH: Spinach salad	LUNCH: Chef's salad with turkey	LUNCH: Make-your-own salad	LUNCH: Tomato soup and toasted cheese
	SNACK: Hot chocolate and strawberries	SNACK: Fruit salad and yogurt	SNACK: Crackers and hummus	SNACK: Vegetable juice and soy nuts	SNACK: Edamame	SNACK: Veggie dippers and hummus	SNACK: Fruit (your choice)
	DINNER: Pizza Margherita	DINNER: Pork with apples and onions	DINNER: Chicken pesto with sautéed veggies	DINNER: Salmon and lentils	DINNER: Dine out!	DINNER: Lamb chops and stuffed tomatoes	DINNER: Beef and turkey meatloaf

10

The Feed Your Face Guide to Eating Out

Just because you're making healthier choices and eating for better skin doesn't mean you can't ever eat at TGI Friday's again. You can, but don't go crazy.

The *Feed Your Face* Guide to Eating Out will help you choose the best options available at some of the country's most popular eateries as well as provide you with general guidelines for dining on your favorite cuisine, whether it's at your favorite steak restaurant, the family-style Italian place, or the local sushi bar. However, you can't dine out *every* night and expect to get the same results you would by preparing meals in your own kitchen. That's because you can't control the amount of salt, sugar, cream, or butter that restaurant fare is prepared with, so sometimes food that seems healthy (or *Feed Your Face* friendly) is actually not that good for you.

Restaurant portions are—across the board—way, *way* larger than what's actually appropriate to eat in a sitting. Ask your waiter or waitress to place half your meal in a take-out container *before* bringing it to the table or split an entree with your buddy. Don't eat the whole portion by yourself.

Try to choose foods you could hunt or gather or foods that are as close as possible to their "natural state." That means nothing fried, breaded, or crusted. Remember, the more "unnatural" the food, the more it's been processed, refined, and stripped of essential nutrients (as well as pumped full of Skin Enemies such as salt, sugar, and dairy to make it irresistible).

You'll also still need to stick to the basics of the *Feed Your Face* Diet. If you have acne and you're avoiding all dairy foods, you'll need to ask the waiter to hold the cheese on any sandwiches, salads, or entrees. Likewise, if you have rosacea and you're avoiding vinegar, you'll need to skip commercial salad dressings and opt for olive oil *on the side*.

If You Like to Dine . . .

. . . at the Steak House

It *is* possible to eat a *Feed Your Face*–friendly meal at the neighborhood steak house, but you'll have to watch it. Steak houses are particularly good at making healthy foods (such as salads and spinach) really *unhealthy* (think: an iceberg lettuce wedge smothered in blue cheese dressing, or creamed spinach).

If you're opting for steak (and why wouldn't you, since beef is a good source of zinc, which is essential for building healthy collagen and elastin as well as fighting acne), choose the leanest cut you can find (like sirloin or tenderloin rather than rib eye or prime rib). Also, ask for any and all sauces *on the side*. Extra points if you can skip the sauce altogether. If you must have the sauce, try dipping just your fork in it, for a hint of flavor. Avoid drowning your steak.

Remember that whenever you're eating a meal that is relatively high in saturated fat (particularly beef), you'll want to add plenty of green and yellow veggies. (People who eat a lot of sat fat *and* green and yellow veggies have fewer wrinkles than those who don't.) For an extra antioxidant boost, enjoy a glass of red wine (preferably cabernet sauvignon, pinot noir, or merlot).

Your Best Bets
- Shrimp cocktail, but go easy on the cocktail sauce, which is usually high in sugar.

- Spinach or mixed green salad; hold the egg, bacon, and cheese, and ask for oil and vinegar on the side
- Sides of steamed or sautéed spinach, asparagus, broccoli, or tomatoes
- Fresh lobster; get the butter on the side and use it *sparingly*!
- Lamb chops (roasted or grilled is better than panfried). Cut off any visible fat.

Steer Clear of

- Iceberg wedge salads, which taste good only because they come loaded with blue cheese dressing and bacon bits. Even though it's a "salad," the iceberg wedge is often packed with saturated fat and sugar (and little to no protein or fiber).
- Potatoes
- Anything "creamed" or "au gratin"
- Sauces on your salad, entree, or veggies

. . . At an Italian Ristorante

You may equate Italian restaurants with a heaping plate of pasta, but there are *Feed Your Face*–friendly options available. Since very few establishments offer whole wheat pasta and the servings are typically two, three, or even four times the amount you should be eating in a sitting, opt instead for a salad and a nonpasta entree such as grilled or roasted chicken, seafood, or lean meat dishes. If pasta comes on the side (and you just can't resist), limit yourself to a few bites to avoid a major spike in blood sugar. Wash it down with Pellegrino (sparkling mineral water) or a glass of Chianti, Barolo, Barbaresco, or another red wine.

Your Best Bets

- Grilled vegetable antipasto
- Green or spinach salad
- Thin-crust (instead of thick-crust) pizza; add extra sun-dried tomatoes and/or chopped tomatoes
- Pomodoro (tomato) sauce
- Anything with sun-dried tomatoes or chopped tomatoes

Steer Clear of
- Fried mozzarella and calamari
- Creamy sauces (Alfredo, carbonara)
- Cheesy dishes (lasagna, ziti)
- Breaded dishes (parmigiana dishes)
- Risotto and gnocchi

. . . At the Chinese Buffet

The majority of Chinese restaurants do not serve traditional Chinese fare. Instead they offer westernized dishes my grandmother wouldn't even recognize—entrees dripping with duck sauce, packed with salt and MSG, and served on a towering mound of white rice or greasy noodles. Keep your meal *Feed Your Face*-approved by asking for brown rice (or skipping the rice altogether), choosing grilled or steamed entrees, and using sauce sparingly, if at all. (I'll admit that even I have problems avoiding the fried rice—it smells so good!—so I often mix just a *little* bit of fried rice in with my brown rice for a kick of flavor.) For a healthy helping of antioxidants (and a boost in UV protection) drink hot or iced green tea.

Your Best Bets
- Lettuce wraps (go easy on the sauce)
- Steamed dumplings (instead of deep-fried or pan-fried)
- Grilled or steamed fish or shrimp
- Baked or stir-fried chicken, pork, and lean meat dishes
- Stir-fried vegetables
- Stir-fried green beans

Steer Clear of
- Fried rice
- Noodles
- Egg rolls
- Dishes with sauce (such as sweet and sour, lobster, or hoisin sauce). If you must have one of these dishes, ask for the sauce on the side.

. . . At the American Bar & Grill

A hamburger and fries might seem like the ultimate all-American meal, but it's not going to do much for the health of your skin (or the size of your waistline). "American food" has unfortunately become somewhat synonymous with unhealthy food and unhealthy eating habits (such as smothering your fries in ketchup and chasing your burger with a huge glass of Coke). Avoid the temptation to eat large portions of fried or breaded foods or to drown your salad in a creamy dressing. Opt instead for grilled or baked lean meats and fresh or steamed vegetables (preferably not smothered in sauce or butter). When possible, choose fruit for dessert.

Your Best Bets
- Grilled chicken, fish, and lean meats
- Steamed veggies, especially green beans
- Salads with green, yellow, and red veggies

Steer Clear of
- The bread basket
- Potatoes
- Creamy dips, sauces, and dressings
- Anything battered, breaded, or crusted
- Anything not in its original shape—such as popcorn shrimp, onion "blossoms," fish sticks, "chicken fries," etc.

. . . At the Sushi Bar

A sushi or Japanese restaurant can be one of the healthiest options when dining out *if* you know your way around a menu. Japanese food tends to have a lot of salt, so avoid foods prepared in sauces (which are typically high in sodium) and use low-sodium soy sauce for dipping. Avoid white rice.

If you're hungry for traditional sushi rolls, opt for brown rice rolls or no-rice rolls (which can be prepared with avocado). Or, alternatively, you can ask that the rolls be prepared with less rice than usual. And if you suffer from regular breakouts, ask for rolls with soybean paper rather than seaweed (since seaweed contains iodine, which can aggravate acne).

Your Best Bets

- Edamame
- Sashimi (raw fish with no rice)
- Fresh and steamed shellfish
- Fresh tofu
- Yakitori (grilled chicken, shrimp, or scallops)
- Sautéed string beans (ask for any sauces on the side)
- Iced or hot green tea, sake, or shochu

Steer Clear of

- Foods that are baked or marinated with sauce (such as baked cod or teriyaki anything), which tend to be high in sugar and salt
- Deep-fried dishes, such as tempura or fried soft-shell crab (found in "spider" rolls)
- Miso and seaweed, which are high in sodium. If you have acne, avoid them entirely.

Part IV

Feed Your Face *Extras*

11

Food on Your Face

(Food-Based Ingredients and Easy Recipes
for Make-at-Home Remedies)

In medicine, as in fashion, sometimes what's old becomes new again. And food has been used for beauty purposes for thousands and thousands of years:

- In the 16th century B.C., high-ranking Egyptians only appeared in public when wearing perfectly curled or braided wigs of human hair, held in place with honey. And it's thought that many years later the Egyptian queen Cleopatra bathed in sour milk, which contains lactic acid and milk proteins that loosen and soften dead skin.
- The ancient Greek physician Galen wrote that ladies could lighten their complexion by mixing a substance from seagull nests with honey and spreading it on the face. To make a cleanser, he instructed women to combine chickpea flour and wheat. And for ladies of luxury, crocodile excrement was used to eliminate freckles and growths (so, yeah, they put animal poo on their faces).
- The Roman poet Ovid wrote about using a facial mask made of Libyan barley and honey to fight wrinkles.
- Herbalists in ancient China during the Han dynasty (circa 200 B.C.) recommended taking a powder composed of tangerine peel, white melon seeds, and peach blossoms three times a day for paler

skin. And in an ancient Chinese medical textbook you can find a prescription for a wrinkle-removing facial mask made from beeswax and sheep bone marrow.

- There are whole collections of recipes from the Renaissance that solve all sorts of beauty problems. One of the most gruesome involved boiling pure white animals—chickens, pigeons, or puppies—and mixing the broth with eggs and lemon juice to make a skin-lightening paste. (So, yeah, they killed puppies.)

It has been only in the last 40 years or so, since the 1960s and 1970s, that large cosmetics and pharmaceutical companies started selling us everything we use on our skin (and telling us that we need a whole slew of new products every season).

But these days the pendulum has begun to swing the other way. While many of my patients are interested in the latest "high-tech" ingredients and the newest cosmetic procedures, an increasing number are looking for ways to simplify their beauty routines (and to use fewer synthetic chemicals). Similarly, these women are becoming more mindful of what they eat, and trying to consume fewer processed and prepackaged foods. I've noticed this trend even among women who use Botox. Many of my patients who get their lips plumped and their wrinkles smoothed would *also* like their skin-care products to include more natural ingredients.

Food *on* Your Face: The Good, the Bad, and the Messy

If centuries of experience don't convince you, maybe more recent research will. Scientists are regularly discovering the true power of natural, topical botanicals, and skin care manufacturers are racing to incorporate ingredients like green tea, shiitake mushroom extract, and soy into increasingly eco-friendly products. This "new" trend proves that skin care doesn't have to be expensive or fancy or even high-tech to be effective. In fact, you can find some of the purest (and certainly cheapest) skin-care ingredients right in your kitchen cupboard or fridge.

There are plenty of advantages other than price, however, when it comes to using food on your face. Natural, food-based ingredients are great for sensitive skin since they don't contain any preservatives, additives, artificial fragrances, or synthetic dyes—all of which can irritate the skin, or even trigger an allergic reaction. (That's provided you don't have a food allergy or sensitivity, of course.) Likewise, food products are easier on your skin than many prescription-strength treatments, and you won't have to worry about potential drug or chemical interactions. (For example, certain prescription-strength topical products such as benzoyl peroxide and sulfur-derived acne lotions shouldn't be used at the same time—when used together, they can turn your skin orange.) Natural products are also safe to use during pregnancy (unlike antibiotics and retinoids). And when you're concocting a face cream from products in your pantry, you won't be contributing to environmental waste (from packaging that winds up in a landfill), nor will you have to worry about animal testing.

I will admit that there are some disadvantages to make-at-home skin care: Without preservatives, homemade beauty products will spoil. For example, you can't keep a batch of egg-white eye mask sitting on your bathroom counter. Homemade products can also be messy since they don't come in fancy packaging. And some food-based ingredients don't dissolve as easily as synthetic ingredients, so they might not rinse off or go down the drain quite as quickly. But even though we've spent ten chapters talking about ways that eating certain foods can benefit the skin, some foods just work better when you smear them on your face. (Remember the poor woman who smeared tomato paste on her face while vacationing in Mexico? Tomatoes aren't one of these foods.) In this chapter I'll give you a crash course in the foods and food-based ingredients that work best when applied topically as well as a number of recipes for easy make-at-home treatments. Let's get cooking.

The Best Foods to Put on Your Skin

One challenge with food-based ingredients (as with natural ingredients) is that they contain many different compounds (unlike synthetic ingredients, which have been developed in a lab to have one specific effect). Since the use of botanical extracts and food-derived ingredients in commercial skin care is still quite new (and researchers are discovering more organic compounds that can protect against sun damage, fight wrinkles, or soothe dry skin nearly every day), we're just at the beginning of the natural skin care revolution. That's why some of the foods I recommend for topical use can literally be pulled from your pantry (and even eaten, but try to restrain yourself), while others have already been incorporated into a number of commercial products (which makes them easier to tote around in your purse or beach bag). Whether you have wrinkles, sun spots, or flaky patches, the following foods work best when you smear them *on* your skin.

For Younger-Looking Skin

Mushrooms have been used medicinally in Asia for centuries as well as in traditional Chinese medicine to treat heart disease, asthma, insomnia, and ulcers. More recent studies show, however, that mushrooms are also great for the skin.

While all mushrooms contain proteins, lipids, and other compounds that fight free radical damage, shiitake and reishi (mannetake) mushrooms have especially strong antioxidant activity as well as the ability to inhibit matrix metalloproteinases (MMPs), the enzymes that break down collagen and elastic tissue. Research shows that skin-care products containing shiitake and mannetake mushroom extract can improve skin texture as well as reduce fine lines, sun spots, and overall sun damage in as little as 4 weeks. And since mushrooms also have anti-inflammatory potential, they're a great option for people with sensitive skin or who can't tolerate prescription-strength products. Find mushroom extract in Aveeno Positively Ageless Lifting and Firming Night Cream.

Pomegranate extract contains a high level of polyphenol antioxidants, including ellagic acid, as well as anti-inflammatory potential, so it makes a great anti-aging ingredient for sensitive skin. Look for it in Korres Pomegranate Balancing Moisturizer or Weleda Pomegranate Regenerating Hand Cream.

Mangosteen is a tropical fruit native to Southeast Asia that is still relatively rare in the produce sections of supermarkets in Europe and America. Like the pomegranate, mangosteen contains a high concentration of polyphenol antioxidants. Both fruits are available in juice form at your local health food shops, but they are increasingly included in skin-care products. One study found that a commercial skin cream containing a mixture of mangosteen and pomegranate improved facial wrinkling and sun damage after daily use for 60 days.

Rosemary, which contains several antioxidants including carnosic acid, has also been shown to fight the MMP enzymes that break down collagen and elastin after sun exposure. Try Clinique Youth Surge Night Age Decelerating Night Moisturizer, or Kiehl's Midnight Recovery Concentrate.

For Dark Patches and Discoloration

Several years ago I had a satellite office in Malibu, right across the street from the beach. In fact, some of my patients would come to their appointments still shaking sand from their shoes. As you can imagine, I saw lots of folks with sun damage, brown spots, and problems with uneven skin tone, including melasma, which produces dark patches on the forehead, cheeks, and upper lip.

Back then I used to recommend prescription-strength fading creams and in-office treatments to correct sun damage, but many of my (hippie) Malibu patients weren't interested. They told me they preferred to use skin-care products with natural ingredients. And while these natural products produced more gradual results than prescription-strength creams, there was no doubt many of them were effective. These days recent research has confirmed what my Malibu patients knew all along.

Soy is one of the most studied food-derived ingredients in skin care, so you can find it in a large number of over-the-counter products. It's particularly effective at correcting brown spots and improving overall skin tone. Soybeans contain enzymes called protease inhibitors, which have been shown to block a series of chemical reactions that produce melanin skin pigment. Soybeans also contain wrinkle-fighting vitamins A and E, both strong antioxidants that help protect and strengthen the skin's collagen and elastic tissue. Since soy is also an anti-inflammatory, it's a great option for people who have sensitive skin or rosacea in addition to blotchiness and discoloration.

While prescription-strength fading creams typically contain such ingredients as tretinoin (found in Retin-A) and hydroquinone—both of which can irritate sensitive skin—moisturizers with soybean extract are mild. Even my patients who can tolerate stronger products often benefit from using milder soy-based creams and cleansers in the morning and saving their prescription treatments for nighttime. You can find soy in Fresh Soy Face

Cream, Philosophy When Hope Is Not Enough, and Aveeno Positively Radiant Anti-Wrinkle Cream.

Arbutin, a natural extract found in bearberry, wheat, and certain types of pears, is one of the newest ingredients available to improve skin tone. Like prescription hydroquinone, arbutin has been shown to block the enzymes that cause excess pigmentation. Find it in Chantecaille Vital Essence with Arbutin.

Licorice extract contains compounds that have been shown to lighten melasma in as little as 4 weeks. Licorice is also anti-inflammatory, so it's safe for those with sensitive skin. Try Eucerin Redness Relief Daily Perfecting Lotion SPF 15.

For Sun Protection and Sunburn Relief

Green or white tea. You already know that drinking green tea before heading outdoors can help ward off sun damage, but for extra protection look for skin-care products that contain green or white tea extract.

Green tea has a high concentration of catechins, which have strong anti-inflammatory, antioxidant, and anti-aging effects. Topical green tea can also help thicken the epidermis, speed up the healing of wounds, and inhibit an enzyme in your skin that causes uneven pigmentation (helping to fight blotchiness and sun spots). In fact, applying green tea to the skin 30 minutes before exposure to UV rays has been shown to *reduce* the resulting sunburn and lessen the amount of DNA damage (one of the first steps to skin cancer) as well as protect against UVA (aging) rays. Why is this important? If you know you're going to be outside for several hours and won't be able to reapply sunscreen as diligently as you'd like (if you're in the middle of a long tennis game or competing in a triathlon, for example), you can boost your skin's UV protection by applying products with green tea before you go out—just apply it on top of your sunscreen (and remember to gulp down your cup of green tea before you head outside, too).

If you've already spent too much time outdoors and you're dreading the inevitable burn, you can lessen the pain and redness by taking care of your skin as soon as you get indoors. Studies have shown that green tea—whether applied topically or taken orally—can protect the skin from sunburn even *after* exposure to UV light. Additional studies have shown that topical application of white tea (which is the least processed of all tea varieties) may be as effective as green tea in protecting the skin from DNA damage after the fact.

As soon as you get indoors, make a large pitcher of iced green or white tea. Drink a tall glass (or two) and soak a thin washcloth or dishcloth in the rest to use as a cool compress. Wring out and apply to the overexposed areas every hour to reduce pain, redness, and blistering.

Berries. Cranberries, raspberries, strawberries, blackberries, and pomegranate seeds (as well as some nuts, including walnuts and pecans) contain high amounts of ellagic acid, a polyphenol antioxidant that's been shown to help prevent wrinkles and premature aging caused by sun damage. They also block the formation of MMPs, which break down collagen and elastin. In a recent study, Korean researchers showed that topical ellagic acid protects skin cells from the damaging effects of UV rays. Additional research shows that skin treated with topical ellagic acid has less wrinkling and less inflammation. What's more, researchers at Ohio State University Medical Center have shown that a topical compound made of black raspberries significantly slowed the growth of squamous cell skin cancer in mice exposed to UVB rays.

If you've been caught out in the sun and want to lessen your risk of burning, consider applying a homemade soothing ointment of mashed ripe berries (which contain more ellagic acid than unripe fruit) and cold yogurt the minute you get inside. The milk proteins will help soothe inflamed skin, the berries will fight DNA damage that leads to sunburn, and the cool temperature will shrink swelling.

For Dry Skin

If you run out of your favorite body lotion during the winter months and don't feel like braving the cold for more, chances are you have products in your kitchen cupboards that can do double duty. These ingredients can relieve chapped, dry skin as well as add a kick of flavor to your favorite recipes. For dry winter skin try the following:

Honey, which was used in the Middle Ages to treat infected wounds, has recently been shown to kill a variety of bacteria, including Staph and *E. coli* (a common cause of food poisoning). In fact, in hospitals and wound care clinics, dressings and topical gels containing medicinal honey are sometimes used to help speed the healing of surgical wounds. Honey has also been shown to soothe burns and help them heal faster.

But that doesn't mean you should reach for the little plastic honey bear next time you get a burn or abrasion. Honey (especially raw, unpasteurized honey) can contain bacteria spores, including the type that causes botulism. Medical-grade honey, on the other hand, has been sterilized and proven to be antibacterial; it's a regulated medical device. A more common use of commercial honey is as a humectant—a substance that hydrates the skin and keeps moisture from evaporating.

If you have sensitive skin, a homemade honey mask is one of the most gentle treatments around. Whisk together avocado and honey until you get a smooth paste. Apply to clean skin and leave on for at least forty-five minutes. This mask can be sticky when it melts, so be sure to wear an old T-shirt and have a cool washcloth nearby to catch the drips. Rinse and pat dry. Your skin will feel soft but not squeaky clean since the treatment is meant to hydrate, not strip your skin of its natural oils.

Vegetable shortening (yes, the same product you use to make flaky pie crusts and crispy fried chicken) is a great remedy for chapped hands and cracked elbows. Back when I was training as a medical resident, one of the supervising doctors taught us that no moisturizer has more emollient power than vegetable shortening—since it's made from soybean and palm oils (and contains no water), it doesn't evaporate like many body lotions. And since it has no chemicals or added fragrances, it won't sting or irritate sensitive skin. Use just a tiny bit, and avoid putting it on your face if you have oily or acne-prone skin, since it can clog the pores.

Macadamia nut oil is commonly used in Australia for baking, frying, and in salad dressings, but it also makes a great moisturizer because it contains high levels of vitamin E, which can soothe irritated skin. It is a heavy oil, however, so while it's great for dry arms and legs, most people find it too greasy to use on their face. You can also try adding a spoonful to your bath.

Sweet almond oil is one of my favorite treatments for hangnails and ragged cuticles. Rub a drop or two onto each fingertip and massage into your nails and cuticles. It's not as heavy as olive or coconut oil, so you can still type and text after applying. Plus, it smells like dessert. (You can find sweet almond oil and macadamia nut oil at specialty food stores as well as online at iherb.com.)

For Scars

Onion extract can be used to make a scar less obvious. Most of us have a scar *somewhere* that we wish was less visible. Mine is on my knee—I got it in a nasty ski accident last winter. (Are you noticing a theme here? Maybe I should lay off the skiing for a while.) Anyway, I ended up tearing a ligament, but I was more concerned with how the ghastly gash was going to heal. I tend to get keloids—thick, raised scars that can be painful, itchy, and dark red. I certainly didn't want one on the front of my leg, so I started using Mederma gel right away. Four months later my scar was barely visible.

Mederma gel contains onion extract, which has been shown to reduce the red discoloration of new scars. Recent studies have indicated that raised, bumpy scars treated with onion extract become less painful, itchy, and bumpy. One study in particular found that onion extract gel—applied two to three weeks after an invasive procedure—significantly improved redness, texture, and the overall appearance of surgery-related scarring.

If you're considering having a tattoo removed, the use of onion extract gel after laser treatments has also been shown to help prevent scarring. And the best news: Researchers have not detected any side effects from the use of onion extract. While not all scars respond as well as mine did (older, raised scars may require a visit to the dermatologist for cortisone injections or laser treatments), Mederma is definitely worth a try. I recommend keeping a tube on hand, especially if you have a tendency to develop keloids.

$E=mc^2$ *Did You Know . . .*

Putting lemon juice in your hair before heading to the beach *will* give you natural, sun-kissed highlights, but you could also develop a blistering scalp rash the minute you go in the sun. (It's called phytophotodermatitis, and you can read more about it in Chapter 6.) Even if you're lucky enough to make it back indoors rash-free, the acid from lemons can dry out your hair and make it unmanageable. Plus, lemon juice highlights are hard to control. You might be aiming for sun-kissed streaks, but end up with bright orange patches. Do yourself a favor and leave hair coloring to the pros.

Homemade Face and Body Scrubs
Yummy Enough to Eat

When we're young, our bodies quickly make new, plump skin cells just as fast as the old dead ones get sloughed off (which is, of course, why children have such soft, smooth skin). As time goes by, however, and the production of new cells slows down, the dead skin doesn't get sloughed off as quickly or as evenly. This dead skin buildup can make your complexion look dull, tired, and blotchy, and your makeup won't go on as smoothly. Dead skin cells can also mix with bacteria and oil, leading to clogged pores, blackheads, and breakouts. That's why exfoliants (or body scrubs) are a great part of any skin care routine. Using a scrub once or twice a week can wash away the dead cells, revealing newer, fresh skin.

Unfortunately, body scrubs can also be expensive (annoying, since they end up getting washed down the drain anyway). Luckily, there's a lot you can do with ingredients that you probably have in your kitchen cupboard (or your fridge, or even your garden). By sticking to actual food ingredients, you'll have a completely all-natural skin-care product (good news for all you eco-friendly girls).

To make your own scrub you'll need two main ingredients: a skin-friendly exfoliant (oatmeal, cornmeal, sugar, salt, and coffee are all good options) and secondary ingredients such as honey and yogurt to help bind the scrub together and make it easier to massage into the skin. I also like to add fragrant herbs or a few drops of essential oil or extract to make my homemade scrubs smell delicious. (Since I love dessert, my favorite flavorings are vanilla, coconut, and almond oils, but you can also use rose oil, peppermint, or jasmine.) If you have sensitive skin (or a sensitive nose), skip the added fragrance.

The following recipes are all excellent (and simple!) for first-timers, but feel free to tweak them depending on what you have in your kitchen on any given day. Start by scrubbing once a week to see how your skin reacts. If your skin is sensitive, scrubbing too hard or too frequently will make you red and irritated. On the other hand, if your skin is oily, acne-prone, or otherwise resilient, you can probably benefit from scrubbing twice a week. And remember to rinse well whenever you use food ingredients so that your drain doesn't get clogged. (In fact, if your bathroom drain is temperamental, I'd suggest using a drain trap.)

Oatmeal Cookie Scrub
(for oily skin and acne)

¼ cup rolled oats
½ teaspoon cinnamon
1 teaspoon vanilla extract
2 teaspoons honey
1 tablespoon plain yogurt

This yummy scrub is particularly effective for girls with oily skin. Oats naturally contain proteins called saponins that help dissolve oil as well as loosen dirt and makeup from your pores. (Just avoid instant oatmeal. It'll turn into a gummy mess as soon as it gets wet.) The yogurt contains lactic acid (a mild, naturally occurring form of alpha-hydroxy acid), which will also loosen dead skin cells and unclog the pores. Oats can soak up a lot of liquid, so if the scrub feels too dry to massage into the skin, continue adding honey until it becomes easier to work with.

Cranberry Cornbread Scrub
(for younger, smoother skin)

¼ cup cornmeal
2 tablespoons crushed cranberries (or substitute raspberries, blackberries, strawberries, or pomegranate seeds)
1 tablespoon buttermilk
2 teaspoons honey

You'll remember that cranberries (as well as raspberries, strawberries, blackberries, and pomegranate seeds) contain ellagic acid, a compound that's been shown to help prevent wrinkles and premature aging caused by sun damage, as well as block the formation of MMPs, which break down collagen and elastin. Just make sure to use ripe berries, which contain more ellagic acid than unripe fruit.

The addition of buttermilk gives this scrub a dose of lactic acid, which, according to recent research, can stimulate your skin's collagen-producing cells, leaving you with softer, smoother skin.

Relaxing Guacamole Body Scrub

1 cup sugar
¼ cup mashed avocado
1 tablespoon sour cream
1 tablespoon olive oil
1 tablespoon honey
A few drops of lavender or ylang ylang essential oil (optional)

If you have large dry patches or "chicken skin" on the backs of your arms or the tops of your thighs, try scrubbing with sugar or salt. It's the one time that sugar can actually be *good* for your skin! If your skin is sensitive, use white granulated sugar for a finer scrub. Brown sugar and turbinado sugar ("Sugar in the Raw") have larger crystals, so they'll make a coarser scrub. Salt is better for the arms or legs since it can be scratchy.

Avocado and olive oil both contain fatty acids to replenish your skin's natural protective barrier without stinging or irritating dry skin or aggravating rashes. In fact, pure olive oil is sometimes the only product that won't make an existing rash worse. (Even some prescription-strength creams can sting or make the skin even more red and inflamed.) Olive oil is also great for treating eczema and winter itch. If you tend to get acne on your chest or back, however, the natural oil may clog your pores and aggravate breakouts, so skip the oil and stick with honey or yogurt.

Both lavender and ylang ylang are relaxing aromatherapy scents that have been shown to help you have a more restful sleep. Consider adding a few drops of essential oil if you scrub before bedtime. You can find essential oils at your local health food store.

Peppermint Patty Foot Scrub

1 cup coarse sea salt
5 tablespoons olive or coconut oil
1 tablespoon cocoa powder
½ cup fresh mint, minced
3 drops peppermint essential oil (optional)

Whether your feet have been trapped in winter boots or you want to show them off in summer sandals, a weekly foot scrub will prevent thick calluses from building up, keeping your feet looking soft and sexy. Coarse sea salt is too scratchy to use on your face, but it's perfect for sloughing the dead skin off your feet, while olive and coconut oils can help repair dry, cracked, callused skin. For best results soak your feet in warm water for 10 to 15 minutes before scrubbing, and apply a rich foot cream immediately afterward.

Natural Face Masks

If a crazy schedule has derailed your skin care routine, a facial mask can get you back on track in just 10 minutes a week. (Just make sure to warn your spouse or roommate before you put it on. You don't want to give anyone a heart attack when they walk in the room and find you covered in goo.) The following are some of my favorite masks that contain food-derived ingredients for softer, smoother skin:

- If you have dry, flaky patches, look for a hydrating mask with oils and emollient ingredients. Origins Drink Up Intensive Mask contains avocado and apricot kernel oils, while Laura Mercier Intensive Moisture Mask contains sweet almond and sunflower seed oils as well as sodium hyaluronate (which helps hold moisture in the skin).
- If you have rosacea, look for water-based gel masks that contain skin soothers, such as cucumber and chamomile. These masks cool you off as they dry, helping to reduce redness and irritation. For best results store the mask in the fridge.
- If you have fine lines around the eyes, try this make-at-home tightening mask: Whisk together egg whites and fresh carrot juice. Then lie down and apply the mask around and under your eyes and let it dry for 20 to 30 minutes. Egg whites contain proteins that form a tight film across your skin when they dry (kind of like how glue dries into a film). Meanwhile, carrot juice contains beta-carotene, which penetrates the epidermis and is converted into retinol (the same stuff found in anti-aging skin-care products), which has been shown to soften fine lines and wrinkles. Repeat this mask at least once a week, and you'll actually feel the delicate skin around your eyes start to firm and tighten.

DERMATOLOGY 911: FAKE A GOOD NIGHT'S SLEEP

*A*s a med student and, later, a medical intern, you're expected to work very long days and then be on call every second or third night. The brutal schedule leaves little time for sleep, let alone a personal life. (One year I celebrated both Thanksgiving *and* Christmas in the hospital with a sad little bowl of instant noodles.)

Being on call is always tough, but it did train me to get by on about 4 hours of sleep a night. And these days I'm still a bit of a night owl. Even though I leave the office by 6 or 7 PM, I use the wee hours of the morning—when the phone has stopped ringing and my BlackBerry has stopped buzzing—to write medical articles and daily email newsletters. In the mornings, however, I sometimes wake up with puffy red eyes (especially if I've forgotten to pop out my contacts before collapsing into bed) even when I otherwise feel awake and rested. On those days I use my secret weapon: soy milk.

At any given time you can open my fridge, and right there on the top shelf (next to my personal stash of Botox) you'll find a small carton of soy milk. I don't drink it—nothing that comes in a carton compares to the fresh soy milk my mother used to make. Instead, I use it on my eyes. Soy is a strong anti-inflammatory, so it can help reduce swelling, and the soy proteins help hydrate the skin, so crow's-feet will look softer. Studies have also shown that applying soy milk extract to the skin can improve elasticity, boost your natural levels of hyaluronic acid, and thicken the skin. Plus, the cold temperature will help shrink swollen under-eye tissue and constrict the veins to make your eyes look less bloodshot. Here's how to de-puff your eyes the next time you need to look well rested on little to no sleep:

- Pour a small amount of soy milk into a bowl.
- Dunk two cotton balls into the milk and squeeze out the excess.
- Hold the cotton balls over your eyes for five minutes. (Ideally, you'll do this while lying down.)
- For extra-puffy eyes, repeat this two or three times.

Recap of Chapter 11

The Best Foods to Put on Your Face

* Food has been used on the skin for thousands and thousands of years. (Hey, if it was good enough for Cleopatra, it's good enough for me.)
* For younger-looking skin, choose products with mushroom, pomegranate, mangosteen, or rosemary extract.
* To fight discoloration, choose products with soy, arbutin, or licorice.
* For dry, cracked skin, apply honey, vegetable shortening, olive oil, macadamia nut oil, or sweet almond oil.
* To prevent and treat sunburns, try topical green or white tea and crushed berries.

12

Aging Gracefully

(With a Little Help from Botox, Injectables, Lasers, and Peels)

Many of my patients—especially the ones who eat organically, exercise regularly, and take really good care of their bodies in general—feel guilty even talking about cosmetic procedures like Botox. A lot of women feel it's better to "age gracefully" without resorting to help from a doctor.

But really, what does it mean to *age gracefully*? If the implication is that we should let nature take its course—i.e., do nothing—then shouldn't we stop dyeing our gray hair? What about brushing our teeth or wearing deodorant? Is shaving your legs a revolt against nature? I don't think so. (If aging gracefully meant that we should just let ourselves go, we'd all be walking around with hairy legs and smelly pits.) I believe you can age gracefully by working to look and *feel* your best at any age, rather than throwing in the towel once you reach some arbitrary birthday. Even my ninety-eight-year-old grandmother gets up every day and draws on her eyebrows.

For some people aging gracefully might mean having a light chemical peel to lighten freckles and treat sun damage. In fact, I often perform chemical peels to remove actinic keratosis precancerous growths (AKs), so there can be health benefits as well as cosmetic advantages to periodic treatments. For others, minor procedures performed over the years may be a way to maintain your looks without resorting to more drastic measures. You know those actresses who look better now than they did 10 years ago but who still look like *themselves*? I can tell you that those women eat well, exercise, and protect and care for their skin. But many of them also have little things done along the way (such as noninvasive laser treatments or tiny amounts of Botox or fillers) rather than opt for an extreme procedure later on that renders them unrecognizable. Their secret to looking ageless is that they go to doctors who make sure their treatments look natural. In fact, it takes much more expertise and experience to give someone a natural "undone" look than it does to overtreat them.

This is one of the reasons why my medical practice has such a large and loyal following. Over the 15+ years that I've been performing cosmetic injections, laser treatments, and chemical peels, I've developed a reputation for giving my patients natural-looking results. (You won't ever see someone leave my office and gasp, "What did she *do* to herself?") In fact, one of my laser patients, a British rock star, told me that he did a photo shoot with some band members that he hadn't seen in a few years. They couldn't believe how great he looked and wanted to know his secret, but my patient insisted that he was just taking better care of himself. (And they believed him!) I was so proud that they couldn't tell he had had any procedures. Many first-timers are also amazed that most treatments I do in the office are relatively painless, with little to no bruising or after-effects. This, too, takes years of experience as well as patience and a willingness to go slowly. Clinics that specialize in what I call "drive-by Botox" (in and out in 2 minutes, and everyone ending up with the same stunned look) are often staffed by practitioners who take a weekend course to "learn" how to do cosmetic procedures. Would you go to a hairstylist who took a weekend course to learn how to cut hair?

In fact, it's always shocked me that people seem to spend more time choosing a hairdresser than someone to do their cosmetic procedures. There's actually a place on the Venice Beach boardwalk in California that advertises "Tattoos, Toe Rings, and Botox." (No joke; I have the photos to prove it.) They may be perfectly qualified to do tattoos and toe rings, but how much experience do you suppose they have doing Botox? Like any medical procedure, these treatments should be performed only in a medical setting. You need to know that the needles are sterile, the syringes are clean, and your doctor is prepared for any unexpected effects. You also want someone who's experienced and performs the procedure often. Remember: It's not the procedure that makes some people look strange and others look ageless. It's the

CHOOSING A COSMETIC DOCTOR
(HINT: NOT FROM A BILLBOARD)

There's a disturbing trend of cosmetic "spas" popping up, advertising bargain basement procedures—often *literally* in someone's basement! (How do you think they can afford to charge you so little?) Real experience and expertise don't come cheap. When it comes to your health, bargain hunting could end up hurting you. If you're considering cosmetic treatments, here's the best way to find a good doctor:

• Select a doctor who has specialist training in dermatology, plastic surgery, ophthalmology, or cosmetic surgery. These types of physicians have most likely received specific training in facial anatomy and cosmetic treatments. Ask a doctor you trust, such as your family doctor or GP, for a recommendation.

• Check the doctor's credentials. Professional bodies such as the British Association of Plastic, Reconstructive, and Aesthetic Surgeons (BAPRAS) list their member doctor's qualifications. Or you can call the doctor's office and ask how long he has been performing the procedure you're interested in and how often. A doctor who performs a treatment every day, for example, probably has more experience than someone who does it only once a month.

• Beware of so-called medispas that provide medical services in addition to massages and facials. While some of these have doctors on site, many are associated with a doctor in name only; your treatment could end up being done by a nonqualified practitioner with questionable experience. Nurses are permitted to do injections under a doctor's supervision, but estheticians and nonmedical staff are not permitted to do injectable treatments with botulinium toxin or fillers, because these are considered prescription-only medicines (POMS).

• If you feel pressured by the facility or doctor, turn around and walk out. I always tell my patients that if they're not 100 percent sure about a particular procedure, it's best to wait. Trust your instincts. You can always reschedule or go somewhere else.

doctor doing the treatment. (No one ever blames the scissors for a bad hair-cut or praises the blow-dryer for an awesome blowout—it's all in the tech-nique. Same with cosmetic procedures.)

This is why I've made it a personal mission to share my knowledge with the medical community. I'm routinely asked to give lectures at local and na-tional medical conferences on the topic of cosmetic dermatology, particu-larly with regard to injectables and other noninvasive treatments. I've been invited to speak at the annual American Academy of Dermatology meeting every year since 2004. I also teach these techniques to young doctors and medical students at the University of Southern California School of Medi-cine, where I hold the title of Assistant Clinical Professor of Dermatology.

Being a Type A overachiever, I'm always looking for ways to give my pa-tients better results. As Principal Investigator in a number of research studies, I've been fortunate to work with brand-new treatments and topical products years before they're available to most doctors. For example, I participated as an investigator in the clinical trials that led to FDA approval of Juvéderm in-jectable wrinkle filler and Latisse (a brush-on liquid that grows eyelashes). It's pratically a full-time job to stay on top of the latest research, however, so I've chosen a subset of procedures to specialize in. Here are the most common noninvasive cosmetic procedures that I perform in my office:

Botox: The World's Most Popular Cosmetic Procedure?

My father has a high, distinguished forehead—some might call it a fivehead—with several deep, horizontal lines that extend from ear to ear. While I'm proud to have inherited my dad's intellect, I also inherited his wrinkles. For as long as I can remember I had four pronounced lines deeply creased across my forehead. And then one day (many, many years ago) I went to visit my parents for the holidays. My mother took one look at me and ex-claimed, "Your forehead! You're turning into your father." I decided I had to do *something*, and that's when I turned to Botox.

Botox, which is a purified version of a protein that's produced by the bac-teria *Clostridium botulinum*, is arguably the world's most popular antiwrinkle treatment. And if you're wondering why anyone would inject bacteria into her face, well, she wouldn't. Consider this: The antibiotic penicillin is actually produced by a type of mold. While you wouldn't eat a piece of moldy bread, you would take penicillin if you had, say, strep throat. Similarly, there's no actual bacteria in Botox, and despite the rumors, Botox won't give you botulism (which typically occurs after ingesting large amounts of bacteria from spoiled foods).

Although most people might think of Botox as a relatively new "invention," the active ingredient has been studied for more than 100 years. In the 1950s, scientists discovered that it could be used to relax "overactive" muscles. In the 1960s, doctors began using it to treat young children with strabismus, also known as lazy eye. (Until then the only treatment to correct crossed eyes was a surgical procedure performed on the eye muscles themselves.) Since the 1990s, Botox has been widely used for cosmetic reasons, but has also been used to treat a variety of medical problems such as migraine headaches, severe muscle spasms, and even overactive bladder.

What's It Like to Get "Botoxed"?

The next time you're in a crowd, take a look at the way people squish and scrunch their faces when they speak. We raise our eyebrows to emphasize a point or to show surprise. We frown and furrow our foreheads while concentrating or when staring at a computer screen for hours on end. We squint in bright sunlight or while trying to read the proverbial fine print. We also use our faces to project emotion, good or bad. But every time you frown or squint or smile, your skin gets pinched and creased. When you're young (with lots of collagen and elastin), your face springs back into place and smoothes out between squints. As time goes by, however, you lose collagen and elastin, so the wrinkles stay creased. Botox works by relaxing the facial muscles, allowing the overlying skin to smooth out and the wrinkles to soften.

Botox is most often used to treat wrinkles in the upper part of the face (above the cheekbones) because most of these wrinkles, like the frown lines between the eyebrows, horizontal lines across the forehead, and crow's-feet, are produced when the facial muscles squish the skin. While I also use it to reduce vertical lines above the lips ("smoker's lines"), to lift the eyebrows or the tip of a droopy nose, and to smooth vertical muscle "bands" on the neck,

RED CARPET RULE #1: DON'T LET THEM SEE YOU SWEAT

*E*very year, a few weeks before the Academy Awards, my phone starts ringing off the hook with nervous nominees who want Botox injections in their armpits. Why? Because aside from ironing out wrinkles, Botox tells the sweat glands to, well, stop sweating. (And when you're posing for the cover of *People* magazine in a $10,000 gown, you sure as hell don't want to be photographed with sweaty pits.)

Bacteria thrive in warm, moist areas (such as sweaty armpits), and produce B.O. But by injecting tiny amounts of Botox right under the skin, you can stay dry (and therefore odor-free) for up to 6 months: *no deodorant necessary.* The underarms aren't particularly sensitive, so most people barely feel the injections. And since you have millions of sweat glands all over your body, "switching off" a few hundred under your arms won't interfere with your natural ability to regulate temperature. (Botox is also effective for treating sweaty palms and feet.)

If you have a major problem with sweating but Botox just isn't practical, try these tips:

• Make sure you're using an antiperspirant (which will help keep you dry), not just a deodorant (which will keep you smelling fresh). For extra protection try a stronger formula such as Dove Clinical Protection Antiperspirant Deodorant or Secret Clinical Strength.

• Apply your antiperspirant at night. That might sound strange, but after a steamy morning shower, your sweat glands are working overtime. If you apply antiperspirant right away, the sweat can wash it off your skin. A better option: Before going to sleep, blow-dry your (clean) armpits with a hairdryer set on cool. Apply antiperspirant and blow-dry again.

• If you're still sweating through your clothes, see a dermatologist who can examine you for possible underlying causes (such as a thyroid condition) as well as recommend a prescription-strength antiperspirant called Driclor. (Beware, this stuff can irritate sensitive skin.)

these areas can be tricky. Too much Botox or wrong placement in the lower face can make it hard to eat or speak. If your doctor suggests treating you in these areas, be sure he or she has a ton of experience—and don't do it right before an important meeting or a big dinner date just in case you have some trouble sipping your soup, which can happen the first time you get it done.

Since the entire treatment takes about 15 minutes, many of my patients come in for Botox treatments during their lunch hour. I use a tiny needle so that most patients barely feel it. To minimize discomfort and bleeding, I apply an ice pack on the area before the treatment, and for those who are very sensitive or apprehensive, I'll also use a numbing cream so they don't feel the pinprick as much. Right afterward the skin may look a little pink and swollen (as if you just got waxed), but that subsides within an hour or so. The most important advice I give people is to avoid rubbing the affected areas for 4 hours after treatment because it takes that long for the Botox to bind to the muscle. If you massage or rub the area vigorously before then, you can push the solution away from where I precisely placed it, leading to an uneven eyelid or eyebrow. After the treatment it takes up to a week for Botox to take effect, and it lasts for an average of 4 months, depending on the area that's treated.

How Much Botox Is Too Much: Will I Look as If I've Been Frozen in Time?

The very first time I had Botox (which was right after my mother pointed out my growing resemblance to dear old Dad), I let a male colleague inject it into my forehead. Well, that turned out to be a mistake. He jabbed the needle into my face, and there was a loud "crunch" with every injection. The worst part was that I couldn't raise my eyebrows to put on eye shadow for the next 3 months.

Since that first horrific treatment more than 15 years ago, I've been performing Botox injections on myself because I just don't trust anyone else. People are always surprised to find out, however, that I've had any treatments at all. That's because, frankly, I look *normal.* I can raise my eyebrows, smile, and express real emotion. (And those four deep creases on my forehead are gone—yay!)

Botox is, hands down, the most popular treatment I perform in the office. In fact, I perform the procedure multiple times every day. But there's a reason why Botox has gotten a bit of a bad rap and why actresses are so afraid to admit to using it: If you get too much, it looks strange and unnatural. In fact, I have several celebrity patients who actually started to lose work because their previous doctors had made them look too stiff and plastic-y.

The thing is that we all look better (and younger) when we can actually move our faces. After all, even teenagers have some lines when they raise their eyebrows. And for some people—men in particular—a few lines can actually *add* to your appeal. George Clooney, for instance, just wouldn't be as sexy without the crinkles around his eyes. And Meryl Streep—who has publicly vowed never to use Botox—seems to get more and more beautiful with each passing year.

CELEBRITY SKIN SECRETS—

A Hip-Hop Mogul's Fear of Needles

For my patients who are wary of looking unnatural and stiff, seeing the results in my face firsthand tends to put them at ease. In fact, one of my patients—an uber-famous hip-hop mogul—came into the office a few weeks ago for his first Botox injection. I knew he was having a rough day; the paparazzi had been even more aggressive than usual, and he'd been on the phone yelling at his publicist while riding in my tiny elevator with his usual large entourage of five—a driver, a very large bodyguard, two assistants, and his girlfriend. Anyway, we get down to business, I hold up the Botox needle, and this powerful, successful, intimidating man—a guy who makes his living managing talent from "the streets"—starts *completely freaking out*. All of a sudden he's squeezing his eyes shut and flailing his arms around, telling me how much he hates needles and can't I give him something for the pain? So my nurse grabbed his hand and held it tightly, while his girlfriend (who's also a patient) teased him for being a baby. And when I finally got him to hold still, he turned to me and asked, "So, you're really good at this, right?"

"Yes," I told him. "The best in the country."

He thought about that for a minute.

"Do you mind if I ask . . . do *you* get Botox?"

"Of course," I said. "I've been getting Botox for fifteen years now. I'm actually 60."

He jumped out of his chair and threw his hands in the air. "Shut the f*** up! NO WAY!" he yelled.

"You know we Asians age well," I said with a wink. Luckily, everyone cracked up. (Tense moment defused.)

The point of Botox shouldn't be to freeze your face into submission or even to resist the aging process. Looking stiff actually ages you. Besides, most women will tell you that their 30s were better than their 20s, their 40s were better than their 30s, and so on. Rather, Botox should help you look refreshed and relaxed, as if you (finally) managed to get a really good night's sleep. The best compliment I can get as a doctor is for one of my patients to be hailed as a "natural beauty." And as I always say, if I'm doing my job right, you shouldn't be able to see my work at all.

There are plenty of other doctors out there, however, who are heavy-handed with the Botox, so their patients end up looking stiff and motionless. Why? The answer is simple: Many doctors don't take the time to study a patient's face, to watch them scrunch and squint their eyebrows, to get a feel for a person's unique muscle makeup. That's the only way to determine where to place the injections, how much Botox to use, and how to keep everything looking natural. While it takes patience and thoughtfulness to get excellent results, some doctors just can't be bothered. They're out the door before you can even ask a question. And here's something really scary: Some unscrupulous practitioners have even been caught using cheap bootleg products labeled "Not for human use" and passing them off as the real thing. If you feel rushed or you aren't happy with the results of your "drive-by Botox," be honest and tell your doctor. If he can't (or won't) stand by his work, it's time to find someone else.

FROM THE (**CELEBRITY**) FILES OF *Dr. Wu*

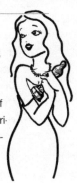

Patient: Kelly Wearstler—Interior Designer to the Stars, Author, Style Guru

Skin Concerns: Fine lines, UV protection

In Kelly's Words: I decided to try Botox after I saw a picture of myself with frown lines. I looked angry, and I didn't like it. My experience has been great, and I strongly recommend Botox as an anti-aging tool. (It's preventive, so if you start early, you'll never get those wrinkles.) But a little goes a long way, and you don't want to overdo it.

About 4 years ago I decided I needed to change my diet for health reasons. I started by cutting out white bread. A year later I stopped eating refined sugar. Right away I felt better and had more energy. I haven't had refined sugar in 3 years.

I'm always on the go, so it can be challenging to eat right. But I've learned to plan ahead, to pack my own food, and to be organized. I always have nuts in the car, and I travel with snacks. (I like apples with almond butter and green tea with manuka honey.) If it's that time of the month and I want something sweet, I'll have one date, which usually satisfies the craving.

This is what I'll eat on a typical day:

Breakfast: Three hard-boiled eggs (only one yolk) and an apple.

Snack: Freshly squeezed veggie drink (made with beets, kale, spinach, half an apple, lemon, and 3 ounces of ginger).

Lunch: Salad greens, grilled organic chicken, and sliced apple.

Snack: If I'm hungry, I'll have almonds or occasionally a brown rice cake or a banana.

Dinner: Grilled salmon or organic chicken, roasted Brussels sprouts, half a baked sweet potato, green salad, ¼ glass of red wine (Syrah or Malbec). On Saturdays I'll have a whole glass.

Dr. Wu's Diagnosis: Kelly has a flawless porcelain complexion, and she works hard at keeping her skin protected. She's already doing a lot right, such as planning ahead, traveling with snacks, and avoiding sugar. But since she lives in sunny SoCal (and travels to places like Florida, the Caribbean, and Aspen, where her husband's boutique hotels—which she decorates—are located), she should definitely add more cooked tomatoes to her diet. This shouldn't be hard since she likes Italian food. (Her favorite restaurant is Madeo, a celeb haunt in Beverly Hills.) She could try having grilled fish or chicken with tomato sauce or grilled or stuffed tomatoes on the side; she could also sprinkle sun-dried tomatoes on her salads. I'd also encourage her to try cabernet, since it has more polyphenol antioxidants (and therefore more UV protection). And instead of a date, she can satisfy a craving for sweets with dark chocolate which contains a dose of anti-oxidants.

Other Alternatives to Botox

In the U.K. and the rest of the E.U., Botox is also known by the name Vistabel. Vistabel was approved in the U.K. by the MHRA (Medicines and Healthcare Products Regulatory Agency) in 2006. It's exactly the same products as Botox, but has been licensed specifically for the cosmetic improvement of frown lines between the eyebrows. Other brands of botulinum toxin that are available in the U.K. are: Dysport (licensed for cosmetic use as Azzalure in 2009); and Xeomin (licensed as Bocouture in 2010). These all work in the same way, to relax overactive muscles. Botox, Dysport, and Xeomin are licensed for medical use (to treat eyelid spasm, for example), while Vistabel, Azzalure, and Bocouture are licensed for cosmetic use, but U.K. practitioners may use either formulation.

Hey, Dr. Wu

Q: My boyfriend is a hunk, but you could plant a flower in his frown line. Should a guy get Botox?

A: While Botox is definitely more popular with women, more and more men are trying it, especially when they see the results on their wives or girlfriends. I actually have a patient whose husband threatened to divorce her if she ever had Botox, so she secretly planned her appointments for when he was out of town on business. (Hey, I'm a dermatologist, not a marriage counselor.) After several rounds of injections, her husband looked through her wallet (though why was he snooping?), found a receipt from my office, and flew into a rage. Fortunately, they worked things out, and 6 months later he decided he wanted Botox, too, because he was tired of being mistaken for his wife's father!

When I'm treating a man with Botox, I'm particularly careful and conservative. Too much, and he could end up looking feminine or slightly Asian or a bit like Spock. If your man is considering getting a treatment for the first time, be sure to choose a doctor who has experience not only with Botox in general but also with treating men in particular.

Fillers: Will I Look Like a Blowfish?

Every day, all day, women come into my office fretting about a particular wrinkle or dreaming about having a plumper, fuller pout. But as soon as I start talking about fillers (such as Restylane and Juvéderm), most women get nervous, insisting that they'd never get anything injected because they don't want that overstuffed "blowfish" look. (You know those women, the ones who slowly transform themselves into life-size versions of Barbie or Jessica Rabbit.) Most women are terrified of having an elective procedure and ending up looking fake, phony, or downright weird. So when I tell them I've had filler in my smile lines for years (thanks again, Dad!), they're usually shocked. "But you don't have any smile lines," they say. "You don't need filler." And then I explain that my smile lines are smoother now *because* I use filler— usually every 6 to 9 months.

How Will I Know Which Filler Is Right for Me?

I always tell my patients that the goal with an injectable filler should be to look softer and more refreshed but still natural—in other words, like the best version of yourself. The way to do that is to be conservative; for example, I inject only a small amount of filler at a time, especially if it's someone's first treatment. (I can always add more, and if I do it gradually no one will suspect that you're having anything done.) If you've ever seen someone who looked like an alien (or a fish) after getting filler, it's not because of the actual product; it's because of poor technique or overinjection. It takes time and thoughtfulness to figure out the right placement and amount of filler to use, so if the doctor seems too busy to listen to your concerns (or if he wants to give you Angelina lips when all you wanted was to fill a chicken pox scar), then you may end up being unpleasantly surprised when you look in the mirror. You need to choose your doctor carefully and make sure he or she understands the look *you* want to achieve.

I like to hand patients a mirror *before* their treatment so we can take a look at everything together and prioritize what to do. In fact, I encourage patients to bring in photos of themselves or pictures from magazines to help illustrate what type of result they're aiming for. Then I can estimate the amount of plumping we can expect to achieve. (In addition, my staff and I discuss fees with patients prior to the treatment so there's no sticker shock when it comes time to pay.)

Since all fillers are not created equal, you'll also want to discuss the pros and cons of different products with your doctor. In some patients I use a combination of products at the same time, depending on the thickness of the skin, the location of the treatment, and the amount needed.

Juvéderm is the most popular filler I use in my office. It's a softer, more malleable substance than many other fillers. In the U.K. it comes in several different versions, such as Juvéderm Ultra, Voluma, Hydrate, and Ultra Smile. Your doctor can choose from among these different formulations depending on your skin type and where it's being injected. For example, I often use Juvé-derm Ultra to fill in nasolabial folds, which are the wrinkles that run from the side of your nose to the corners of your mouth. Voluma is a substance with more lift, so it's typically used to enhance the cheekbones or chin, where it can last 18 months or longer. Juvéderm Ultra Smile is specifically formulated for the lips, since it contains lidocaine, a local anesthetic that numbs the sensitive lip area as it's injected. Ultra Smile can be used along the lip border to provide definition and soften the lines above the lip; it can also be used to plump the lips. (Full disclosure: Although I was Principal Investigator in the U.S. clinical trial that led to approval of the product, and did receive a research grant to help fund the study, I'm not an employee of the company or a paid spokesperson, nor do I get any compensation for using it in my private practice.)

Hey, Dr. Wu

Q: I had a wrinkle filler injected in my face, and now I look lumpy! This is not what I signed up for! Help!

A: Not to worry! Sometimes swelling can make the filler appear lumpy. If it has only been a day or two since treatment, the swelling should go down within a few days. If it has been longer than a few days, however, you should notify your doctor. Although most patients have a smooth, natural-looking result from hyaluronic acid (HA) fillers, every so often the filler can clump together and form a visible bump that you can see or feel. This is more common in the lips since the filler gets squished together every time you pucker or chew. Luckily, there is a liquid enzyme called hyaluronidase (brand name Vitrase or Wydase) that can smooth away HA lumps within 24 hours. Ask your doctor if this might work for you.

What to Expect with Injectable Wrinkle Fillers

Certain body parts (like the lips, boobs, and earlobes) tend to shrink over time, while others—like the nose and feet—grow. While I can't give a patient back her perky teenage breasts, I *can* restore her 18-year-old lips. In fact, that's what most of my patients request—not someone else's lips but their own. (This is yet another reason why you should bring a photo to your consultation; it's important to be clear about your expectations.)

Injectable wrinkle fillers aren't terribly painful, but it's not a bad idea to discuss your pain tolerance with your doctor before the actual treatment. (Are you the type who went through labor without drugs, or do you need to be put under just to get your teeth cleaned?) For many patients I use a numbing cream to help reduce the discomfort of the pinprick injection. For others I also use a "dental block," which is the same type of numbing injection you get at the dentist. This numbs your lip, cheeks, and chin. It can take hours to wear off, so you probably won't want to schedule an injection right before an important business lunch. (The same goes for people with very sensitive skin or people who break out in hives easily, because reactions and swelling may be worse for these patients.) I also use lots of ice before the treatment to minimize the risk of bruising.

The procedure itself can take anywhere from 15 to 30 minutes, depending on exactly what you're having done. For the next few days you may be a little pink and slightly swollen (not unlike how your skin looks after getting waxed). Most of my patients experience little or no bruising and go right back to work. You can also apply makeup, eat, drink, and even kiss immediately after injections.

When it comes to lip injections, using ice is especially important because the lips are particularly vulnerable to swelling and bruising. (Think about it: Your lips are pink because they have many blood vessels and plenty of circulation, which means a higher risk of bleeding and bruising.) For this reason it's often wise to stop taking aspirin, ibuprofen, vitamin E, and fish oil for a week before filler injections. If you're taking prescription blood thinners, be sure to check with your doctor before stopping. Since the lips are also extremely sensitive, the ice helps alleviate the sting, too.

REPAIRING STRETCHED EARLOBES

Chandelier earrings may look elegant, but they can really do a number on your poor little ears. That's because there's very little connective tissue in the earlobes (just a thin layer of skin and a bit of fat), so the holes can stretch into long, unsightly slits. The earlobes also tend to get thinner with age, which makes them even less able to support the weight of heavy jewelry. As a result, larger earrings don't sit correctly on the earlobe. Instead of facing forward for everyone to admire, your grandmother's pearls flop down and face the ground. If left untreated (or if you continue to wear heavy pieces), the earlobes can eventually split open completely. And the only way to fix ripped earlobes is to sew them back together and repierce after several months.

Luckily, a few drops of Restylane helps to stiffen the earlobes, making them better able to support heavy earrings (as well as help prevent the earlobe from tearing apart in the first place). The best part? The results can last for a year or longer.

One of my patients, a well-known pop princess, "cheated" on me with another doctor. Well, the next day she showed up in my office looking like Marge Simpson (you know, all top lip). She finally had to admit to her boyfriend that she'd been getting her lips done. When I'd done her previous injections, her lips always looked soft and natural, so he never knew the difference—even when they kissed. After that painful episode, she came back to my office, and I made sure to ice her lips thoroughly beforehand so she wouldn't bruise. It's also important to give yourself a few days for the swelling to subside and to "adjust" to your lips again.

Non–hyaluronic Acid Fillers: Sculptra and Radiesse

Occasionally, one of my patients will request a longer-lasting alternative to an HA filler. Sculptra and Radiesse are two types of non–hyaluronic acid filler that typically last for a year or longer. While I've used both to treat patients, they're not usually my first choice. Non-HA fillers tend to be less forgiving than Juvéderm and Restylane and, unlike HA fillers, there's no way to "reverse" the treatment if you end up with lumps or an uneven appearance. Sculptra and Radiesse are useful in certain situations, but if you're considering either treatment, it's especially important to choose your doctor carefully and make sure he or she has plenty of experience since you'll be living with the results for a while.

Sculptra

Picture the face of a baby or toddler—soft, round, and smooth. A thick layer of subcutaneous tissue, which is common to all babies, keeps their skin smooth and wrinkle-free. But as time passes, the "baby fat" in our bodies redistributes: Our faces become more angular, our cheeks and temples hollow out, and the skin under our eyes sinks in. For some (genetically blessed) people, this isn't a problem. (Think of Sophia Loren and her stunning sculpted cheekbones.) But for others, particularly people who are naturally thin or who have lost a lot of weight, the effect can leave them looking gaunt, unhealthy, and suddenly older. This is where Sculptra can help.

Sculptra is made of poly-L-lactic acid, a synthetic material that's also used in dissolvable stitches and facial implants. Like the HA fillers, it's not an animal or human product, so no allergy testing is necessary. Unlike Restylane and Juvéderm, however, Sculptra doesn't plump the skin immediately, nor is it meant to fill in individual wrinkles or scars or to plump the lips. Instead, the Sculptra liquid is injected in a layer underneath the skin, where it stimulates the skin to produce its own collagen. The point is to gradually replace the facial volume that's been lost over time, leaving you with thicker, plumper skin and a rounder, softer face. (Think of it as a facial "volumizer.") You'll start to see improvement in a few weeks, but most people need an average of three treatments spread over a period of a few months to see real results.

Sculptra works best when it's used to fill in facial hollows or to make the face appear fuller, but you must be careful not to overdo it or you'll look like a bobble-head doll. And unlike Juvéderm and Restylane, there isn't a treatment that can "reverse" the effects of Sculptra, so it's wise to go slowly. Common side effects include pain, redness, bruising, and swelling. Some patients may also develop firm bumps underneath the skin that can last as long as the period of treatment, which is typically around two years.

Radiesse

Radiesse is a type of filler made from calcium hydroxylapatite, which is basically synthetic bone. When injected, it stimulates the body to produce scar tissue—that's what "fills" the wrinkles. Because it's very firm when it sets, Radiesse must be injected deep within the skin; otherwise, you'll be able to see and feel small, pebble-like lumps. Likewise, it should never be used under the eyes or in the lips where it can form hard nodules. Radiesse can be especially visible in people with thin or fair skin; in some cases you can feel the bumps even if you can't see them.

Some doctors prefer to use this product when filling deep smile lines. While the results can last as long as one to two years, the procedure itself can be tricky to perform. Radiesse is a thick, pasty substance, so it must be injected through a large needle and then massaged vigorously to minimize the risk of lumps. This comes with a greater risk of bruising and bleeding. Like Sculptra, there's also no "reversal" treatment if you do develop bumps, so if you're interested in Radiesse, you'll want a physician with oodles of experience.

DERMATOLOGY 911: PERMANENT FILLERS = PERMANENT PROBLEMS

One of my patients, a popular soap actress, recently went to a "party" where a South American man was performing lip injections. My patient—let's call her Vicky—is usually very picky about what products she uses on her skin, but on this day she let the man perform the procedure. (It was probably because he promised permanent results, and Vicky was tired of getting Juvéderm injections twice a year.) Vicky looked great for 2 weeks, but then her lips started to get hard and lumpy. By the time she came to see me a month later, she had developed bumpy nodules. When she smiled, she had four little peas bulging from her upper lip. The worst part was that she didn't ask what she was getting, so she didn't even know what was in her mouth.

If Vicky had gotten an HA filler (like Restylane or Juvéderm), we could have fixed the problem by injecting a solution that smoothes out bumps within 24 hours. But when I tried that, nothing happened. That means the injection Vicky received was most likely silicone or another permanent filler that's not approved in the U.S. Sure, it can be annoying (and expensive) to keep repeating your filler injections once or twice a year, but if you get a permanent filler and there's a problem, the only way to fix it is with surgery—that's right, cutting it out. *Ouch.*

Laser Treatments: Is High-Tech the Way to Go?

Every so often, I get asked to appear on talk shows or news segments to discuss some new trend in dermatology or to demonstrate a new procedure— and every time I get seriously excited. (I'm such a dork.) So when a producer from the medical talk show *The Doctors* asked me to perform a laser treatment in front of a live studio audience, I enthusiastically agreed. Unfortunately, when she called back the following week—2 hours before I was supposed to leave for the set—she had some bad news. Apparently, the Muppets (you know, Kermit, Elmo, the whole gang) were scheduled to appear before me, and since they take so long to set up, the show was way behind schedule. Turns out they wouldn't need my services after all. So, yeah, I got bumped for the *Muppets*. Humiliating.

There is some good news, though: When they finally invited me back to the show, the laser treatment turned out to be a pretty popular segment. The audience got a kick out of wearing orange goggles while I shot a beam of laser light right there on the stage! As I explained to the guests that day, lasers are basically different wavelengths (or colors) of light that react with the skin in various ways. Some lasers improve skin texture and zap discoloration; others can diminish wrinkles and promote collagen growth; still others react with the pigment in hair follicles and make the hair fall out. The very first cosmetic laser treatments (conducted in the early 1990s) utilized carbon dioxide (CO_2) lasers that literally burned off layers of skin, leaving the face bloody, oozing, and raw for several weeks. Once the skin healed, sun damage and wrinkles would be gone, but the face could remain bright red for several months to several *years;* eventually, the skin on the face could end up a completely different color from the rest of the body. Some of the first people to be treated with CO_2 lasers ended up looking waxy and white. These days we have much less invasive treatments that can improve the skin without such drastic side effects. (Besides, who has the time to hide out for several weeks or months while her face heals?)

What Are Lasers Used For?

One of the most common treatments I perform in my office is the "photofacial," which uses a type of low-level laser called Intense Pulsed Light (IPL) to shrink red patches, tiny blood vessels, and certain types of brown spots and sun damage. While there are several brands of IPL machines, I use one called the Aurora. It's commonly used to treat redness associated with rosacea, as well as freckles and sun spots. (Though I don't typically use it for melasma, since the photofacial can actually make that condition worse.)

Before the treatment (which lasts about 20 minutes) I give my patients a pair of protective eye goggles to wear, and I spread a cold gel all over the treatment area. Then, while my assistant holds a cool fan, I treat the face with a series of light pulses. Each pulse of the laser feels like a quick, hot sting, kind of like a small drop of hot oil that jumps onto your skin when you're cooking—annoying but tolerable. Afterward it looks and feels a bit like a mild sunburn, a little pink and warm for a few hours but not uncomfortable. The skin might be a little sensitive for a few days, so I tell patients to avoid anything abrasive such as facial scrubs and scratchy washcloths. Otherwise, they can resume normal activity, including wearing makeup. Over the following week, freckles and sun spots will become smaller and darker as the pigment gets broken down; they'll look like tiny specks of black pepper or coffee grounds. A week later these spots will fall off, and your skin will appear softer, smoother, and more even-toned. Many people also notice that their pores are smaller. For best results most people need three to five treatments, spaced a month apart. Photofacials can also be performed on the neck, chest, and back (so when you wear an open-necked blouse or spaghetti straps, your chest will match your face).

Another popular noninvasive treatment I use is the Affirm laser, which uses a wavelength of light that interacts with the collagen in your skin. The heat of the laser makes the collagen tighten (kind of like how a piece of bacon shrinks when you heat it in a pan). Over the next several weeks this brief episode of laser stimulates the skin's fibroblast cells to produce more collagen.

The Affirm laser is more painful than a photofacial; I use a fan to help dissipate the heat, but it still feels intense. Luckily, each flash covers about the size of a nickel, so I can treat the entire face in about 15 minutes. Immediately after the treatment you will look red and welted, as if you had gotten stung by bees all over your face. I send patients home with cold aloe vera gel and mineral water spray. They feel a little tender (like a bad sunburn) for the rest of the day, but the redness and tenderness are usually gone by the next morning—or in 3 or 4 days in patients who are very sensitive or who have very fair skin. Some patients also feel immediate tightening and firming, but it's more common to see and feel results after a series of three treatments. The Affirm laser is especially good for treating crow's-feet and fine lines under the eyes as well as for tightening the upper eyelid skin. I also use it to smooth out chest creases and soften vertical wrinkles above the upper lip.

Another laser that I use quite frequently is the Diolite laser, which uses a fine beam of light, similar to a laser pointer, to zap individual dark brown freckles (like those on the chest and the backs of the hands), capillary veins on the sides of the nostrils, and cherry-colored angiomas, those tiny red blood vessel bumps that we all start to get once we reach our 30s and 40s. Each spot takes seconds to treat, during which the laser feels like a hot pinprick. Immediately following the treatment, the area looks pink and a little swollen, like a mosquito bite. Then it turns dark and may crust or scab, which takes up to a week to fall off. Depending on the size and number of spots that are being treated, it may take several sessions; the veins or brown spots may return, so patients often come back once or twice a year to clean up new and recurring growths.

With any laser it's safest to get a treatment when you're not tan since your skin's excess pigment may react very strongly with the laser light, giving you deeper results than you or the doctor intended. I'll often send a patient home who has forgotten, and comes in for a laser treatment with a golden glow. For the same reason, if you have a darker skin tone, you should seek a doctor who has experience treating those with more skin pigment since some lasers can leave unwanted darker or lighter patches.

Chemical Peels: Will I Look Like a Burn Victim?

For treating melasma and certain kinds of deep sun damage, I find that chemical peels are often safer and more effective than lasers. But people tend to get a little nervous when I suggest this type of procedure, and often ask for laser treatments instead. For some reason people assume that lasers, being more high tech, are somehow less painful or less aggressive forms of treatment—as if I can wave my magic laser wand and make years of sun damage disappear with zero pain and no recovery time. (Sorry, that's not how it works.) The truth is that some lasers can be more aggressive and more damaging to the skin than chemical peels depending on the condition we're treating and a person's skin type.

I think a lot of the hesitation is that people are scared by the word *acid*, as in "I'm getting an alpha-hydroxy acid peel." You can think about it like this: Lemonade has ascorbic acid (better known as vitamin C) and balsamic vinegar has acetic acid, but nobody is afraid of *those*. Others worry about what a chemical peel will feel like, how long the recovery will be, and what they'll look like afterward. (And that episode of *Sex and the City*—the one where Samantha shows up at Carrie's book party after a chemical peel, her face a crusty, oozing mess—probably hasn't helped allay anyone's fears.) If you're considering a chemical peel, you should weigh your options carefully, as with any cosmetic treatment. The results will depend on the doctor's expertise and experience as well as how diligently you follow instructions on prepping your skin and caring for it after the peel. If you have a darker skin tone, you'll want to be especially careful about choosing a doctor who is experienced with treating more richly pigmented skin. Here's everything else you need to know before deciding if a chemical peel is right for you.

Chemical peels are performed by applying an acidic solution to the face that causes dead, damaged skin cells to slough and peel off. They can improve your skin tone and texture, and they're particularly beneficial for treating uneven skin pigmentation, acne blemishes and discoloration, and fine lines and wrinkles. For best results I usually insist that my patients start using a retinoid cream (such as Retin-A) for a month or so before getting a peel. This preps the surface of your skin by sloughing off dead skin cells so that the peel solution penetrates more evenly and you're more likely to get a uniform result. It also minimizes the risk that brown spots or discoloration will come back after the chemical peel is performed.

There are four types of peels that I perform in my office:

1. Glycolic peels, also known as alpha-hydroxy peels, are the most superficial type of chemical peel that I perform. During a glycolic peel, the acid will dissolve the "glue" that holds the top layers of the skin together, helping the dead cells to slough off and the pores to unclog. They usually feel warm, they may sting for the first few minutes, and your face may be pink for the next few hours, but there's little to no visible peeling. Glycolic peels are most useful for mild acne and mild sun damage. And while some facialists may use a glycolic solution, they're permitted much weaker formulas than what a doctor can use in a medical office.

2. Jessner peels, which penetrate deeper into the skin than glycolic peels, are a combination of salicylic acid (to unclog the pores) and lactic acid (to exfoliate). I often use this type of peel to treat moderate acne and discoloration, mild sun damage, and mild melasma on the face, neck, chest, back, and the backs of the hands. It's also helpful for keratosis pilaris (chicken skin) on the backs of the arms and tops of the thighs. Jessner peels will sting or feel itchy for the first few minutes, and your face will appear red for several hours to several days. Some flaking of the skin over the next three to five days is also common (as if you're peeling from a mild sunburn). After about a week, acne is smoother and discoloration is lighter, although it may take a series of peels for best results.

3. Trichloroacetic acid peels (TCA) are the strongest type of chemical peel I perform as well as the most involved. They are best for treating melasma, acne scars, moderate sun damage, and fine lines under the eyes and above the upper lip. TCA peels require advance planning on the part of the patient since they can produce a lot of peeling for a week or longer. They also sting more and feel "hotter" than other peels; for this reason my assistant holds a fan angled at your face to keep you cool during the treatment, which takes about 15 to 20 minutes. By the end your face will feel hot and sensitive, but rarely do any of my patients need pain medication. You can resume your normal activity and even wear makeup the same day as long as you don't use anything abrasive (such as a scrub) to wash your face. It's also important to use sun protection when you're healing from the peel.

By the second or third day the redness subsides, and your skin looks shiny and dark; then it cracks and peels (very similar to a bad sunburn). It's important not to pick or peel off the skin, which could lead to bleeding, infection, or scarring. During the peeling phase (which can last anywhere from seven to ten days), it's best to avoid makeup and stay out of the sun. Once the peeling phase ends, your skin will appear fresh and new. You may still be a little pink, but that will fade in a week or two. At that point you can resume using retinoid cream, but you must be diligent about using sunscreen. Brown spots can come back darker if your newly peeled skin is exposed to UV rays.

It's important to note that none of the chemical peels I perform in my office (including those listed above) are as deep as a "phenol peel." These utilize a heavy-duty solution containing a chemical called "phenol," which peels away *many* layers of living skin. The procedure itself requires mild sedation and monitoring by an EKG machine since there's a risk of irregular heartbeat. (Scary, right?) While the results can last for decades, they also turn your skin white and waxy *forever*. No, thanks.

When Is It Time for Plastic Surgery?

Noninvasive procedures such as injectables, laser treatments, and chemical peels are little beauty secrets that can help you look "fresher" and more relaxed without surgery. They can even help delay the need for more invasive treatments. But it's important to start early: It's much easier to keep your skin firm with an injectable than to lift it once it has fallen.

Here are some things I can do with injectables and lasers as an alternative to plastic surgery:

Instead of	*I can do*
Surgical brow lift	Botox brow lift: a drop under the end of the eyebrow pops up the brow and lifts the lids; or Restylane brow lift: a bit of filler along the brow bone props up the brows
Facelift	Filler in the hollow area along the jaw (in front of the jowl) to reduce the jowl and make the jawline sharper
Lower eyelid surgery	Juvéderm to fill in under-eye hollows
Asian eyelid surgery	Botox in the under-eye muscles to make the eyes wider and more open
Nose job (rhinoplasty)	Filler to soften a bump on the nose
Neck surgery	Botox to soften vertical neck bands

Keep in mind that no amount of Botox or filler can lift very loose skin. I'm very honest with patients about the results that they can expect with injectables, lasers, and peels. Sometimes the results won't be noticeable enough to validate the expense. When that's the case, it's time to see a surgeon. For example, if you can pinch an inch of skin on your neck or jawline, a wrinkle filler won't be enough to sharpen the jawline, so surgery may be the most effective option. A plastic surgeon can tighten and remove the extra skin with a neck lift (called a cervicoplasty). If you have a hereditary fat collection under the chin and jaw, Botox is unlikely to help. Instead, a surgeon can remove the fat deposit with liposuction. Similarly, if your under-eye bags need their own Zip code or if your eyelids are falling onto your eyelashes (or starting to impair your vision), Botox and fillers alone are unlikely to lift your lids enough to make a noticeable difference. When this is the case, I refer patients to an ophthalmic (eye) plastic surgeon who can better discuss your options.

If there's some aspect of your appearance that bugs you, go ahead and see a dermatologist now rather than waiting until the problem gets worse. If you get started earlier rather than later, you'll look better along the way—plus you're less likely to need something drastic down the road.

Afterword

ome people might define "aging gracefully" as letting nature take its course, just as some people might define a doctor as a stuffy, stodgy old guy in a white coat. But you know what? I understand—because that used to be me (well, not the old guy part).

Even though I've always had a love of fashion, a mild obsession with *Vogue,* and a torrid affair with my Visa card, I used to think that being a doctor meant dressing like a "serious" medical professional: drab navy suits, sensible shoes (i.e., "orthopedic pumps"), and a big white lab coat. I longed to buy fashionable clothes; instead, I skulked around in polyester stretch. And that was fine for a while—until I got bored.

By the summer of 2004, I had built a booming business in Los Angeles, doling out advice to editors at the magazines I've always worshipped and treating some of the most famous faces in Hollywood. Every day these glamorous women would parade in and out of my office, all of them having fun with fashion, really reveling in being strong, successful, beautiful women, while I was stuck in a dull uniform, feeling frumpy and boyish and blah. I was tired of trying to be the perfect doctor; I just wanted to enjoy being *me.* And if that meant wearing a Prada blouse to the office, then, damnit, I was going to. Still, it took me a long time to—as I like to

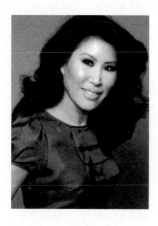

say—"cast off the white coat." And although it has certainly been liberating, embracing my true self hasn't come without challenges:

Picture if you can the ballroom at the Four Seasons, awash in ill-fitting suits and bad comb-overs. This is the Friday-night cocktail reception, standard at national conferences of the American Academy of Dermatology. (We're not traditionally a fashion-forward bunch.) I've already mentioned that I've been a featured speaker every year since 2004. Despite this, I'm usually ignored for the first few hours. As a well-dressed woman in stiletto heels, I'm often mistaken for someone's wife or girlfriend. Don't believe me? One year I was seated near a prominent dermatologist in his 70s, a native of Manhattan's Upper East Side. He formally introduced himself to every single person at our table . . . except me.

This kind of thing drives me crazy. There's nothing more annoying (or more self-confidence-crushing) than being ignored or excluded because of the way you look—whether that's because you're a geek in glasses who can't roll with the cool kids (that was me in high school) or because you've embraced your love of Louboutins and, subsequently, people think you're an airhead. (Sometimes that's me now.) But you know what? Every year when it comes time to pack for the AAD Conference, I don't reach for my most conservative duds. Instead, I pack the hottest thing I own and a kick-ass pair of heels, because when they call the featured speaker to the stage, I can hold my head up high. There is nothing like that long walk from the back of the room to the podium, the moment when 8,000 doctors realize they've flown thousands of miles and shelled out hundreds of dollars to listen (and learn!) from me: the petite woman from the party, the one who just doesn't look like a doctor. Knowing that I've earned the right to speak as a medical expert (and look damn good doing it) is the best feeling in the world (right up there with graduating from Harvard Medical School and getting paid to examine half-naked celebrity hunks).

I love what I do: counseling my patients on the best diets for their skin, searching for the best skin care, and experimenting with makeup—in short, helping women look and feel their best—because that journey has been so important in *my* life. I know that following the *Feed Your Face* Diet will help your skin look clearer, smoother, and healthier. It will also give you *control* over your skin and the confidence to look and feel your best without apology. If your version of aging gracefully means eating all organic foods, then good for you. And if it means giving yourself permission to consider Botox (or some other cosmetic procedure), then you go, girl. Because whatever you do, being true to yourself may be hard, but it's the only way to be happy. And that's advice that won't go out of style.

Dr. Jessica Wu

Where to Find Me

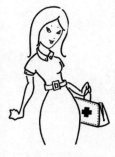

FeedYourFace.com
JessicaWu.com

For more tips, tricks, product picks, and celeb gossip:
Jessica Wu.com/newsletter

References

1. Getting to Know Your Skin

Norval M, Wulf HC. Does chronic sunscreen use reduce vitamin D production to insufficient levels? *Br J Dermatol* 2009;161(4):732–6.

2. What's Food Got to Do with It

Bett DG, Morland J, Yudkin J. Sugar consumption in acne vulgaris and seborrhoeic dermatitis. *Br Med J* 1967;3:153–5.

Burton JL. Diet and dermatology. *BMJ* 1989;298(6676):770–1.

Campbell TM, Neems R, Moore J. Severe exacerbation of rosacea induced by cinnamon supplements. *J Drugs Dermatol* 2008;7(6): 586–7.

Dormire S, Howharn C. The effect of dietary intake on hot flashes in menopausal women. *J Obstet Gynecol Neonatal Nurs* 2007;36(3):255–62.

Fulton EF, Plewig G, Kligman AM. Effect of chocolate on acne vulgaris. *J Am Med Assoc* 1969;210:2071–4.

Karppanen H, Karppanen P, Mervaala E. Why and how to implement sodium, potassium, calcium, and magnesium changes in food items and diets? *J Human Hypertension* 2005;19:S10–S19.

Melnik BC, Schmitz G. Role of insulin, insulin-like growth factor-1, hyperglycaemic food and milk consumption in the pathogenesis of acne vulgaris. *Exp Dermatol* 2009;18:833–41.

Smith R, Mann N, Makelainen H, Roper J, Braue A, Varigos G. A pilot study to determine the short-term effects of a low glycemic load diet on hormonal markers of acne: a nonrandomized, parallel, controlled feeding trial. *Mol Nutr Food Res* 2008;52:718–26.

Stahl W, Heinrich U, Aust O, Tronnier H, Sies H. Lycopene-rich products and dietary photoprotection. *Photochem Photobiol Sci* 2006;5(2):238–42.

Strauss JS, Krowchuk DP, Leyden JJ, et al. Guidelines of care for acne vulgaris management. *J Am Acad Dermatol* 2007;56:651–63.

4. Understanding Acne

Adebamowo CA, Spiegelman D, Berkey CS, et al. Milk consumption and acne in teenaged boys. *J Am Acad Dermatol* 2008;58:787–93.

Bechelli LM, Haddad N, Pimenta WP, et al. Epidemiological survey of skin diseases in schoolchildren living in the Purus Valley (Acre State, Amazonia, Brazil). *Dermatologica* 1981;163(1):78–93.

Capitanio B, Sinagra JL, Ottaviani M, Bordignon V, Amantea A, Picardo M. Smoker's acne: a new clinical entity? *Br J Dermatol* 2007;157(5):1070–1.

Cappel M, Mauger D, Thiboutot D. Correlation between serum levels of insulin-like growth factor 1, dehydroepiandrosterone sulfate, and dihydrotestosterone and acne lesion counts in adult women. *Arch Dermatol* 2005;141:333–8.

Ciotta L, Calogero AE, Farina M, De Leo V, La Marca A, Cianci A. Clinical, endocrine and metabolic effects of acarbose, an alpha-glucosidase inhibitor, in PCOS patients with increased insulin response and normal glucose tolerance. *Hum Reprod* 2001;16(10):2066–72.

Collier CN, Harper JC, Cantrell WC, Wang W, Foster KW, Elewski BE. The prevalence of acne in adults 20 years and older. *J Am Acad Dermatol* 2008;58:56–9.

Cordain L, Lindeberg S, Hurtado M, Hill K, Eaton B, Brand-Miller J. Acne vulgaris: a disease of Western civilization. *Arch Dermatol* 2002;138:1584–90.

Cupisti S, Häberle L, Dittrich R, et al. Smoking is associated with increased free testosterone and fasting insulin levels in women with polycystic ovary syndrome, resulting in aggravated insulin resistance. *Fertil Steril* 2010;94(2):673–7.

Dreno B, Foulc P, Reynaud A, Moyse D, Habert H, Richet H. Effect of zinc gluconate on propionibacterium acnes resistance to erythromycin in patients with inflammatory acne: in vitro and in vivo study. *Eur J Dermatol* 2005;15(3):152–5.

Dreno B, Moyse D, Aliresai M, et al.; Acne Research and Study Group. Multicenter randomized comparative double-blind controlled clinical trial of the safety and efficacy of zinc gluconate versus minocycline hydrochloride in the treatment of inflammatory acne vulgaris. *Dermatology* 2001;203(2):135–20.

Farage MA, Neill S, MacLean AB. Physiological changes associated with the menstrual cycle: a review. *Obstet Gynecol Surv* 2009;64(1):58–72.

Grid AH, Nilsson M, Holst JJ, Bjorck IM. Effect of whey on blood glucose and insulin responses to composite breakfast and lunch meals in type 2 diabetic subjects. *Am J Clin Nutr* 2005;82(1):69–75.

Liljeberg EH, Bjorck I. Milk as a supplement to mixed meals may elevate post-prandial insulinaemia. *Eur J Clin Nutr* 2001;55:994–9.

Logan AC. Omega-3 fatty acids and acne. *Arch Dermatol* 2003;139(7):941.

Melnik BD, Schmitz G. Role of insulin, insulin-like growth factor-1, hypergly-caemic food and milk consumption in the pathogenesis of acne vulgaris. *Exp Dermatol* 2009;18:833–41.

Roh M, Han M, Kim D, Chung K. Sebum output as a factor contributing to the size of facial pores. *Br J Dermatol* 2006;155(5):890–4.

Rubin MG, Kim K, Logan AC. Acne vulgaris, mental health and omega-3 fatty acids: a report of cases. *Lipids Health Dis* 2008;7:36.

Smith RN, Mann NJ, Braue A, Mäkeläinen H, Varigos GA. The effect of a high-protein, low glycemic-load diet versus a conventional, high glycemic-load diet on biochemical parameters associated with acne vulgaris: a randomized, investigator-masked, controlled trial. *J Am Acad Dermatol* 2007;57(2):247–56.

Smith R, Mann N, Mäkeläinen H, Roper J, Braue A, Varigos G. A pilot study to determine the short-term effects of a low glycemic load diet on hormonal markers of acne: a nonrandomized, parallel, controlled feeding trial. *Mol Nutr Food Res* 2008;52(6):718–26.

Spencer EH, Ferdowsian HR, Barnard ND. Diet and acne: a review of the evidence. *Int J Dermatol* 2009;48:339–47.

Stoll S, Shalita AR, Webster GF, Kaplan R, Danesh S, Penstein A. The effect of the menstrual cycle on acne. *J Am Acad Dermatol* 2001;45(6):957–60.

Strauss JS, Krowchuk DP, Leyden JJ, Lucky AW, Shalita AR, Siegfried EC, Thiboutot DM, Van Voorhees AS, Beutner KA, Sieck CK, Bhushan R. Guidelines of care for acne vulgaris management. *J Am Acad Dermatol* 2007;56:651–63.

Treloar V. Comment on acne and glycemic index. *J Am Acad Dermatol* 2008;58(1):175–7.

. . . .

5. Redness, Itching, and Flaking

Anderson P, Dinulos, J. Atopic dermatitis and alternative management strategies. *Curr Opin Pediatr* 2009;21(1):131–8.

Behnam SM, Behnam SE, Koo JY. Smoking and psoriasis. *SKINmed* 2005;4(3):174–6.

Callaway J, Schwab U, Harvima I, et al. Efficacy of dietary hempseed oil in patients with atopic dermatitis. *J Dermatolog Treat* 2005;16(2):87–94.

Campbell TM, Neems R, Moore J. Severe exacerbation of rosacea induced by cinnamon supplements. *J Drugs Dermatol* 2008;7(6):586–7.

Collier PM, Ursell A, Zaremba K, Payne CM, Staughton RC, Sanders T. Effect of regular consumption of oily fish compared with white fish on chronic plaque psoriasis. *Eur J Clin Nutr* 1993;47(4):251–4.

Dantzig PI. A new cutaneous sign of mercury poisoning? *J Am Acad Dermatol* 2003;49(6):1109–11.

Dormire S, Howharn C. The effect of dietary intake on hot flashes in menopausal women. *J Obstet Gynecol Neonatal Nurs* 2007;36(3):255–62.

Farkas A, Kemény L. Psoriasis and alcohol: is cutaneous ethanol one of the missing links? *Br J Dermatol* 2010;162(4):711–6.

Fortes C, Mastroeni S, Leffondré K, et al. Relationship between smoking and the clinical severity of psoriasis. *Arch Dermatol* 2005;141(12):1580–4.

Grimalt R, Mengeaud V, Cambazard F. The steroid-sparing effect of an emollient therapy in infants with atopic dermatitis: a randomized controlled study. *Dermatology* 2007;214:61–7.

Jansen T, Reomiti R, Kreuter A, Altmeyer P. Rosacea fulminans triggered by high dose vitamins B6 and B12. *J Eur Acad Dermatol Venereol* 2001;15:484–5.

Koch C, Dolle S, Metzger M, et al. Docosahexaenoic acid (DHA) supplementation in atopic eczema: a randomized, double-blind, controlled trial. *Br J Dermatol* 2008;158(4):786–92.

Magerl M, Pisarevskaja D, Scheufele R, Zuberbier T, Maurer M. Effects of a pseudoallergen-free diet on chronic spontaneous urticaria: a prospective trial. *Allergy* 2010;65(1):78–83.

Maintz L, Novak N. Histamine and histamine intolerance. *Am J Clin Nutr* 1007;85(5):1185–96.

Malanin G, Kalimo K. The results of skin testing with food additives and the effect of an elimination diet in chronic and recurrent urticaria and recurrent angioedema. *Clin Exp Allergy* 1989;19(5):539–43.

Matsumomo M, Aranami A, Ishige A, Watanabe K, Benno Y. LKM512 yogurt consumption improves the intestinal environment and induces the T-helper type 1 cytokine in adult patients with intractable atopic dermatitis. *Clin Exp Allergy* 2007;37(3):358–70.

Michail SK, Stolfi A, Johnson T, Onady GM. Efficacy of probiotics in the treatment of pediatric atopic dermatitis: a meta-analysis of randomized controlled trials. *Ann Allergy Asthma Immunol* 2008;101(5):508–16.

Miyake Y, Sasaki S, Tanaka K, et al. Relationship between dietary fat and fish intake and the prevalence of atopic eczema in pregnant Japanese females: baseline data from the Osaka Maternal and Child Health Study. *Asia Pac J Clin Nutr* 2008;17(4):612–9.

Morse NL, Clough PM. A meta-analysis of randomized, placebo-controlled clinical trials of Efamol evening primrose oil in atopic eczema. Where do we go from here in light of more recent discoveries? *Curr Pharm Biotechnol* 2006;7:503–24.

Rokaite R, Labanauskas L, Balciunaite S, Vaideliene L. Significance of dietotherapy on the clinical course of atopic dermatitis. *Medicina* 2009; 45(2):95–103.

Rosenfeldt V, Benfeldt E, Nielsen SD, et al. Effect of probiotic Lactobacillus strains in children with atopic dermatitis. *J Allergy Clin Immunol* 2003;111(2):389–95.

Sidbury R, Sullivan AF, Thadhani RI, et al. Randomized controlled trial of vitamin D supplementation for winter-related atopic dermatitis in Boston: a pilot study. *Br J Dermatol* 2008;159:245–7.

Stuckert J, Nedorost S. Low-cobalt diet for dyshidrotic eczema patients. *Contact Dermatitis* 2008;59(6):361–5.

Veien NK, Hattel T, Laurberg G. Low nickel diet: an open, prospective trial. *J Am Acad Dermatol* 1993;29(6):1002–7.

Wolk K, Mallbris L, Larsson P, Rosenblad A, Vingård E, Ståhle M. Excessive body weight and smoking associated with a high risk of onset of plaque psoriasis. *Acta Derm Venereol* 2009;89(5):492–7.

Wolters M. Diet and psoriasis: experimental data and clinical evidence. *Br J Dermatol* 2005;153(4):706–14.

Worm M, Ehlers I, Sterry W, Zuberbier T. Clinical relevance of food additives in adult patients with atopic dermatitis. *Clin Exp Allergy* 2000;30(3):407–14.

Worm M, Fiedler EM, Dolle S, et al. Exogenous histamine aggravates eczema in a subgroup of patients with atopic dermatitis. *Acta Derm Venereol* 2009;89(1):52–6.

6. To Tan or Not to Tan

Aust O, Stahl W, Sies H, Tronnier H, Heinrich U. Supplementation with tomato-based products increases lycopene, phytofluene, and phytoene levels in human serum and protects against UV-light-induced erythema. *Int J Vitam Nutr Res* 2005;75(1):54–60.

Biesalski HK, and Obermueller-Jevic UC. UV light, beta-carotene and human skin-beneficial and potentially harmful effects. *Arch Biochem Biophys* 2001;389: 1–6.

Black HS, Herd JA, Goldberg LH, et al. Effect of a low-fat diet on the incidence of actinic keratosis. *N Engl J Med* 1994;330(18):1272–5.

Black HS, Rhodes LE. The potential of omega-3 fatty acids in the prevention of non-melanoma skin cancer. *Cancer Detect Prev* 2006;30(3):224–32.

Camouse MM, Santo Domingo S, Swain FR, et al. Topical application of green and white tea extracts provides protection from solar-simulated ultraviolet light in human skin. *Exp Dermatol* 2009;18(6):522–6.

Chiu AE, Chan JL, Kern DG, Kohler S, Rehmus WE, Kimball AB. Double-blinded, placebo-controlled trial of green tea extracts in the clinical and histologic appearance of photoaging skin. *Derm Surg* 2005;31(7 Pt 2):855–60.

Elmets CA, Singh D, Tubesing K, et al. Cutaneous photoprotection from ultraviolet injury by green tea polyphenols. *J Am Acad Dermatol* 2001;44:425–32.

Fazekas Z, Gao D, Saladi RN, Lu Y, Lebwohl M, Wei H. Protective effects of lycopene against ultraviolet B-induced photodamage. *Nutr Cancer* 2003;47(2):181–7.

Gärtner C, Stahl W, Sies H. Lycopene is more bioavailable from tomato paste than from fresh tomatoes. *Am J Clin Nutr* 2007;66:116–22.

Hakim IA, Harris RB, Ritenbaugh C. Fat intake and risk of squamous cell carcinoma of the skin. *Nutr Cancer* 2000;36:155–62.

Heinrich U, Neukam K, Tronnier H, Sies H, Stahl W. Long-term ingestion of high flavanol cocoa provides photoprotection against UV-induced erythema and improves skin condition in women. *J Nutr* 2006;136(6):1565–9.

Hesterberg K, Lademann J, Patzelt A, Sterry W, Darvin ME. Raman spectroscopic analysis of the increase of the carotenoid antioxidant concentration in human skin after a 1-week diet with ecological eggs. *J Biomed Opt* 2009;14(2):24–39.

Hsu S. Green tea and the skin. *J Am Acad Dermatol* 2005;52:1049–59.

Hughes MC, van der Pols JC, Marks GC, Green AC. Food intake and risk of squamous cell carcinoma of the skin in a community: the Nambour skin cancer cohort study. *Int J Cancer* 2006;119(8):1953–60.

Hughes MC, Williams GM, Fourtnaier A, Green AC. Food intake, dietary patterns, and actinic keratoses of the skin: a longitudinal study. *Am J Clin Nutr* 2009;89(4):1246–55.

Ibiebele TI, van der Pols JC, Hughes MC, Marks GC, Williams GM, Green AC. Dietary pattern in association with squamous cell carcinoma of the skin: a prospective study. *Am J Clin Nutr* 2007;85(5):1401–8.

Institute of Medicine, Food and Nutrition Board. *Dietary Reference Intakes: Calcium, Phosphorus, Magnesium, Vitamin D, and Fluoride.* Washington, DC: National Academy Press, 1997.

International Agency for Research on Cancer Working Group on Artificial Ultraviolet (UV) Light and Skin Cancer. The association of use of sunbeds with cutaneous malignant melanoma and other skin cancers: A systematic review. *Int J Cancer* 2006;120(5):1116–22.

Janjua R, Munoz C, Gorell E, et al. A two-year, double-blind, randomized placebo-controlled trial of oral green tea polyphenols on the long-term clinical and histologic appearance of photoaging skin. *Dermatol Surg* 2009;35(7):1057–65.

Jasinghe VJ, Perera CO. Ultraviolet irradiation: The generator of Vitamin D_2 in edible mushrooms. *Food Chemistry* 2006;95(4):638–43.

Katiyar SK, Elmets CA. Green tea polyphenolic antioxidants and skin photoprotection. *Int J Oncol* 2001;18:1307–13.

Ljunggren B. Severe photoxic burn following celery ingestion. *Arch Dermatol* 1990; 126:1334–36.

McKenzie RL, Liley JB, Björn LO. UV Radiation: balancing risks and benefits. *J Photochem Photobiol* 2008;85(1):88–98.

McNaughton S, Marks G, Green A. Role of dietary factors in the development of basal cell cancer and squamous cell cancer of the skin. *Cancer Epidemiol Biomarkers Prev* 2005;14:1596–607.

Nichols JA, Katiyar SK. Skin photoprotection by natural polyphenols: anti-inflammatory, antioxidant and DNA repair mechanisms. *Arch Dermatol Res* 2010;302(2):71–83.

No JK, Soung DY, Kim YJ, et al. Inhibition of tyrosinase by green tea components. *Life Sci* 1999;65:241–6.

Orengo IF, Black HS, Wolf JE. Influence of fish oil supplementation on the minimal erythema dose in humans. *Arch Dermatol Res* 1992;284:219–21.

Pathak MA. Phytophotodermatitis. *Clin Dermatol* 1986;4(2):102–21.

Puig L, deMoragas JM. Enhancement of PUVA phototoxic effects following celery ingestion: cool broth also can burn. *Arch Dermatol* 1994;130:809–810.

Rhodes LE, O'Farrell S, Jackson MJ, Friedmann PS. Dietary fish-oil supplementation in humans reduces UVB-erythemal sensitivity but increases epidermal lipid peroxidation. *J Invest Dermatol* 1994;103:151–54.

Stahl W, Heinrich U, Aust O, Tronnier H, Sies H. Lycopene-rich products and dietary photoprotection. *Photochem Photobiol Sci* 2006;5(2):238–42.

7. Stop Wrinkles Before They Start

Adlercreutz H. Phytoestrogens: epidemiology and a possible role in cancer protection. *Environ Health Prospect* 1995;103:101–12.

Boelsma E, van de Vijver PL, Goldbohm A, et al. Human skin condition and its associations with nutrient concentrations in serum and diet. *Am J Clin Nutri* 2003;77(2):348–55.

Brincat M, Kabalan S, Studd JW, Moniz CF, de Trafford J, Montgomery J. A study of the decrease of skin collagen content, skin thickness, and bone mass in the post-menopausal woman. *Obstet Gynecol* 1987;70:840–5.

Brincat M, Moniz CJ, Studd JWW, et al. Long-term effects of the menopause and sex hormones on skin thickness. *Br J Obstet Gynaecol* 1985;92:256–9.

Cosgrove MC, Franco OH, Granger SP et al. Dietary nutrient intakes and skin-aging appearance among middle-aged American women. *Am J Clin Nutr* 2007;86:1225–31.

Dunn LB, Damesyn M, Moore AA, Reuben DB, Greendale GA. Does estrogen prevent skin aging? Results from the first National Health and Nutrition Examination Survey (NHANES I). *Arch Dermatol* 1997;133:339–42.

Escoffier C, de Rigal J, Rochefort A, et al. Age-related mechanical properties of human skin: an in vivo study. *J Invest Dermatol* 1989;93:353–7.

Fenske NA, Lober CW. Stuctural and functional changes of normal aging skin. *J Am Acad Dermatol.* 1986;15(4 pt 1):571–85.

Fisher GJ, Varani J, Voorhees JJ. Looking older: fibroblast collapse and therapeutic implications. *Arch Dermatol* 2008;144(5):666–72.

Guinot C, Malvy DJM, Ambrosine L, et al. Relative contribution of intrinsic vs extrinsic factors to skin aging as determined by a validated skin age score. *Arch Dermatol* 2002;138:1454–60.

Henry F, Pierard-Franchimont C, Cauwenbergh G, Pierard GE. Age-related changes in facial skin contours and rheology. *J Am Geriatr Soc* 1997;45:220–2.

Kronenberg F. Hot flashes: epidemiology and physiology. *Ann NY Acad Sci* 1990;592:52–86.

Liao H, Zakhaleva J, Chen W. Cells and tissue interactions with glycated collagen and their relevance to delayed diabetic wound healing. *Biomaterials* 2009;30(9):1689–96.

Miquel J, Ramírez-Boscá A, Ramírez-Bosca JV, Alperi JD. Menopause: a review on the role of oxygen stress and favorable effects of dietary antioxidants. *Arch Gerontol Geriatr* 2006; 42(3):289–306.

Nagata C, Nakamura K, Wada K, et al. Association of dietary fat, vegetables, and antioxidant measurements with skin ageing in Japanese women. *Br J Nutr* 2010;103(10)1493–8.

Pageon H. Reaction of glycation and human skin: the effects on the skin and its components, reconstructed skin as a model. *Pathol Biol* (Paris) 2010;58(3)226–31.

Pierard GE, Letawe C, Dowlati A, Pierard-Franchimont C. Effect of hormone replacement therapy for menopause on the mechanical properties of skin. *J Am Geriatr Soc* 1995;43:662–5.

Purba MB, Kouria-Blazus A, Wattanapenpalboon N, et al. Skin wrinkling: can food make a difference? *J Am Coll Nutri* 2001;20:71–80.

Shah MG, Maibach HI. Estrogen and skin: an overview. *Am J Clin Dermatol* 2001;2:143–50.

Yin L, Morita A, Tsuji T. Alterations of extracellular matrix induced by tobacco smoke extract. *Arch Dermatol Res* 2000;292(4):188–94.

8. Eating for Stronger, Healthier Hair and Nails

Arck PC, Overall R, Spatz K, et al. Towards a "free radical theory of graying": melanocyte apoptosis in the aging human hair follicle is an indicator of oxidative stress induced tissue damage. *FASEB J* 2006;20(9):1567–9.

Barel A, Calomme M, Timchenko A, et al. Effect of oral intake of choline-stabilized orthosilicic acid on skin, nails and hair in women with photodamaged skin. *Arch Dermatol Res* 2005;297(4):147–53.

Dawber RP, Rundegren J. Hypertrichosis in females applying minoxidil topical solution and in normal controls. *J Eur Acad Dermatol Venereol* 2003;17(3):271–5.

Hunt JR. Bioavailability of iron, zinc, and other trace minerals from vegetarian diets. *Am J Clin Nutr* 2003;78(3 Suppl):633S–639S.

Jugdaohsingh R, Anderson SH, Tucker KL, et al. Dietary silicon intake and absorption. *Am J Clin Nutr* 2002;75(5):887–93.

Kantor J, Kessler LJ, Brooks DG, Cotsarelis G. Decreased serum ferritin is associated with alopecia in women. *J Invest Dermatol* 2003;121(5):985–8.

Legakis JE, Koepke JI, Jedeszko C, et al. Peroxisome senescence in human fibroblasts. *Mol Biol Cell* 2002;13(12):4243–55.

Li N, Jia X, Chen CY, et al. Almond consumption reduces oxidative DNA damage and lipid peroxidation in male smokers. *J Nutr* 2007;137(12):2717–22.

Mosley JG, Gibbs AC. Premature grey hair and hair loss among smokers: a new opportunity for health education? *BMJ* 1996;313(7072):1616.

Sarink KY, Artandi SE. Aging, graying and loss of melanocyte stem cells. *Stem Cell Rev* 2007;3(3):212–7.

Scheinfeld N, Dahdah MJ, Scher R. Vitamins and minerals: their role in nail health and disease. *J Drugs Dermatol* 2007;6(8):782–7.

Sealey WM, Teague AM, Stratton SL, Mock DM. Smoking accelerates biotin catabolism in women. *Am J Clin Nutr* 2004;80(4):932–5.

Sripanyakorn S, Jugdaohsingh R, Dissayabutr W, Anderson SH, Thompson RP, Powell JJ. The comparative absorption of silicon from different foods and food supplements. *Br J Nutr* 2009;102(6):825–34.

Stern DK, Diamantis S, Smith E, et al. Water content and other aspects of brittle versus normal fingernails. *J Am Acad Dermatol* 2007;57(1):31–6.

Trost LB, Bergfeld WF, Calogeras E. The diagnosis and treatment of iron deficiency and its potential relationship to hair loss. *J Am Acad Dermatol* 2006;54(5):824–44.

Van de Kerkhof PC, Pasch MC, Scher RK, et al. Brittle nail syndrome: a pathogenesis-based approach with a proposed grading system. *J Am Acad Dermatol* 2005;53(4):644–51.

Wickett RR, Kossmann E, Barel A, et al. Effect of oral intake of choline-stabilized orthosilicic acid on hair tensile strength and morphology in women with fine hair. *Arch. Dermatol Res* 2007;299(10):499–505.

Wood JM, Decker H, Hartmann H, et al. Senile hair graying: H_2O_2-mediated oxidative stress affects human hair color by blunting methionine sulfoxide repair. *FASEB J* 2009;23(7):2065–75.

Yaemsiri S, Hou N, Slining MM, He K. Growth rate of human fingernails and toenails in healthy American young adults. *J Eur Acad Dermatol Venereol* 2010;24(4):420–3.

11. Food on Your Face

Aiyer HS, Vadhanam MV, Stoyanova R, Caprio GD, Clapper ML. et. Al. Dietary berries and ellagic acid prevent oxidative DNA damage and modulate expression of DNA repair genets. *Int J Mol Sci* 2008;9:327–41.

Antille C, Tran C, Sorg O, Saurat SH. Topical beta-carotene is converted to retinyl esters in human skin ex vivo and mouse skin in vivo. *ExpDermatol* 2004;13(9):558–61.

Azoulay E, Demian A, Frioux, D, eds. *100,000 Years of Beauty*. Paris: Editions Babylone, 2009.

Bae JY, Choi JS, Kang SW, Lee YJ, Park J, Kang YH. Dietary compound ellagic acid alleviates skin wrinkle and inflammation induced by UV-B irradiation. *Exp Dermatol* 2010;19(8):e182–90.

Camouse MM, Santo Domingo S, Swain FR, et al. Topical application of green and white tea extracts provides protection from solar-simulated ultraviolet light in human skin. *Exp Dermatol* 2009;18(6):522–6.

Duncan FJ, Martin JR, Wulff BC, et al. Topical treatment with black raspberry extract reduces cutaneous UVB-induced carcinogenesis and inflammation. *Cancer Prev Res* 2009;2(7):665–72.

Fu B, Li H, Wang X, Lee FSC, Cui S. Isolation and identification of flavonoids in licorice and a study of their inhibitory effects on tyrosinase. *J Agric Food Chem* 2005;53(19): 7408–14.

Jimenez F, Mitts TF, Liu K, Wang Y, Hinek A. Ellagic and tannic acids protect newly synthesized elastic fibers from premature enzymatic degradation in dermal fibroblast cultures. *J Invest Dermatol* 2006;126(6):1272–80.

Lee JH, Talcott ST. Fruit maturity and juice extraction influences ellagic acid derivatives and other antioxidant polyphenolics in muscadine grapes. *J Agric Food Chem* 2004;52(2):361–6.

Martin R, Pierrard C, Lejeune F, Hilaire P, Breton L, Bernerd F. Photoprotective effect of a water-soluble extract of Rosmarinus officinalis L. against UV-induced matrix metalloproteinase-1 in human dermal fibroblasts and reconstructed skin. *Eur J Dermatol* 2008;18(2):128–35.

Mau JL, Lin HC, Chen CC. Antioxidant properties of several medicinal mushrooms. *J Agric Food Chem* 2002;50(21):6072–7.

Miyazaki K, Hanamizu T, Sone T, Chiba K, Kinoshita T, Yoshikawa S. Topical application of Bifidobacterium-fermented soy milk extract containing genistein and daidzein improves rheological and physiological properties of skin. *J Cosmet Sci* 2004;55(5):473–9.

Munne-Bosch S, Alegre L. Subcellular compartmentalization of the diterpene carnosic acid and its derivatives in the leaves of rosemary. *Plant Physiol* 2001;125:1094–1102.

No JK, Soung DY, Kim YJ, et al. Inhibition of tyrosinase by green tea components. *Life Sci* 1999;65:241–6.

Omi T, Sato S, Numano K, Kawana S. Ultrastructural observations of chemical peeling for skin rejuvenation (ultrastructural changes of the skin due to chemical peeling). *J Cosmet Laser Ther* 2010;12(1):21–4.

Puttaraju NG, Venkateshaiah SU, Dharmesh SM, Urs SM, Somasundaram R. Antioxidant activity of indigenous edible mushrooms. *J Agric Food Chem* 2006;54(26):9764–72.

Shimogaki H, Tanaka Y, Tamai H, Masuda M. In vitro and in vivo evaluation of ellagic acid on melanogenesis inhibition. *Int J Cosmet Sci* 2000;22(4):291–303.

Wallo W, Nebus J, Leyden JJ. Efficacy of a soy moisturizer in photoaging: a double-blind, vehicle-controlled, 12-week study. *J Drugs Dermatol* 2007;6(9):917–22.

Yoshimura M, Watanabe Y, Kasai K, Yamakoshi J, Koga T. Inhibitory effect of an ellagic acid-rich pomegranate extract on tyrosinase activity and ultraviolet-induced pigmentation. *Biosci Biotechnol Biochem* 2005;69(12):2368–73.

Zhu W, Gao J. The use of botanical extracts as topical skin-lightening agents for the improvement of skin pigmentation disorders. *J Investig Dermatol Symp Proc* 2008;13(1):20–24.

Acknowledgments

....

Writing this book has truly been a labor of love (at times with no anesthesia). A big hug and sincere thanks to everyone who supported and encouraged me along the way. I'm especially grateful to:

My patients, who willingly tested the *Feed Your Face* Diet back when it was a stapled stack of pages, and gave me their honest feedback.

Maria Bello, Roma Downey, Katherine Heigl, Kelly Hu, Lisa Ling, Kris McNichol, Kelly Meyer, Christa Miller, Kelly Packard, Kimora Lee Simmons, Marina Sirtis, Nikki Sixx, Nicole Sullivan, Kat Von D, Kelly Wearstler, Adrienne, Anna Liza, Ariane, Diena, Hilla, Jasmin, Michelle, Pamela, and Vanessa, for generously contributing your stories and experiences. You give hope and inspiration to my readers.

Mike Keriakos and Steven Petrow, who, over lunch at the Ivy many moons ago, saw the potential in my idea and thought that it could someday be a book. Here's to many more meals and projects.

Richard Pine, my agent at Inkwell Management, for believing in me and finding a home for this book. Thank you for your critical eye, sound advice, and for keeping me on my toes—to this day, I always have a joke prepared.

Sally Richardson, my editor Kathryn Huck, Alyse Diamond, John Murphy, and the entire team at St. Martin's Press, for believing in my vision, enthusiastically welcoming me into your family, and patiently guiding me through the often-bewildering process of writing my first book. You had me at the pizza.

Courtney Hargrave, my talented and invaluable writing partner and illustrator, who worked tirelessly to make the manuscript the best it could be. Thank you for your creativity, diligence, and willingness to spend many hours and late nights on the phone and e-mail.

Jessica Levinson, RD, who evaluated the meal plan and made sure it was as nutritious as it was delicious.

Marc Chamlin, my attorney and trusted adviser, for making sure I'm always protected.

Heidi and Erik Murkoff, for your generous and thoughtful advice and reassurance that it's OK to be compulsive. I appreciate you so much and treasure our friendship.

Scott Barnes, dear friend and a kindred spirit—you truly understand what it's like to juggle five bowling balls at once.

Bari Medgaus and Janet D'Oliveira, for your friendship, honesty, loyalty, and enthusiasm. Thank you for being on my side from the beginning, and for your helpful comments on the manuscript.

My staff: Jennifer Spencer, Lisa Roberts, and Kaylie Alexander, for keeping my office running smoothly when I was buried in pages of manuscript.

Most of all, my family and friends, for loving me and always supporting my many projects, even when it means I don't spend as much time with you as I would like.

Index